DATE DUE

DEC - 2 2003	

BRODART   Cat. No. 23-221

THE NEW
CIVIL
WAR

PSYCHOLOGY OF WOMEN
BOOK SERIES

CHERYL B. TRAVIS, Series Editor

Bringing Cultural Diversity to Feminist Psychology: Theory, Research, and Practice
    Hope Landrine, Editor
The New Civil War: The Psychology, Culture, and Politics of Abortion
    Linda J. Beckman and S. Marie Harvey, Editors
Shaping the Future of Feminist Psychology: Education, Research, and Practice
    Judith Worell and Norine G. Johnson, Editors

THE NEW CIVIL WAR

THE PSYCHOLOGY, CULTURE, AND POLITICS OF ABORTION

EDITED BY

LINDA J. BECKMAN
S. MARIE HARVEY

AMERICAN PSYCHOLOGICAL ASSOCIATION
WASHINGTON, DC

Published by
American Psychological Association
750 First Street, NE
Washington, DC 20002

Copies may be ordered from
APA Order Department
P.O. Box 92984
Washington, DC 20090-2984

In the UK and Europe, copies may be ordered from
American Psychological Association
3 Henrietta Street
Covent Garden, London
WC2E 8LU England

Typeset in Goudy by EPS Group Inc., Easton, MD

Cover designer: Minker Design, Bethesda, MD
Front cover photo: Copyright 1998 by PhotoDisc, Inc.
Printer: United Book Press, Baltimore, MD
Technical/production editor: Tanya Y. Alexander

Library of Congress Cataloging-in-Publication Data
The new civil war : the psychology, culture, and politics of abortion / Linda J.
   Beckman and S. Marie Harvey, editors.
       p.   cm.
   Includes bibliographical references and index.
   ISBN 1-55798-517-0 (casebound : alk. paper)
   1. Abortion—United States.   2. Pregnancy, Unwanted—United States.
   3. Abortion services—United States.   I. Beckman, Linda J.
   II. Harvey, S. Marie.
   HQ767.5.U5N45   1998
   363.46'0973—dc21   98-3553
                                                                        CIP

British Library Cataloguing-in-Publication Data
A CIP record is available from the British Library.

Printed in the United States of America
First edition

CONTENTS

List of Contributors ix

Foreword xi
Henry P. David

Acknowledgments xvii

Introduction xix

Part I: The Sociopolitical Context of Abortion 1

Chapter 1   Federal Abortion Policy and Politics:
              1973 to 1996 3
              Brian L. Wilcox, Jennifer K. Robbennolt, and
              Janet E. O'Keeffe

Chapter 2   Why Is Abortion Such a Controversial Issue in
              the United States? 25
              Nancy Felipe Russo and Jean E. Denious

Chapter 3   Barriers to Access to Abortion Services 61
              Stanley K. Henshaw

Chapter 4   The Impact of Antiabortion Activities on Women
              Seeking Abortions 81
              Catherine Cozzarelli and Brenda Major

Part II: The Cultural Context of Abortion 105

Chapter 5   Black Women and the Question of Abortion 107
              Karen Dugger

Chapter 6   Latinas and Abortion 133
                Pamela I. Erickson and Celia P. Kaplan

Chapter 7   Abortion and Asian Pacific Islander Americans.... 157
                Sora Park Tanjasiri and Sono Aibe

Part III: Intrapersonal and Interpersonal Contexts of Abortion   187

Chapter 8   The Acceptability of Medical Abortion
                to Women 189
                Linda J. Beckman and S. Marie Harvey

Chapter 9   Understanding the Relationship of Violence
                Against Women to Unwanted Pregnancy and
                Its Resolution 211
                Nancy Felipe Russo and Jean E. Denious

Chapter 10   Testing a Model of the Psychological
                Consequences of Abortion 235
                Warren B. Miller, David J. Pasta, and
                Catherine L. Dean

Chapter 11   Men and Abortion: The Gender Politics of
                Pregnancy Resolution 269
                William Marsiglio and Douglas Diekow

Chapter 12:   Abortion Among Adolescents 285
                Nancy E. Adler, Lauren B. Smith, and
                Jeanne M. Tschann

Part IV: Abortion in the Context of Practice 299

Chapter 13   A Cognitive Approach to Patient-Centered
                Abortion Care 301
                Barbara Fisher, Mary Ann Castle, and
                Joan Mogul Garrity

Chapter 14   Abortion Issues in Psychotherapy 329
                Maria J. Rivera

Chapter 15   Bringing Lessons Learned to the United States:
                Improving Access to Abortion Services 353
                Saba W. Masho, Francine M. Coeytaux, and
                Malcolm Potts

Part V: Conclusion 367

Chapter 16   Where Do We Go From Here? Recommendations
              for Abortion Practice, Policy, and Research 369
              S. Marie Harvey, Linda J. Beckman, and
              Sheryl Thorburn Bird

Author Index 383

Subject Index 395

About the Editors 405

CONTRIBUTORS

Nancy E. Adler, Health Psychology Program, University of California,
   San Francisco
Sono Aibe, Asians and Pacific Islanders for Reproductive Health,
   Oakland, CA
Linda J. Beckman, California School of Professional Psychology,
   Los Angeles; Pacific Institute for Women's Health, Los Angeles
Sheryl Thorburn Bird, Center for the Study of Women in Society,
   University of Oregon; Pacific Institute for Women's Health,
   Los Angeles
Mary Ann Castle, New York, NY
Francine M. Coeytaux, Pacific Institute for Women's Health,
   Los Angeles
Catherine Cozzarelli, Department of Psychology, Kansas State
   University, Manhattan
Henry P. David, Transnational Family Research Institute, Bethesda, MD
Catherine L. Dean, Private Practice, St. Louis, MO
Jean E. Denious, Department of Psychology, Arizona State University
Douglas Diekow, Department of Sociology, University of Florida,
   Gainesville
Karen Dugger, Department of Sociology and Anthropology, Bucknell
   University
Pamela I. Erickson, Department of Anthropology, University of
   Connecticut, Storrs
Barbara Fisher, Independent Consultant, New York, NY
Joan Mogul Garrity, Garrity-Jones Health Consulting & Training,
   Towson, MD
S. Marie Harvey, Center for the Study of Women in Society, University
   of Oregon, Eugene; Pacific Institute for Women's Health,
   Los Angeles

Stanley K. Henshaw, The Alan Guttmacher Institute, New York, NY

Celia P. Kaplan, Department of General Internal Medicine, University of California, San Francisco

Brenda Major, Department of Psychology, University of California, Santa Barbara

William Marsiglio, Department of Sociology, University of Florida, Gainesville

Saba W. Masho, Department of Maternal and Child Health, School of Public Health, University of California, Berkeley

Warren B. Miller, Transitional Family Research Institute, Sunnyvale, CA

Janet E. O'Keeffe, American Association of Retired Persons, Washington, DC

David J. Pasta, DMA Corporation, Sunnyvale, CA

Malcolm Potts, School of Public Health, University of California, Berkeley

Maria J. Rivera, Jersey City, NJ

Jennifer K. Robbennolt, Center on Children, Families and the Law, University of Nebraska

Nancy Felipe Russo, Department of Psychology, Arizona State University

Lauren B. Smith, Health Psychology Program, University of California, San Francisco

Sora Park Tanjasiri, School of Social Ecology, University of California, Irvine

Jeanne M. Tschann, Health Psychology Program, University of California, San Francisco

Brian L. Wilcox, Center on Children, Families and the Law, University of Nebraska, Lincoln

FOREWORD

HENRY P. DAVID

Reproductive behavior, fertility regulation, and abortion continue to be emotionally charged, divisive issues in American political and cultural life. Although among the most fundamental aspects of human behavior, they have elicited only limited interest among psychologists. Specialists profoundly interested in psychosexual issues and child development have given scant attention to the procreative aspects of sexuality, the possible etiological and epidemiological significance of chance versus planned births, or the resolution of unwanted pregnancy. For these and many other reasons, this volume is particularly timely and welcome. Placing abortion firmly within the context of women's rights, and sexual and reproductive health, this book reflects the diverse aspects of the complex abortion issue and its wide interdisciplinary appeal, echoing the resolutions of the 1994 United Nations Cairo International Conference on Populations and Development ("The Report on the International Conference on Population and Development," 1995).

In accepting the editors' kind invitation to contribute this foreword, it was agreed that the focus would be on the historical roots of the American Psychological Association's (APA) support of women's reproductive rights, particularly abortion and reproductive health. The numerous suggestions for improved practice and research, discussed in this volume, reflect the strength of an interdisciplinary approach to the vexing issue of abortion.

Although nearly all of my research has been in cooperation with colleagues outside the United States, it was my privilege to be involved in the earliest APA activities related to women's reproductive rights. As an APA Council member, I introduced a resolution in October 1969, together with the Association for Women Psychologists, declaring that termination of an unwanted pregnancy was a mental health and child welfare issue, and thus a legitimate concern of APA. The resolution resolved that termination of pregnancy be considered "a civil right of the pregnant woman," to be handled as any other medical and surgical procedure in consultation with the woman's physician (McKeachie, 1970, p. 37). At the request of some Council members, a second resolution was then moved by Division 18 (Public Service), which I represented, resolving that APA establish a Task Force on Psychology, Family Planning, and Population Policy "for the purpose of preparing a review of the current state of psychological research related to family planning and population policy" and making recommendations for "encouraging greater research and professional service participation by psychologists in this emerging area of social concern" (McKeachie, 1970, p. 34). After only brief discussion, both resolutions passed by a substantial margin, thus placing APA firmly in support of women's reproductive rights well before the January 1973 Roe vs. Wade Supreme Court Decision (*Roe v. Wade*, 1973).

The context in which APA Council approved the resolutions is worth recalling. Most of the morning had been devoted to bitter debates about what APA's public position should be on the Vietnam War. Each of the proposed resolutions and suggestions for action was defeated. After our resolutions were introduced, it was apparent that Council members were wary of debate and wanted to show the association's awareness that professional expertise should be applied to topics of current social significance. The two resolutions passed, and the task force was established.

The initial members of the task force were James T. Fawcett, Deborah Matory, Sidney H. Newman, Edward T. Pohlman, and Vaida Thompson, with Miriam Kelty as APA staff liaison. I served as chair. Nancy Russo joined us later. When the task force convened its organizational meeting on December 17, 1969, fewer than a dozen of the nation's more than 31,000 psychologists were estimated to be working primarily in population-related endeavors. Through the efforts of Jim Fawcett, APA obtained a small grant from the Population Council to supplement the task force budget. A workshop was convened in Washington, DC, on March 6, 1970; several symposia were organized at APA conventions in 1970 and 1971; and a close relationship was established with the Center for Population Research at the National Institute of Child Health and Human Development. A conference on Psychological Measurement in the Study of Population Problems was held in February 1971 at the Institute of Personality Assessment and Research of the University of California at Berkeley. Designed to be interdisciplinary, the conference attracted participants from anthropology, demography, sociology, obstetrics–gynecology, psychiatry, and public health, as well as from subspecialties of psychology. The conference proceedings were edited by Harrison Gough (1972) and published by the

Institute of Personality Assessment and Research (IPAR). Warren B. Miller and Nancy Russo contributed papers to the conference, as they have to this volume.

In October 1971, the task force joined with the Center for Population Research at the National Institute for Child Health and Human Development in sponsoring a workshop at the University of North Carolina, Chapel Hill, on ideas for developing and educating psychologists to work in the field of population. A summary of the workshop proceedings, edited by co-chairs Vaida Thompson and Sidney Newman (1972), was disseminated to chairs of psychology departments, noting that practically none of the psychologists working in the field entered it directly after completing their doctorates. Not a single U.S. institution of higher learning had a psychology department with an undergraduate, graduate, or postdoctoral program explicitly dealing with population or reproductive behavior. That situation has changed little over the past 25 years.

During its existence, the task force published resource information on family planning (Newman & Kelty, 1972), facilitated the coordination of a special issue of the *Journal of Social Issues* (Back & Fawcett, 1974), and encouraged the publication of several books devoted to the topic area (e.g., Fawcett, 1970, 1972). It also distributed an occasional newsletter to over 750 individuals and organizations, established a liaison with the Association of Women Psychologists, stimulated inclusion of the category of population and family planning in the 1972 *National Register of Science and Technical Personnel* in the field of psychological science, and worked with Brewster Smith (1972) on psychological perspectives related to the complex ethical implications of population policy.

In reflecting on the field in 1972, the task force noted that the chief contribution of psychologists had been the identification of personal and attitudinal variables related to fertility. Some studies focused on fertility-regulating behavior and on couple decision-making processes. Others emphasized the normative rather than the pathological sequelae of contraception and pregnancy termination. Increasingly sophisticated, these studies promised to deepen understanding of the determinants of human fertility while extending the research parameters of motivation theory, decision making, and assessment. It was argued that new measures were needed of variables that were both theoretically and empirically relevant to family planning. Also needed were new methods of analysis that gave greater attention to the powerful interpersonal determinants of fertility-regulating behavior. Thought to be particularly desirable were measures that were "relatively simple, brief, easily administered, and transnationally adaptable" (APA Task Force, 1972, p. 1102). The chapters in this book indicate how much has been accomplished 25 years later.

Among the recommendations of the task force was the establishment of an APA Division of Population Psychology. On meeting the necessary requirements and approval by APA Council, the Division was duly organized in August 1974, with Vaida Thompson as president. The four subsequently elected presidents had all been members of the task force (Fawcett, Russo, David, and Kelty). The fifth president is another contributor to this volume, Nancy Adler.

An important by-product of task force efforts was the convening of an interdisciplinary Abortion Research Workshop on the day before the 1973 meeting of the Population Association of America. Over the next two decades, the workshop expanded its scope of interest, and, in 1982, it was renamed the Psychosocial Workshop. Its annual sessions attract a coterie of anthropologists, demographers, economists, psychologists, psychiatrists, sociologists, and other health professionals. Happily informal, it has no bylaws or elected officers and requires no dues. Annual program chairs organize the 2-day meeting. Several contributors to this book have served as program chairs, and more have participated in the workshop. A review of the topics discussed during the quarter century reflects many of the areas further developed in this volume (David, 1986, 1997).

The APA task force was a timely catalyst within psychology and between psychology and other professions that shared the aim of attaining a better understanding of the complex psychosocial variables interacting in the process of human fertility behavior. Now, 25 years later, APA is publishing a book on abortion in the United States as part of the Division 35 book series. It is a strong affirmation of women's reproductive rights and a major contribution to the advancement of reproductive health, related research, and the roles and responsibilities of health professionals. I am happy to commend the editors and congratulate them and their 30 colleagues on broadening the scope in which the still very controversial topic of abortion needs to be considered within the profession, among professions, and with the public. APA and Division 35 lend further credence to the goals expressed in 1969 and extended in the recommendations of the 1994 International Conference on Population and Development.

REFERENCES

American Psychological Association Task Force on Psychology, Family Planning, and Population Policy. (1972). Report of the Task Force on Psychology, Family Planning, and Population Policy. *American Psychologist, 27,* 1100–1105.

Back, K. W., & Fawcett, J. T. (Eds.). (1974). Population policy and the person: Congruence or conflict [Special issue]. *Journal of Social Issues, 30*(40), 1–295.

David, H. P. (1986, fall). Reflections on the psychosocial workshop. *P.A.A. Affairs,* pp. 2–3.

David, H. P. (1997). *The psychosocial workshop: A personal perspective.* Unpublished manuscript, Transnational Family Research Institute, Bethesda.

Fawcett, J. T. (1970). *Psychology and population: Behavioral research issues in fertility and family planning*. New York: The Population Council.

Fawcett, J. T. (Ed.). (1972). *Psychological perspectives on population*. New York: Basic Books.

Gough, H. (1972). *Conference proceedings: Psychological measurement in the study of population problems*. Berkeley: Institute of Personality Assessment and Research, University of California.

McKeachie, W. J. (1970). Proceedings of the American Psychological Association of the year 1969: Minutes of the annual meeting of the Council of Representatives. *American Psychologist, 25*, 13–37.

Newman, S. H., & Kelty, M. F. (1972). Support for psychologists in the population and family planning areas. *American Psychologist, 27*, 31–36.

The Report of the International Conference on Population and Development, Cairo, September 15–19, 1994. (1995). New York: United Nations.

Roe v. Wade, 410 U.S. 113 (1973).

Smith, H. B. (1972). Ethical implications of population policies: A psychologist's view. *American Psychologist, 27*, 11–15.

Thompson, V. D., & Newman, S. H. (1972). *Education psychologists for work in the population field: A workshop*. Unpublished manuscript, Washington, DC.

ACKNOWLEDGMENTS

Any undertaking of this magnitude involves the goodwill and cooperation of many. Without the assistance and contributions of other individuals this book would not have come to fruition. First and foremost, we are deeply grateful to the authors of the book chapters. Some are good colleagues whom we have known and collaborated with for many years, whereas others came to this endeavor as strangers, known to us only by their work and reputations. We are especially indebted to Henry David, who wrote the foreword to the book; on numerous occasions during the last 20 years he has served as a role model, mentor, and most enthusiastic supporter.

Throughout the almost 2 years that it took to complete this volume, Cheryl Travis, the current editor of the Division 35 Book Series, provided solid advice, confidence, patience, and many uplifting email messages written at strange hours of the night. The editors and staff of APA Books, especially Andrea Phillippi and Mary Lynn Skutley, also have provided invaluable support in guiding us through the maze of tasks that are necessary for completion of a volume of this magnitude. In addition, they helped us deal with thorny editorial issues with skill and grace. Our students and colleagues at the California School of Professional Psychology (CSPP), Pacific Institute for Women's Health (PIWH), and Center for the Study of Women in Society (CSWS) at the University of Oregon have provided comments on content areas, editorial suggestions, and other assistance during all phases of book development and preparation, and both CSPP and PIWH have donated student research assistance and staff support to the project.

Two colleagues were critical in the completion of the book, Christy Sherman and Sheryl Thorburn Bird. We extend our heartfelt thanks to Christy for her invaluable assistance, including her organizational efforts in all aspects of manuscript preparation, her cogent comments about our own as well as others' chapters, and her editing and proofreading skills. We are grateful to Sheryl for her significant assistance in preparation and editing of the book's introduction and closing chapter.

Above all we are grateful for the love, encouragement, and support of our parents, Marie's sisters, and especially our partners, Stan and Franz, during the completion of this volume. We dedicate this book to them with our love.

INTRODUCTION

Abortion is one of the most divisive issues in the United States today. Americans disagree about the circumstances under which abortion should be legally permissible and whether it should be permissible under any circumstances. Whereas many vehemently support women's unrestricted right to abortion, others just as strongly affirm the de-legalization of all types of abortion in the United States. The majority, however, probably hold a middle view, concurring that abortion should be available for women, but also believing that some restrictions should apply. Such beliefs and attitudes are rooted in alternative ideologies that structure both the interpersonal context in which abortion decisions are made and the sociopolitical context in which the provision of abortion services is embedded.

Abortion is a common occurrence in the United States today. Half of the 6.4 million pregnancies that occur each year are unintended, and close to half of these unintended pregnancies end in induced abortion (Forrest & Henshaw, 1993). Thus, 1.6 million American women terminate a pregnancy through abortion. Blacks; Latinas; women aged 18–24; women with low incomes; women with no religious identification; and women who live with a partner outside of marriage, are separated, or have never married appear to have a higher likelihood of abortion (Henshaw & Kost, 1996). Although abortion rates have declined in the United States since the early 1980s, in part because of decreasing availability of services (see Henshaw's discussion, chapter 3, this volume), U.S. rates are significantly higher than those of Western European countries.

Women generally want to avoid having an abortion. Yet nearly one half of American women have had at least one abortion (Forrest & Henshaw, 1993), including many women who are ambivalent about or ideologically opposed to the procedure. Often, the circumstances of women's lives make abortion the best option for them, even if they experience social, cultural, or religious proscriptions against abortion.

Despite the widespread use of legal abortion in the United States, the right to abortion is an issue of great controversy, invoking religious, moral, and personal values. Recently this controversy has become even more visible, vitriolic, and violent. The continuing conflict over abortion attests to the continued need and importance of scholarly research and discourse on the topic. Our call for research in this area is not new (e.g., David, 1971). Yet, despite a growing body of knowledge about the antecedents and consequences of abortion, the national debate about abortion often is not informed by empirical evidence. In addition, most of the existing literature on abortion is unidisciplinary, focusing on the historical, legal, or political aspects of the abortion controversy. Few volumes have considered cultural or psychological issues in any detail.

This volume describes the sociopolitical, cultural, and psychological contexts of abortion in the United States as they influence (a) the availability and provision of abortion services, (b) individual and group attitudes and beliefs about abortion, and (c) the consequences of the decision to terminate a pregnancy through abortion. We provide a multidisciplinary perspective rather than a purely psychological one; this approach is evident both across chapters and within many individual chapters. Although we try to provide an unbiased perspective on this controversial issue, our feminist beliefs and feminist scholarship concerning gender roles and women's status in society shape the volume. Thus, the book adopts a broad perspective relating gender roles and women's status in U.S. society to current and emerging issues and policies.

We support public policy; practice; and advocacy for political, economic, and social equality for women. For such equality to be achieved, all women *must* have personal control over reproductive behaviors and events, including whether to terminate a pregnancy. On balance, the research literature strongly supports the conclusion that abortion has many more positive than negative psychosocial and health consequences. The bearing of unwanted children has negative effects for both parents and child (David, 1992). Moreover, the legalization of abortion in the United States has been one of the most significant factors in saving women's lives and improving their quality of life (Tietze, 1984).

Yet, it is becoming more difficult for some women, particularly when they are poor, young, or live in rural areas, to obtain legal abortions in the United States. The intense controversy surrounding abortion and the protest against it have created a social climate in which voluntary termination of pregnancy is regarded as unacceptable for many women. Thus, it is particularly important to understand the context in which the abortion debate is occurring and the multitude of factors that can influence women's access to and use of abortion services.

ORGANIZATION OF THIS VOLUME

This volume is divided into five parts. Part I: The Sociopolitical Context of Abortion examines the complex pattern of variables that influence the heated debate surrounding abortion in the United States. Part II: The Cultural Context of Abortion describes racial, ethnic, class, religious, and other sociodemographic differences in abortion attitudes and behaviors. Part III: Intrapersonal and Interpersonal Contexts of Abortion covers the intrapersonal and interpersonal contexts of abortion, including method and service delivery system characteristics that influence accessibility, acceptability, and psychological consequences of abortion for women and their partners. Other diverse issues considered include the role of violence against women, the ability of adolescents to make informed decisions about abortion, and men's role in pregnancy resolution decisions and abortion.

Scholarly analyses can inform individual decision making, service provision, and social policy as well as integrate and extend research knowledge. Therefore, the last two sections of the book examine applied issues. Part IV: Abortion in the Context of Practice considers diverse issues including pre- and postabortion counseling strategies, patient-sensitive provision of services, use of psychotherapy to help women better understand and cope with their abortion experience, and the application of experiences in other countries to improve service delivery in the United States. The volume concludes with recommendations for improving abortion services, legislation, social policy, advocacy, and research efforts.

Part I: The Sociopolitical Context of Abortion

The first chapter provides a historical overview of national abortion policies and politics in the United States since the legalization of abortion in 1973 and, thus, is an appropriate introduction to Part I as well as the entire volume. Wilcox, Robbennolt, and O'Keeffe review the legislative actions and extra-legislative initiatives undertaken by the federal government as well as key Supreme Court decisions related to abortion policy from 1973–1988, 1989–1992, and 1993–1996. During these years, numerous attempts were made to change abortion policy in the United States, the majority of these being in the direction of restricting abortions. Although abortion opponents have been successful in limiting federal funding for abortions, the basic right to abortion remains intact. Wilcox, Robbennolt, and O'Keeffe discuss the role of psychology in addressing abortion policy issues, suggesting that psychologists must try to ensure that empirical data are not misused by pro-life or pro-choice proponents, that psychologists continue to testify as expert witnesses, and that the American Psychological Association continues to provide Congress with analyses of research on specific abortion issues such as parental notification.

In chapter 2, Russo and Denious examine a wide variety of factors within the broad sociopolitical context of abortion. By addressing the question of why abortion is a controversial issue in the United States, these authors demonstrate the complexity of abortion as a social issue. They discuss the connections among attitudes toward abortion and feminist perspectives, women's roles, female sexuality, religious ideology, government, beliefs about prenatal life, and the health professions. They also examine how attitudes toward abortion are affected, manipulated, and distorted by research methodology, including the wording of survey questions.

The general sociopolitical context ultimately affects the availability and quality of abortion services. Access may decrease because of changes in federal and state abortion policy, activities of abortion opponents, and the lack of training for health care providers. The Alan Guttmacher Institute's (AGI) periodic surveys of known abortion providers in the United States contain information about who is providing abortions and the number of abortions being performed. In chapter 3, Henshaw reports findings from the 1993 AGI Abortion Provider Survey. At the national and state levels, abortion rates are decreasing. Henshaw presents data suggesting that one reason for declining abortion levels is that abortion services have become increasingly unavailable; in particular, there are fewer and fewer abortion providers. In addition, barriers such as gestational limits on when abortions can be performed and harassment by antiabortion protestors make accessing abortion services even more difficult. Moreover, the increasing isolation of abortion services from mainstream medical care may decrease physicians' willingness to perform abortions. Henshaw concludes his chapter by offering a variety of recommendations for improving access to abortion services.

A more specific arena in which the politics of abortion have been carried out in the United States includes the activities of pro-life activists that are directed at abortion clinics, their clients, and staff. Such activities may have a range of influences on the accessibility of abortion services and the psychological well-being of women seeking abortions. In chapter 4, Cozzarelli and Major consider several pathways through which antiabortion activities may impact women seeking an abortion and women who obtain an abortion. Although antiabortion organizations have been in existence since the 1960s, the membership and activities of such organizations have changed over time. Cozzarelli and Major suggest that antiabortion activities may have indirect effects on women seeking abortions through reducing the number of abortion providers. They also discuss the potential impact of antiabortion activities on women's decisions to abort and the psychological effects on women who enter an abortion clinic. In addition, the authors examine the influence of pro-choice escorts and injunctions designed to limit antiabortion activities. Little research has been conducted that examines the effects of antiabortion activities on women wanting to obtain an abortion. Finally, Cozzarelli and Major identify several important research questions in this area. In particular, they recognize the need for theoretical models that identify the paths by which antiabortion demonstrators influence women's postabortion adjustment.

These four chapters demonstrate the complex interaction between social context, availability of abortion services, and attitudes toward abortion. The general sociopolitical context, activities of pro-choice activists, specific legislation, and extra-legislative initiatives all affect availability of services for specific groups of women. The social context also influences acceptability, that is, a woman's willingness to have an abortion as well as her choice of specific abortion methods. In addition, these chapters suggest that not only are attitudes of women seeking abortion and the general public important in sifting through the complexity of issues surrounding this topic, but also it is essential to consider the attitudes, beliefs, and values of health professionals who perform or potentially could provide such services. Moreover, the behaviors and strategies of those who oppose abortion may strongly impact both women with unintended pregnancies and health care providers.

Part II: The Cultural Context of Abortion

Part II examines the abortion attitudes and behavior of African American, Latina, and Asian and Pacific Islander women. In chapter 5, Dugger examines six explanations for Black–White differences in abortion attitudes. In short, these differences are thought to reflect sociodemographic, cultural, and religious distinctions; generational and life cycle factors; and perceptions among Black communities that birth control and abortion are forms of Black genocide. Given the history of coercive reproductive policies toward African American and poor women in this country, concern among African Americans about how abortion might be used to limit or decrease the Black population is not surprising. Dugger also discusses African Americans' involvement in a multiracial reproductive rights movement and why this movement is separate and different from the mainstream pro-choice movement. Dugger concludes that African American women support abortion as a practical necessity. She also points out that most research on the abortion attitudes of Black women has focused on Black–White comparisons. In-depth studies of African American women are needed to better understand abortion attitudes and behavior among this population.

Chapter 6 explores abortion among Latina women in the United

States. Erickson and Kaplan describe the sociodemographic and fertility characteristics of the U.S. Latino population. A theme introduced in this section and reinforced throughout the chapter is that Latinos are not homogeneous. In addition to differences between Latinos and non-Latinos, the limited data on Latino subgroups suggest that considerable variation in the use of abortion among Latina subgroups (i.e., Mexican, Puerto Rican, and Cuban women) also exists. Mexican women appear to use abortion less than Puerto Rican and Cuban women; Cuban women are the most likely to use abortion. Although the few studies that examined abortion attitudes among Latinos suggest that their attitudes differ from those of non-Latinos, differences among Latino subgroups are not known. Erickson and Kaplan point out that important changes in Latino gender and fertility beliefs have occurred. Contrary to what is commonly believed, Latino attitudes toward abortion more closely resemble those of the general American population than those of the Catholic Church. Further research on Latino attitudes toward abortion and abortion behavior, particularly studies that examine Latino subgroups separately, are needed.

Tanjasiri and Aibe begin chapter 7 by describing the nativity and immigration history of Asian and Pacific Islander Americans (APIAs). This description is followed by a discussion of the sociodemographic characteristics of APIAs. Similar to Latinos, there is substantial heterogeneity within the APIA population. Because many APIA women are born outside the United States and have only recently immigrated, Tanjasiri and Aibe describe the differences in abortion policies and practices of APIA women in their countries of origin, providing background for understanding the abortion attitudes and behavior of APIA women. Very limited information exists on use of and attitudes toward abortion among APIAs. The data that are available suggest that fertility and abortion patterns vary considerably by APIA subgroups. Factors that likely influence the abortion practices and attitudes of APIAs include reluctance to discuss sex and reproduction, misperceptions about contraceptive methods, gender and family roles, lack of power in relationships, and barriers to reproductive health services. In conclusion, Tanjasiri and Aibe emphasize the lack of data on APIA women and the need for research that addresses the demographic, cultural, and immigration characteristics of APIA subgroups.

The chapters in Part II clearly suggest that research needs to go beyond the description of racial and ethnic differences in abortion attitudes and practices. Researchers must examine and test various explanations for such differences, including culture, poverty, and religious beliefs. It will be clear from these chapters that data on African American, Latina, and APIA women are severely limited. Considerable variation within these large racial and ethnic categories exists, and future research must recognize and address these within-group differences. The abortion attitudes and behavior of all women must be examined within the broader cultural context. Acculturation and ethnic identity may help to explain variation in abortion attitudes and behavior within more narrowly defined racial and ethnic categories.

Part III: Intrapersonal and Interpersonal Contexts of Abortion

The chapters in Part III examine the diverse intrapersonal and interpersonal factors that influence women's and men's abortion decisions and behavior, as well as the consequences they experience. The topic of chapter 8 by Beckman and Harvey is the acceptability of medical abortion among women. The authors begin by describing the characteristics and history of medical abortion. Although mifepristone (RU 486) is used in France and other countries as an abortifacient, it has yet to be approved by the Food and Drug Administration for use in the United States. Beckman and Harvey present findings from their own research on the acceptability of mifepristone among American women. Their findings generally concur with studies from other countries, which indicate that women choose medical abortion over surgical abortion because of anxiety about surgery and fear of general anesthesia. In addition to a focus group study of women in three cities in the United States, the authors investigated the characteristics of 262 women who chose medical abortion as part of a national clinical trial, the reasons those women chose mifepristone rather than surgical abortion, their expectations with regard to the method and how these compared to their actual experiences, and their satisfaction with medical abortion. Beckman and Harvey conclude with recommendations for educational materials and counseling about medical abortion and for the provision of medical abortion services in the United States. They note that among American women a large obstacle to choice of medical abortion is lack of knowledge and misconceptions about the method.

In chapter 9, Russo and Denious explore the relationship between violence against women and unwanted pregnancy and its resolution. The authors begin their discussion by describing the prevalence of male violence against women and its consequences. Russo and Denious then discuss the linkages between gendered violence and unintended and unwanted pregnancy and high-risk sexual behavior. They also examine the extent to which violence exists in the lives of women who have abortions. The authors conclude that research that has linked unintended pregnancy with violence has important implications for family planning and abortion policies and programs as well as society. In addition, reproductive health professionals have critical roles to play in addressing the problem of violence against women and its effect on women's health.

Several theoretical approaches have been used to study the psychological effects of induced abortion. The model presented by Miller, Pasta, and Dean in chapter 10 integrates the major components of six approaches commonly used: the stress approach, the decision-making approach, the norm violation approach, the loss approach, the crisis approach, and the learning approach. The authors test their model with data from a sample of 145 women participating in a clinical trial of mifepristone at one location. The women were interviewed immediately prior to the administration of mifepristone, with follow-up interviews occurring 2 weeks and 6 to 8 months later. The findings are of both research and clinical significance. Psychological consequences 6 to 8 months after a medical abortion are not necessarily related or similar to those experienced 2 weeks after the abortion. The factor that had the greatest effect on stress and regret 6 to 8 months after abortion was wantedness of the child. Attitude toward abortion and using positive thinking to cope also had major effects on chronic stress after abortion. A failed medical abortion was associated with less relief and increased regret.

In chapter 11, Marsiglio and Diekow examine men's roles in pregnancy resolution decisions and abortion within the larger context of gender politics. Legally, men can neither force women to have an abortion nor require that they carry a pregnancy to term. They are, however, financially responsible for their offspring whether or not they wanted them. Men's involvement (or lack thereof) in decisions about abortion and their responsibility (or lack thereof) for their offspring are viewed quite differently by conservative and progressive philosophies of family life and reproductive issues. Marsiglio and Diekow describe these two philosophies, their relationships to feminist and men's rights ideologies, and their implications for men's roles in abortion decisions and child support. They also discuss men's personal and interpersonal experiences with abortion. As these authors indicate, research is needed that examines men's beliefs and attitudes about abortion and fatherhood as well as their involvement in pregnancy resolution decisions.

The topic of chapter 12 by Adler, Smith, and Tschann is abortion among adolescents, in particular the issue of parental consent legislation. Two assumptions underlie the perceived need for parental consent. First, it assumes that abortion has negative psychological consequences for adolescents. Second, it assumes that adolescents are unable to make informed decisions about the risks associated with abortion. Adler, Smith, and Tschann review the empirical evidence and find that the research to date supports neither of these assumptions. The authors conclude with recommendations for further research on adolescence and abortion.

Overall, the chapters in this section examine a large number of macro- and microlevel variables that influence abortion decisions and their consequences. Interpersonal and social factors not only restrict women's access to abortion services but also restrict women's control over their own sexual and contraceptive behaviors. Several of these chapters also question common assumptions about abortion and support the rights and involvement of groups other than adult women, such as adolescents who are often assumed unable to make informed decisions about abortion and men who are often perceived as irrelevant to the abortion decision. An equally important emphasis is placed on the psychological outcomes of abortion, in particular, new abortion technology. As suggested by Miller, Pasta, and Dean in chapter 10, these consequences are complex and fluid, change over the course of time since the abortion procedure, and are dependent on the meaning of abortion to an individual woman and her ability to cope with stress.

Part IV: Abortion in the Context of Practice

Chapters in Part IV raise numerous issues and offer many suggestions about how best to provide abortion services and counsel women who seek abortion, both before and after the procedure. In chapter 13, Fisher, Castle, and Garrity propose a cognitive approach to patient-centered abortion care. In contrast to the focus on psychopathological reactions to abortion in the literature, these authors propose an abortion counseling strategy that is based on cognitive social psychological theory. The cognitive approach to patient-centered abortion care (a) recognizes that the social psychological elements within the clinic need to be managed; (b) is time limited, goal oriented, and problem focused; (c) restructures how patients think about their decision; and (d) focuses on the pregnancy resolution decision. To illustrate how the cognitive approach works in the clinical setting, Fisher, Castle, and Garrity provide specific examples of techniques that can be used in the pre- and postabortion counseling of women seeking a first trimester abortion and in patient–staff interactions during the procedure. In addition to addressing the patient's psychological needs, this approach can positively influence the ease of conducting the abortion and the woman's postabortion experience.

In chapter 14, Rivera discusses clinical issues related to the abortion experience that may be considered during psychotherapy. In contrast to abortion counseling, which focuses on decision making around having an abortion, in psychotherapy women are seeking to better understand their abortion experience and how it relates to their perceptions of themselves. This chapter offers suggestions for treating women who raise abortion as an issue. According to Rivera, psychotherapy must address three interdependent phases of the abortion experience: the pregnancy acknowledgment phase, the pregnancy resolution phase, and the postabortion response phase. Rather than focusing only on the emotional aftermath of having an abortion, therapists should address the entire abortion experience and the larger context within which the woman's abortion occurs. Rivera also considers the danger of therapist bias, especially when therapists' views are based on traditional gender roles or a pro-life ideology, and the need for therapists' awareness of how their views may affect the psychotherapeutic process.

Chapter 15, by Masho, Coeytaux, and Potts, examines how the practices of other countries can be applied in the United States to improve access to and the quality of abortion services. Following the examples set by other countries, abortion services in the United States can be improved in a variety of ways. First, abortion training must be incorporated into existing medical school training curricula and made available for currently practicing health professionals. Second, nonphysicians such as physician assistants, nurse-midwives, and nurse practitioners can be trained to perform abortions. Third, abortion services can be decentralized through the use of manual vacuum aspiration. Fourth, new abortion technologies must be explored and made available. Finally, the United States must recognize that restrictive abortion policies have adverse consequences for the lives of women and children.

These chapters describe a plethora of ways to improve the provision of abortion services. Models and programs already available both internationally and nationally provide direction for such efforts. It is imperative to provide adequate mental health services for women at all stages of the abortion process. Appropriate counseling can help women make better informed decisions about pregnancy termination. Psychotherapy techniques, particularly feminist methods, can help alleviate possible negative consequences of abortion such as guilt and regret that are experienced by some abortion patients. Emerging abortion technologies such as medical abortion will create new challenges for provider and patient education and appropriate counseling of women regarding choice among methods.

Part V: Conclusion

In chapter 16, Harvey, Beckman, and Bird discuss recommendations to strengthen the availability and quality of abortion services, promote legislation and public policy that both protect women who seek abortion and reduce the societal need for abortion, and provide empirical support for policy and legislative initiatives. Although the authors believe that it is important to acknowledge and be respectful of differing values about the acceptability of abortion, they emphasize that empirical data support the need for access to safe, legal abortion. They emphasize that abortion and other reproductive health services need to be considered within the larger context of women's role in society. The broader issues of sexism, racism, and classism must be addressed if the long-term health and well-being of women in the United States are to be improved significantly. They recommend that the pro-choice movement build partnerships with pro-life feminists and the multiracial reproductive rights movement to achieve common goals that promote women's health and improve their social, economic, and political status.

This volume is particularly timely because of the many policy issues involving abortion currently being debated, the changing political and social context of abortion as we approach the 21st century, and the development and introduction of new medical methods such as mifepristone and methotrexate that may transform the future provision of abortion services. We have tried to provide a fresh look at issues and controversies surrounding abortion in the United States today, discussing the implications of research for the improvement of women's mental and physical health.

REFERENCES

David, H. P. (1971). Abortion: Public health concerns and needed psychosocial research. *American Journal of Public Health, 61,* 510–516.

David, H. P. (1992). Born unwanted: Long-term developmental effects of denied abortion. *Journal of Social Issues, 48*(3), 163–181.

Forrest, J., & Henshaw, S. (1993). Providing controversial health care: Abortion services since 1973. *Women's Health Issues, 3*(3), 152–157.

Henshaw, S., & Kost, K. (1996). Abortion patients in 1994–95: Characteristics and contraceptive use. *Family Planning Perspectives, 28,* 140–147, 158.

Tietze, C. (1984). The public health effects of legal abortion in the United States. *Family Planning Perspectives, 16*(1), 26–28.

I

THE SOCIOPOLITICAL
CONTEXT OF ABORTION

1

FEDERAL ABORTION POLICY AND POLITICS: 1973 to 1996

BRIAN L. WILCOX, JENNIFER K. ROBBENNOLT,
AND JANET E. O'KEEFFE

Few policy issues have created as much political turmoil as abortion (Steiner, 1983). In the two plus decades since the U.S. Supreme Court held, in *Roe v. Wade* (1973; hereafter, *Roe*), that the Constitution protects a woman's decision whether to terminate a pregnancy and, in *Doe v. Bolton* (1973), that a state may not unduly burden the exercise of that right through regulations that prohibit or limit access to services necessary for the exercise of that right, the debate surrounding abortion has continued at a steady boil, representing what one constitutional scholar called a "clashing of absolutes" (Tribe, 1990).

This article reviews the legislative branch actions triggered in large part by these two decisions and examines the extra-legislative initiatives undertaken by the executive branch designed to alter abortion policy. This discussion explores several different areas of policy and provides some indications of the extent to which abortion politics have influenced the course of policy discussions and decisions on a wide variety of issues. The periods 1973–1988, 1989–1992, and 1993–1996 are all discussed separately. The first period represents the 15 years following *Roe*, a time span that saw abortion opponents gaining the clear upper hand in the legislative arena. We examine the second period to ascertain the impact of the Supreme Court's decision in *Webster v. Reproductive Health Services* (1989) on policy making during the Bush presidency. The discussion of the final period reviews the abortion policy landscape as influenced by the pro-choice administration of President Clinton. Finally, we examine the role to be played by psychology in addressing these policy questions.

ABORTION-RELATED LEGISLATION: 1973 TO 1988

In the years since *Roe*, over 1,000 bills addressing abortion in one manner or another have been introduced by members of the U.S. Congress. Generally, these bills fall into one of three categories: (a) constitutional amendments, (b) statutes prohibiting or restricting abortion, and (c) appropriation amendments limiting funding for abortion services.

Constitutional Amendments

Opponents of legalized abortion have sponsored dozens of constitutional amendments designed to reverse the effects of *Roe*. These amendments tend to fall into two distinct classes: right-to-life or human life amendments and states' rights amendments. The former would grant a new right to the fetus—personhood—which the Supreme Court has declared is not guaranteed under the Constitution. Right-to-life amendments attempt to extend Fifth and Fourteenth Amendment protections to the unborn fetus. These proposals use a variety of terms to define the point at which this new right would attach to the fetus: at the moment of fertilization, at any state of biological development, at conception, and so forth. Some of these amendments have been crafted to allow for certain exceptions to the general ban on abortions (e.g., in cases of rape or incest, to prevent the death of or protect the health of the mother); others allow no exceptions. States rights amendments would give states the option of setting their own abortion standard, much as was the case prior to the decision in *Roe*.

The only time a constitutional amendment addressing abortion was considered on the floor by either the House or the Senate was in 1983. The Human Life Federalism Amendment (S. J. Res. 3), introduced by Senator Orrin Hatch (R-UT), was debated by the Senate after having been considered by the Senate Committee on the Judiciary and sent to the Senate floor without recommendation. An amendment by Senator Thomas Eagleton (D-MO) stripped the bill of enforcement provisions, leaving a straightforward bill: "A right to abortion is not secured by this Constitution." This language was designed to return complete authority for abortion policy to the state legislatures—in essence, a reversal of *Roe*.

Passage of a constitutional amendment is complex, first requiring affirmation by a supermajority (two thirds) of each chamber of Congress prior to ratification by the states. Senator Hatch's legislation received only 50 votes—far short of the 67 needed (Carr, 1991).

In recent years, pro-choice members of Congress have virtually abandoned this strategy. Although members continue to introduce constitutional amendments, no serious attempt to bring such legislation to a vote has occurred since the defeat of the Hatch amendment in 1983.

Abortion-Related Statutes

Partly because of the difficulty of achieving the supermajority necessary for the passage of a constitutional amendment, members of Congress have more often attempted to achieve the same ends through legislation, with somewhat more limited aims. Some of these bills are quite broad and others are very narrow. An example of a broad bill is one introduced by Representative Henry Hyde (R-IL) during the 98th Congress. This bill, H.R. 618, would have broadly prohibited federal involvement in abortions, except when the mother's life might be endangered. Prohibited activities would have included (a) use of federal funds to perform, reimburse, or refer for abortion; (b) performance of abortion by any federal agency; (c) contracting for health insurance that covers abortions; (d) supporting, financially or otherwise, the performance of abortions in other countries; and (e) discrimination against persons on the basis of their opposition to abortion. No action was taken on this legislation.

There are several examples of more narrowly tailored legislation designed to limit access to abortion. During debate on the Tax Reform Act of 1986 in the 99th Congress, Senator Gordon Humphrey (R-NH) offered an amendment designed to deny tax-exempt status to organizations that directly or indirectly performed or financed abortions. Humphrey withdrew the amendment after considerable pressure was placed on him by Senator Robert Dole (R-KS), then the majority leader of the Senate, and the Reagan administration, which had agreed on a "no amendment" strategy for passing the tax bill.

Another example occurred during consideration of the Civil Rights Restoration Act in 1988. The threat of abortion-related amendments held up consideration of this bill for 2 years. Once the bill was finally brought up, Senator John Danforth (R-MO) offered an "abortion neutral" amendment that stated that

> Nothing in this title shall be construed to require or prohibit any person, or public or private entity, to provide or pay for any benefit or service, including the use of facilities, related to an abortion. Nothing

in this section shall be construed to permit a penalty to be imposed on any person because such person has received any benefit or service related to a legal abortion.

According to Danforth, the amendment was designed to protect church-affiliated colleges and universities from sex discrimination suits under Title IX should those institutions choose not to provide, fund directly or indirectly, or provide facilities for abortions. This amendment passed by a vote of 56 to 39.

On the international front, the abortion battle has been fought out in the foreign aid authorizations for family planning programs. These include (a) measures to reverse the Reagan administration's Mexico City policy—effective since 1985, which prohibits U.S. family planning aid to foreign nongovernmental organizations that use non-U.S. funds to provide abortion and information and referrals for abortion—and (b) measures that would reverse the ban on U.S. support to the United Nations Fund for Population Assistance (UNFPA), originally cut off due to concern over reports of coerced abortions under China's family planning program. Attempts to reverse these two policies have repeatedly failed.

Appropriations Bill Amendments

The principal strategy of pro-life legislators has been the "Hyde-type" amendments to appropriation bills, named after their originator, Representative Hyde. The first version of these amendments, attached to the fiscal year 1977 (FY77) Labor–Health, Education, and Welfare (Labor–HEW) Appropriation Act, stated the following:

> None of the funds contained in this Act shall be used to perform abortions except where the life of the mother would be endangered if the fetus were carried to term.

Later versions of this type of amendment have been extended to other appropriation bills, including the Department of Defense bill, the District of Columbia bill, the Treasury–Postal Service bill, and the Department of Justice bill. The funding ban attached to the Treasury–Postal Service bill was one of the broadest in terms of impact because it prohibited coverage for abortion services in the Federal Employees Health Benefits Program. The Department of Defense abortion funding prohibition was codified in 1984, making it unnecessary to revisit the issue during the annual appropriation process. The restrictions imposed by the District of Columbia bill were broadened in 1989 to preclude the District from using its own non-federal funds to finance abortion services.

Some of these bills contain language identical to the original Hyde amendment; others include exceptions for pregnancies resulting from rape or incest (such as the Department of Justice bill). During the 97th, 98th and 99th Congresses and the first session of the 100th Congress, the Labor–HEW (later to become the Labor–Health and Human Services, HHS) bill contained the original Hyde language. In 1988, however, the Senate passed its Labor–HHS–appropriation bill with an amendment by Senator Lowell Weicker (R-CT) that would have provided Medicaid funding for abortions in cases of rape or incest. The attempt to expand access to abortion services to poor women failed when the House refused to accept the Senate provision.

Passage of these Hyde amendments has had a significant effect on federal financing of abortions. By 1978, federally financed Medicaid abortions had been reduced by 99%. It is estimated that slightly more than 200,000 abortions that would have been paid for by Medicaid are no longer eligible for federal funds. Nevertheless, the overall trend in abortion numbers and rates increased from 23,000 in 1969 (pre-*Roe*) to about 1.6 million in 1990. The abortion rate (abortions per 1,000 women 15–44 years of age) stabilized at about 29,000 between 1980 and 1990 before declining to 26,000 in 1992 (Alan Guttmacher Institute, 1995). And although sound data are not available, most policy analysts believe that the majority of Medicaid-eligible women desiring abortions find some way of financing the procedure (Steiner, 1983).

Summary

Legislation addressing the issue of abortion has become a constant in Congress. Both sides have experienced victories of various magnitudes. The mixture of victories and defeats has provided incentive for the participants to continue the fight. The most successful tactic for placing restrictions on abortions has been the Hyde-type appropriation amendments. Unless there is a substantial change in the political landscape in the near future, the likelihood for passage of a Constitutional amendment of either of the two types discussed is quite slim. Between 1984 and 1988 even the most ardent pro-life members of Congress ceased anything more than token efforts at securing the passage of legislation that would tip the current policy balance in a significant fashion. Similarly, pro-choice advocates did not seriously entertain notions of overturning the abortion-funding restrictions. It appeared as though a truce had been called within Congress. This seeming truce was shattered in 1989 when the Supreme Court handed down its decision in *Webster v. Reproductive Health Services* (hereafter, *Webster*). This decision significantly expanded the state's ability to place restrictions on a woman's access to abortion. The federal legislative ramifications of this decision are discussed following a review of federal extra-legislative actions affecting abortion policy.

REGULATORY POLICY AND ADMINISTRATIVE ACTIONS: 1989 TO 1992

During his first 6 years in office, President Reagan, like his predecessor President Carter, found little support in Congress for his proposals to radically alter the abortion policy landscape. A new strategy was developed in mid-1987, however, that took a very different tack at the policy dilemma. White House staff members argued that because there is and always will be disagreement about the appropriateness of legal abortion, the debate must be framed in a different way (Victor, 1987). They suggested that because there is fairly widespread agreement among the public that abortion is undesirable, even among individuals who support the continued legality of access to abortion services, much like the growing consensus that smoking is undesirable, the administration should choose a policy approach similar to the one taken in the smoking arena. Among the suggestions offered by the staffers were the following: (a) transfer program funds from groups that promote or otherwise support abortions to those that assist with adoptions, (b) end tax deductions for medical expenses associated with abortions, (c) direct the Surgeon General to develop and disseminate pamphlets warning of the medical hazards of abortion, and (d) veto every bill allowing federal dollars to be spent on abortion.

This approach was adopted by President Reagan and highlighted in his July 30, 1987, remarks to right-to-life activists. In a letter to Surgeon General C. Everett Koop, Reagan ordered Koop to prepare "a comprehensive medical report on the health effects, physical and emotional, of abortion on women" (R. Reagan, personal communication to C. E. Koop, July 30, 1987). It is worth noting that the Surgeon General, an outspoken right-to-life advocate, was extremely displeased about being brought into the abortion debate at a time when he wished to devote his attentions to AIDS and smoking. Nonetheless, Koop conducted a review of the research on the physical and mental health sequelae of abortion for women. In a follow-up letter to the president, Koop (1989) informed President Reagan that his review had concluded that the physical risks associated with abortion were insignificant and that methodological problems characteristic of most studies of the mental health sequelae of abortion prevented any conclusions from being drawn. Consequently, the Reagan administration did not publicly release the Surgeon General's report, hoping to avoid the embarrassment of seeing their "public health strategy" backfire in the media. Congressional hearings (Medical and Psychological Impact of Abortion, 1989) and reports (H. Rep. 101-392, 1989), however, placed the Surgeon General

on record as concluding that there are no long-term physical health sequelae of abortion and that abortion does not represent a public health
problem with respect to the mental health of women. Representative Ted
Weiss later published the "final draft" of the Surgeon General's report in
the *Congressional Record* ("Abortion report," 1989).

Reagan also ordered the Department of Health and Human Services
to issue new regulations for the Title X family planning program that would
deny funding to any group providing abortion counseling or referral as part
of its services. The regulations were to require all Title X grant recipients
to separate all nonfederally funded abortion services both administratively
and physically from Title X programs. Further, Title X funds were to be
denied to any organization promoting, encouraging, or advocating abortions, even with their own funds.

The Office of Population Affairs within HHS was charged with draft-
ing revised regulations for Title X. The proposed regulations were published
on September 1, 1987, and followed the outline just given. Final regulations were issued by HHS on February 2, 1988. Few changes were made
from the draft regulations, despite protests by nearly all national health
organizations and over 200 members of Congress. Several organizations and
states immediately filed suit in Colorado, Massachusetts, and New York to
block implementation of the regulations, scheduled to take effect on March
3, 1988. On that day, the U.S. District Court for Massachusetts issued a
permanent injunction, stating that the regulations as a whole violate both
congressional intent and rights protected by the Constitution. Judges in
Colorado also declared the regulations unconstitutional, but the second
circuit court in New York upheld the regulations. Given this split, the
Bush administration appealed the decision to the Supreme Court, which
agreed to hear the case. On May 23, 1991, the Supreme Court, in *Rust v.
Sullivan* (1991, hereafter, *Rust*), upheld the constitutionality of the regulations.

Finally, the Reagan administration imposed a ban on the use of federal
funds in research using fetal tissue. Over the past decade, researchers have
been exploring the possible use of fetal tissue transplants in treating a
number of diseases, most notably Parkinson's disease. The administration
argued that if research demonstrated that fetal tissue is effective in treating
such disorders, the demand for fetal tissue might lead to an increase in the
abortion rate. President Bush decided to continue the ban in 1989, despite
the recommendations of two advisory committees that ethical safeguards
could easily be put in place to prevent such a consequence (Rovner, 1991).

ABORTION-RELATED LEGISLATION: 1989 TO 1992

Following the Supreme Court decision in *Webster*, handed down in
July 1989, the 101st Congress witnessed a significant shift in the 10-year

pattern of antiabortion votes, particularly in the House of Representatives. This shift has been attributed to the mobilization of support for abortion rights following the *Webster* decision, just as the *Roe* decision mobilized those who were opposed to abortion in 1973. However, although several pro-choice measures were passed in the 101st Congress, they were vetoed by President Bush, and the Congress was unable to gather sufficient votes for an override. The change in the political landscape was significant, nonetheless. Prior to 1989, abortion-related legislation passed or failed to pass with little direct involvement of the executive branch. Following *Webster*, numerous policy vehicles designed to eliminate some prior restrictions on access to abortion have reached the White House, forcing the president to take a more active and visible role in the national debate.

Abortion-Related Statutes

Title X of the Public Health Service Act is the major source of public funds for family planning services. Because of opposition from antiabortion advocates, the program has not been authorized since 1985, although it continues to be funded on a yearly basis. In the second session of the 101st Congress, the reauthorization bill was brought to the Senate floor for the first time in 5 years. At this time, the Senate passed an amendment offered by Senator Chafee overturning the Reagan administration's regulations—widely referred to as the "gag rule"—which prohibited, among other things, abortion counseling and referrals in family planning clinics funded under Title X. The Supreme Court had heard oral arguments in *Rust* but had not yet issued a ruling. However, the Senate failed to table another amendment offered by Senator Armstrong that required Title X programs offering abortion services (with non-Title X funds) to notify a parent of a minor seeking an abortion. As a result, the sponsors withdrew the entire Title X reauthorization bill at the request of the family planning advocacy community.

On May 23, 1991, during the first session of the 102nd Congress, the Supreme Court issued its opinion in *Rust*, ruling 5 to 4 that the Reagan administration regulations barring abortion counseling and referrals did not violate free speech and privacy rights guaranteed by the First and Fifth Amendments. In addition, the decision stated that the HHS regulations were a reasonable interpretation of the statute's prohibition of the use of Title X funds in programs where abortion is a method of family planning. The decision resulted in an immediate public campaign to overturn the regulations. A broad coalition of organizations, ranging from the American Civil Liberties Union to the American College of Obstetricians and Gynecologists, voiced opposition to the regulations on the grounds that they allow the federal government to dictate what physicians and other health care workers may and may not say to their patients. In effect, the regulations require that health care providers violate their professional code of ethics, which require them to give patients complete information regarding all of their options for dealing with a problem pregnancy.

Legislation designed to overturn the Title X regulations had been introduced in both houses in advance of the *Rust* decision, and as soon as the decision was issued, congressional leaders indicated that they would move quickly to pass the bills. The Senate bill, introduced by Senator John Chafee (R-RI), was approved 12 to 5 by the Senate Labor and Human Resources Committee but was never considered by the full Senate. In the House, two measures had been introduced that would have overturned the gag rule: a free-standing bill introduced by Representatives John Porter (R-IL), Henry Waxman (D-CA), and Ron Wyden (D-OR) and language contained in Waxman's Title X reauthorization bill. Initial attempts to mark up these bills in Waxman's Subcommittee on Health and the Environment were unsuccessful because pro-life members threatened to attach parental notice amendments, which the committee chairman did not have the votes to defeat. A second attempt succeeded after the chairman offered a pre-empting parental notification amendment that in essence recognized parental notification law as an issue to be settled at the state level.

Given the problems inherent in passing a bill directly overturning the Title X regulations, pro-choice members in the House attached an amendment to the Labor–HHS appropriation bill prohibiting the Department of Health and Human Services from spending any of its funding on enforcement of the regulations. A parental notice amendment was also included, but because of House of Representatives rules prohibiting the inclusion of authorizing legislation in an appropriation bill, it was struck from the bill on a point of order when it was considered by the entire House. The campaign to repeal the regulations failed when supporters realized they lacked the votes to override President Bush's veto authority.

As in previous Congresses, a number of bills to restrict abortion rights were introduced in the 101st and 102nd Congresses. However, the 101st Congress saw the first-time introduction of a bill that would guarantee the right of a woman to terminate a pregnancy should *Roe* be overturned. On November 17, 1989, Senator Alan Cranston (D-CA) introduced the Freedom of Choice Act, which was designed to codify *Roe*. A companion bill introduced in the House by Representative Edwards (D-CA) would have forbidden states from limiting a woman's right to an abortion prior to fetal viability. Hearings on the bill were held by the Senate Labor and Human Resources Committee, and it was reported out of the House Judiciary Subcommittee on Civil and Constitutional Rights without any weakening amendments, but did not receive further consideration in either the House or the Senate.

A large group of House members reintroduced the Freedom of Choice

Act on the first day of the 102nd Congress. Like its predecessor, this bill was designed to supersede states' authority to limit access to abortion, in effect codifying *Roe*. A companion bill was later introduced in the Senate. However, given the already large number of abortion votes expected in the 102nd Congress and the assurance of a presidential veto of any pro-choice measures, the legislation was never brought up for a vote.

Several bills to restrict abortion rights were introduced in the 101st Congress, including a measure by Representative Robert Dornan (R-CA), which would have declared fetuses to be persons, but none of these measures were seriously considered. In the 102nd Congress, measures designed to limit access to abortion included a bill that would have permanently codified existing abortion restrictions using appropriated funds, a bill that would have prohibited abortions from being performed solely because of the gender of the fetus (the Civil Rights of Infants Act), a bill intended to prohibit federal funding for research on RU-486 (the French-developed abortifacient), and bills designed to establish parental notification requirements for any programs receiving federal financial aid. None of the bills received serious attention by either legislative body.

The issue of minors' access to abortion services has proven to be the major impediment to the passage of pro-choice legislation in the Congress. Because polls show that the majority of Americans support some parental involvement in minors' abortion decisions, even pro-choice members of Congress are reluctant to oppose amendments requiring parental notice. In addition, many members seem to view the issue from their own personal perspective as parents and appear unwilling to consider the problems involved in enforcing such laws and their potentially deleterious consequences for many minors. Because neither side of the abortion debate desires to compromise on this issue, the threat of parental notification provisions virtually guarantees the effective defeat of any legislation to which they might be attached, as happened in the 101st Congress when the Title X bill was pulled from the Senate floor, and in the 102nd, when Representative Waxman chose not to mark up the free-standing reversal of the Title X regulations because he did not have the votes to defeat a parental notification provision.

Appropriations

Because Congress must make appropriations decisions annually, attempts to advance the agenda of both sides in the abortion debate are seen most consistently in this area. Since the Supreme Court's decision in *Webster*, the issue of federal funding has been revisited each year by those attempting to relax the prohibitions and those seeking to maintain or extend them.

In the FY90 District of Columbia appropriations bill, the House rejected an amendment barring federal funds for abortion even to save the life of a woman and prohibiting the District government from using its own locally raised revenue to fund abortions for poor women. This was the first success for pro-choice advocates following the *Webster* decision and the first time the House voted against an abortion-funding restriction since 1980. However, given that the amendment barred federal funding even to save the life of the mother, the 206 votes in support of the amendment indicate the continuing strong antiabortion views of a large number of House members. The Senate also did not include the restrictive language in its final bill, but two vetoes by President Bush ultimately led to the adoption of the restrictive language.

In 1990, during the second session of the 101st Congress, both the House and the Senate passed District appropriations bills adopting this less restrictive language, but the Conference Report was defeated when antiabortion members in the House argued that voting for the Report was tantamount to a vote for abortion rights.

Another post-*Webster* appropriation vote saw the House reverse its long-standing support of the Hyde amendment prohibiting Medicaid funding of abortions, except to save the life of a woman. Instead, the House passed an amendment by Representative Barbara Boxer (D-CA) to the Labor–HHS–Education FY90 appropriations bill that allowed Medicaid to fund abortions for poor victims of rape or incest. The Senate also voted to expand Medicaid coverage in these cases, but President Bush vetoed the appropriations bill and the Congress failed to obtain the votes for an override.

In the second session of the 101st Congress, given general public support for rape and incest exceptions, antiabortion forces in the Senate developed a strategy to prevent negative publicity surrounding another presidential veto of an amendment providing exceptions to the abortion-funding ban in cases where the pregnancy results from rape or incest. To assure that the Labor–HHS FY91 appropriations bill would not reach President Bush with the rape and incest language, Senator Armstrong offered an amendment requiring that any program receiving any federal funds, even though those funds are not used for abortion-related services, require parental notification for minors seeking an abortion. The amendment made no provision for alternatives to parental notification, such as a judicial decision declaring that notification is not in the best interests of the minor. A motion to table this amendment failed on a tie vote, and procedural requirements resulted in the joining of the parental notification provision and the rape and incest provisions in the final bill. Because a majority of the conference committee members did not want to see the parental notification provision pass, the rape and incest as well as the parental notification provisions were dropped.

Congress has also attempted to reshape the Department of Defense's policy on abortion through the annual appropriations bills. For a number of years, the Department of Defense permitted abortions in overseas military hospitals on a private pay basis. This was a necessity for women stationed in countries where abortion was illegal or very difficult to obtain, such as Germany, the Philippines, and Saudi Arabia. It is estimated that approximately 65,000 women in the military and 400,000 dependents of military personnel who serve overseas are affected by the policy, which was rescinded in 1988. In the 101st Congress, the Senate passed but the House defeated a bill to repeal a Defense Department policy prohibiting women in the military and their dependents from having an abortion in a military health facility, even though paid with personal funds. However, in the 102nd Congress, partly as a result of the publicity surrounding deployment of large numbers of women in the Gulf War, the House and Senate included provisions in both the Department of Defense authorization and appropriation bills to repeal the policy, but the provisions were dropped by the conference committees. A free-standing bill to overturn the policy was passed late in 1992 and sent to President Bush, who pocket-vetoed the bill and prevented an override attempt.

REGULATORY POLICY AND ADMINISTRATIVE ACTIONS: 1993 TO 1996

President Clinton took office in January 1993 and almost immediately began to take actions designed to forge a change in abortion policy. On January 22, 1993, just days after taking office, Clinton issued a series of executive orders regarding abortion policy. First, Clinton called an end to enforcement of the gag-rule, which had prohibited facilities receiving federal funds from engaging in abortion counseling or referral. These regulations had been upheld by the Supreme Court in *Rust v. Sullivan* in 1991. Second, Clinton ordered an end to the ban on federal funding for fetal tissue research. This prohibition had been in place since 1988, late in the Reagan administration. Third, Clinton ordered an end to the ban on privately funded abortions in military hospitals overseas that had been in place since 1988. Fourth, Clinton instructed the Department of Health and Human Services to investigate the appropriateness of lifting the "import alert" that had forbidden the importation of the abortifacient RU-486 into the United States. Finally, Clinton overturned the ban against U.S. aid to international organizations that performed or promoted abortions. These changes were thought by many to signal an important shift in abortion politics.

In addition to his appointment of Justices Ginsburg and Breyer to the Supreme Court bench in 1993 and 1994, one Clinton nomination that was notable in terms of abortion policy was his failed nomination of Henry

Foster as Surgeon General. Foster, an advocate of legal access to safe abortions and of access to birth control for adolescents, was nominated to replace Joycelyn Elders as Surgeon General in February 1995. Foster had developed a program to combat teenage pregnancy and had been designated one of President Bush's "points of light" in 1991.

Within days of his nomination, Foster faced trouble from antiabortion groups over his abortion history. Some groups were concerned that there had been "misstatements" regarding the precise number of abortions he had performed as a practicing obstetrician-gynecologist. Others felt that the fact that Foster had performed abortions at all, even though they were legal, should disqualify him from consideration as Surgeon General altogether. This exemplified a shift in strategy for abortion opponents from the earlier persistent attacks on the legality of abortion to challenging "the moral and ethical acceptability of abortion" (Schneider, 1995, p. 462). The hope was that these tactics would appeal to the large number of Americans who, although opposed to making abortion illegal, supported efforts to curtail the number of abortions performed (such as teen pregnancy prevention programs). President Clinton repeatedly expressed this view in his position that abortion should be "safe, legal, and rare." Moreover, these tactics send the message to other physicians that performing abortions "is a risky and controversial activity that imperils your career" (Schneider, 1995, p. 462), furthering the objective of making abortion less accessible.

The Senate Labor and Human Services Committee voted 9 to 7 on May 26, 1995, to support Foster's nomination. However, on June 21 and 22 the Senate blocked a vote on the nomination, effectively ending Foster's chances. In January 1996, President Clinton appointed Foster senior advisor to the president for teen pregnancy prevention and youth development, a position that does not require approval by Congress.

ABORTION-RELATED LEGISLATION: 1993 TO 1996

Discussions in Congress during 1992 through 1996 continued to include a number of debates over abortion rights. Although amendments to the Constitution continued to be introduced, none reached the point of being debated on the floor of either the House or the Senate. Attempts to make abortion illegal were less common than in years past, and the debate centered more strongly around the delineation of the contours of the right. Instead of trying to make abortion illegal, antiabortion activists attempted to make it more difficult to access and finance abortion, attempted to weaken the moral acceptability of doctors and clinics that perform abortions, and attempted to forestall any gains by the pro-choice movement. For their part, abortion-rights supporters attempted to ensure broad access to abortion services and information.

Constitutional Amendments

Opponents of legalized abortions continued to sponsor legislation designed to amend the Constitution of the United States to either protect or to prohibit abortion. An example is the Right to Life Act of 1995. This legislation would direct that "the right to life guaranteed by the Constitution is vested in each human being at fertilization." However, neither this nor any other proposed amendment was debated on the floor of either chamber. Instead, the debate surrounding abortion rights focused on specific statutes and appropriations legislation.

Abortion-Related Statutes

A number of abortion-related statutes were introduced in the 103rd and 104th Congresses by both sides in the abortion debate. Most of these actions had less to do with the legality of abortion per se and more to do with policies that would affect access to abortions or policies argued to encourage or discourage abortions.

Shortly after President Clinton lifted the ban on the use of federal funds for fetal tissue research, the 103rd Congress codified this ruling in the National Institutes of Health (NIH) Reauthorization legislation. Concerned that safeguards be in place to prevent the policy from encouraging women to have abortions, the bill delineated rules intended to prevent abuses (e.g., prohibition of the purchase or sale of fetal tissue). In 1992, President Bush had vetoed a similar measure, but President Clinton signed the NIH reauthorization in June 1993.

Another major issue faced by the 103rd Congress involved women's access to abortion clinics. Abortion rights supporters were spurred to action early in 1993 when the Supreme Court issued a ruling in *Bray v. Alexandria Women's Health Clinic* (1993). The Court ruled that an 1871 civil rights law (commonly known as the Ku Klux Klan Act) could not be used to obtain injunctions against abortion protesters. Concurrently, in 1993, violence surrounding abortion clinics escalated, reaching its height in the fatal shooting of David Gunn outside an abortion clinic in Pensacola, Florida. By the end of the first session of the 103rd Congress, both the House and the Senate had passed bills making it a federal crime to use force, the threat of force, or physical obstruction to intimidate abortion clinic workers or women clients of clinics. The bills also prohibited the destruction of clinic property and provided criminal penalties for violations. An amendment offered by Senator Hatch (R-Utah) was adopted that extended the protections of the legislation to pregnancy counseling centers operated by antiabortion supporters and places of worship as well as to abortion clinics. The legislation was intended to prohibit violent or threatening behavior while permitting free speech and expression of individual viewpoints. President Clinton signed the bill on May 26, 1994. Two Supreme Court cases in 1994 further narrowed the rights of antiabortion protesters outside clinics. In *National Organization for Women, Inc. v. Scheidler* (1994), the Court held that RICO, an organized crime statute that provides for treble damages, could be used to sue those engaged in violence against abortion clinics. Later, in *Madsen v. Women's Health Center* (1994), the Court held that a court-ordered 36-foot buffer zone around an abortion clinic was constitutionally acceptable.

Welfare and health care reforms were the focus of much legislative discussion in 1994 and 1995. The abortion-related controversy in the reform of national health care largely centered around whether coverage for abortion-related services would be included in a mandated package of standard benefits. Abortion-rights supporters advocated the inclusion of abortion coverage, whereas antiabortion activists fought to eliminate abortion from the standard package or, at least, to allow each insurance company to decide whether to cover abortions. No clear winner emerged from the debate and no comprehensive health care reform legislation was completed.

In the summer of 1996 the House and Senate passed the Personal Responsibility and Work Opportunity Act of 1996, which turned over much responsibility for welfare to the individual states but mandated strict guidelines for eligibility. A set of provisions in the welfare reform package that generated objections from both sides of the abortion debate provided for optional denial of cash welfare benefits to unwed teenage mothers and denial of increases in a family's benefits for children conceived while the mother was receiving welfare (known as a "child exclusion" or "family cap"). Some abortion opponents opposed these provisions because they feared that such restrictions would motivate more women to have abortions. Simultaneously, abortion-rights supporters opposed these provisions because welfare benefits were tied to the reproductive choices of mothers. In response to these types of concerns, the legislation included a financial incentive intended to encourage states to reduce their rates of out-of-wedlock births while avoiding any increase in the number of abortions performed. This incentive was known as the "illegitimacy ratio" and was originally equal to the number of out-of-wedlock births plus the number of abortions performed, all divided by the total number of births in the state. States reducing this ratio were to be provided with additional block grant monies. In response to concerns voiced by abortion-rights supporters that such a system would encourage states to restrict access to abortion services, the illegitimacy ratio formula was amended to equal the number of out-of-wedlock births plus the number of additional abortions performed over the number performed in the previous year, all divided by the total number of births. An attempt to strike the illegitimacy ratio from the legislation altogether was unsuccessful. It is unclear how states will calculate their illegitimacy ratios, as many do not collect and report information on abortions.

The 104th Congress also marked the first time an attempt was made to codify language restricting federal funding for abortions as part of the Medicaid statute. Prior to this time, Medicaid funding restrictions, Hyde-amendment language, had always been debated yearly as part of the appropriations process for the Department of Health and Human Services. The Medicaid Transformations Act proposed to revise Title XIX of the Social Security Act (the statute that governs Medicaid) so that prohibitions on Medicaid funding of abortions except in cases of rape, incest, and life endangerment would be directly incorporated into the statute. Although it is significant that the attempt was made, the measure was vetoed by President Clinton as part of the Balanced Budget Act of 1995 in December 1995 and did not become law.

Another new tactic that surfaced in the 104th Congress was the attempt to make the performance of a specific abortion technique subject to criminal sanctions and civil damages. The particular abortion technique, termed *late-term* abortion or *partial-birth* abortion, is a procedure typically performed after the pregnancy has progressed past 20 weeks and involves the partial vaginal delivery of the fetus and the collapsing of the head prior to the completion of the abortion. The passage of this legislation by the House and the Senate marked the first time that Congress had voted to criminalize an abortion method. The legislation was viewed by both sides of the debate as a direct attack on the right to abortion established in *Roe* and a retreat on the deference given to decisions made by a woman and her doctor (Idelson & Palmer, 1995). Bill supporters pointed to what they saw as the "needlessly brutal" nature of the procedure, whereas opponents of the bill emphasized the technique's use as a safer alternative for women whose pregnancies are past 20 weeks and whose lives are in danger or whose fetuses have severe problems. Stating that the "bill does not allow women to protect themselves from serious threat to their health" and as such "is consistent neither with the Constitution nor with sound public policy," President Clinton vetoed the Partial-Birth Abortion Ban Act of 1995 on April 10, 1996 ("Presidential veto message," 1996). An attempt to override the veto failed when the Senate sustained the veto by a nine-vote margin on September 26, 1996.

A final example of the ways in which the abortion debate impacted legislation during 1992 through 1996 is the Comstock Clean-Up Act of 1996. The Comstock Act is a statute passed in 1873 that originally prohibited the mailing, transportation, or importation of materials relating to abortion or contraception. Prohibitions relating to contraception were eliminated by Congress in 1971. Prior to *Roe* prohibitions relating to abortion-related materials were interpreted to mean only materials related to unlawful abortions, and once *Roe* made abortion legal the restrictions remained on the books but were unenforced. The Telecommunications Act of 1996 extended the Comstock Act to apply to the distribution of abortion-related information on computer services such as the Internet. Accordingly, the Comstock Clean-Up Act was introduced in March 1996 and was intended to lift the ban on the distribution of abortion-related materials on the Internet. The bill (H.R. 2272), introduced by Representative Barney Frank (D-MA), was referred to the Subcommittee on Crime of the House Judiciary Committee. As of this writing, the Subcommittee had taken no action on the bill.

Appropriations Bill Amendments

Appropriation legislation continued to be the method of much of the abortion debate during the Clinton administration. However, abortion-related amendments to appropriations bills were inconsistently used during this period. The FY94 appropriations bill for the Departments of Labor and HHS was originally presented without the Hyde-amendment type language, an omission that would have effectively ended the restrictions on Medicaid-financed abortions. However, the final bill continued the Hyde-amendment-type restrictions on the use of Medicaid funds to finance abortions for poor women that had been used since 1981. Nonetheless, the bill expanded the exceptions to include pregnancies that were the result of rape or incest, in addition to those cases in which the life of the mother was endangered. Although abortion opponents had vehemently opposed any relaxation of the restrictions (beyond life endangerment) in prior years, the amendment to allow funding for abortion in cases of rape, incest, or life endangerment was offered by abortion opponents (Hyde, R-IL) to prevent a wholesale elimination of any restrictions. With the focus directed toward health care, this relaxation of restrictions was carried forward to the FY95 appropriations bill with little debate.

However, with the beginning of the Republican-dominated 104th Congress, the debate over the FY96 appropriations bill once again revolved around issues related to abortion. The House adopted an amendment offered by Jim Istook (R-OK) that would require states to use Medicaid funds for abortion only in cases in which the life of the mother was endangered. The Istook amendment would have tightened the restrictions on abortion, returning the bill's language to that which had been in place from 1981 until the FY94 appropriation. Another House-adopted Istook amendment would have prohibited federal grant recipients from using more than a specified proportion of their budgets for political advocacy or lobbying. However, the Senate version did not include either of these restrictions. Finally, in April 1996, President Clinton signed a conference agreement that maintained the FY94 and FY95 exceptions for rape, incest, and life endangerment.

The appropriations legislation for Treasury, Postal Service, and General Government and for Washington, DC, followed a similar pattern over this period, with easing of restrictions for FY94 and FY95 but then a retightening of restrictions for FY96. FY94 was the first year since 1984 that the appropriations bill for Treasury did not impose restrictions on coverage for abortions under the Federal Employees Health Benefits Program. Appropriations bills since 1984 had prohibited the health plan from funding abortions except in cases in which the mother's life was endangered. The conference report that omitted this prohibition was narrowly adopted in the House (207 to 206) but was signed into law by President Clinton on October 28, 1993. Like the Labor–HHS FY95 appropriations legislation, the Treasury abortion funding provisions for FY95 were not debated because of the focus on health care reform; thus, the ban remained lifted.

However, during consideration of the FY96 Treasury appropriations, opposition to abortion coverage by the federal employee's health plan resurfaced. The House approved a bill that would again bar coverage for abortions except in cases in which the mother's life was threatened. However, the Senate rejected similar language, although it did adopt an only slightly more broad amendment introduced by Don Nickles (R-OK) that would bar coverage except in cases of rape, incest, and life endangerment. The final bill that President Clinton signed in November 1995 included the Senate provision and, thus, allowed coverage only for cases of rape, incest, and life endangerment.

The appropriations legislation for Washington, DC, had, since 1980, prohibited the city from spending any federal or locally raised funds on abortions except in cases of rape, incest, or life endangerment. In 1993 this ban was partially lifted in the FY94 District of Columbia appropriations bill; the ban on the use of locally raised funds was eliminated, whereas the ban on the use of federal funds remained. Again, this relaxation of restrictions on abortion was continued in the FY95 bill. Consequently, the District of Columbia was able to use local funds to provide coverage for abortions for women with incomes up to 185% of the poverty level. Again, the debate over these provisions recurred in discussions surrounding the FY96 appropriations for the District of Columbia. Although the Senate version would have continued to allow the use of local funds to finance abortion but to restrict the use of federal funds, the conference committee passed a version similar to that of the House, which prohibited the use of both local and federal funds except in cases of rape, incest, and life endangerment. The omnibus spending bill that was eventually signed by President Clinton in April 1996 did include this restriction.

Clinton's executive order lifting the ban on the performance of abortions at overseas military facilities was also challenged in the 104th Congress. Because there was an existing statutory ban on the use of federal funds for abortions at military facilities absent a threat to the life of the mother, the debate over the Department of Defense's appropriations for FY96 centered around the use of federal military facilities for abortions paid for with private funds. After much contentious debate, the House and Senate agreed to reinstate the ban on privately funded abortions except in cases of rape, incest, and life endangerment. President Clinton, expressing concern about the restrictions on access to abortion contained in the bill, did not sign it, but did allow it to become law without his signature.

Similarly, in FY94 and FY95 the appropriation for the Departments of Commerce, Justice, and State, and the Judiciary did not include restrictions on access to abortions for federal prisoners. However, in discussion of the appropriation for FY96, attempts were made to include restrictions. Both the House and Senate versions of the appropriations legislation prohibited the use of funds for abortions for federal female prisoners except in cases of rape, incest, or life endangerment, but allowed for assistance in scheduling and traveling to obtain an abortion elsewhere. President Clinton vetoed this legislation in December 1995 and the House failed to override this veto in January 1996. However, the omnibus spending bill that was signed in April 1996 did include these restrictions.

PSYCHOLOGY'S CONTRIBUTION

The core of the abortion controversy is essentially a nonscientific one (Callahan, 1982). Most scientists agree that science will not provide answers to some of the central questions in this debate (i.e., when does life begin?). The debate centers around fundamental differences in values, exactly the type of situation that cannot result in an agreement to simply disagree. At this level, at least, psychology's role will be limited.

Nevertheless, psychology must protect against the misuse of psychological research—by either side of the debate. The White House staff policy memo on abortion was clear in its assumption that the Surgeon General's report on the medical and emotional sequelae of abortion would demonstrate significant harms, thereby providing ammunition to the right-to-life movement. Organized psychology, represented by the American Psychological Association (APA), presented testimony to Surgeon General Koop summarizing the research on the psychological sequelae of abortion (APA Public Interest Directorate, 1987; Wilmoth, Bussell, & Wilcox, 1991), and provided testimony on this same issue before a related hearing held by the House Committee on Government Operations (Adler, 1989). In this instance, Koop's failure to draw the conclusions expected by the White House might be due in part to the efforts by psychologists to assure an accurate accounting of the relevant research.

Psychology has also played a role in Congress's debates on the issue of parental notification or consent for minors' abortion decisions. At various points during these debates, members of Congress have made reference to issues such as the capability of minors to make informed, reasoned decisions about their pregnancies, the likely impact of required parental notification or consent on family communications, and the possible effects of such laws on adolescent girls living in violent, dysfunctional families. Again, through the activities of the APA, psychology has provided Congress with analyses of the research on these issues (Maracek, 1991; Melton & Russo, 1987; O'Keeffe & Jones, 1990). Although it remains unlikely that the policy decisions being made regarding parental consent and notification will change, it is critical that policy makers not base their decisions on misconceptions about such psychological issues.

Barring a dramatic and unexpected shift in public opinion, abortion will remain the most divisive of policy issues. In such an emotionally charged arena, careful analysis of the relevant empirical research is needed to assure that all participants in the debate appropriately characterize the results of such research and base policy claims on solid findings rather than assumptions. Psychological research has the potential to play a more direct role in the debate. As psychologists begin directly addressing policy questions and actions in their research, such as the impact of varying state laws regarding parental consent or notification on adolescent sexual behavior, family communications, and so forth, policy makers might well take note.

The political turbulence generated in the aftermath of *Roe v. Wade* (1973) is unlikely to subside. Whereas the strategies and tactics of political activists on both sides of this issue have varied over the past 23 years, the intensity of the battle has remained high. Pro-choice advocates have, with the exception of a brief period following the election of President Clinton, found themselves on the defensive, attempting to safeguard the basic right to abortion. Abortion opponents, although on the offensive, have succeeded primarily in limiting federal funding for abortions but have not had success at the federal level in their more direct attacks on the basic right to abortion. Legislators have shown a reluctance to tackle the fundamental questions surrounding abortion. As we have shown, though, abortion politics have nonetheless affected policy making in a wide array of policy areas. Given the historical experience with this issue and the emotion attached to it, this situation is unlikely to change.

REFERENCES

Abortion report Koop withheld released on Hill. (1989, March 17). *The Washington Post*, p. A12.

Adler, N. E. (1989, March 16). *Testimony before the Subcommittee on Human Resources and Intergovernmental Relations, Committee on Government Operations,*

U.S. House of Representatives. Washington, DC: U.S. Government Printing Office.

Alan Guttmacher Institute. (1995, September). *Fact sheet: Abortion in the United States*. New York: Author.

American Psychological Association Public Interest Directorate. (1987). *The psychological sequelae of abortion*. Washington, DC: American Psychological Association.

Bray v. Alexandria Women's Health Clinic, 506 U.S. 263 (1993).

Callahan, D. (1982). Raw data vs. wisdom. *Society, 19*, 70–72.

Carr, T. P. (1991, April 30). Abortion: Legislative control. *CRS Issue Brief*. Washington, DC: Congressional Research Service.

Doe v. Bolton, 410 U.S. 179 (1973).

H. Rep. No. 101-392: *The federal role in determining the medical and psychological impact of abortion on women*, 101st Cong., 1st Sess. (1989).

Idelson, H., & Palmer, E. A. (1995, November 4). Vote on late-term abortions signals attack on *Roe*. *Congressional Quarterly Weekly Report*, 3375–3378.

Koop, C. E. (1989, January 9). Letter to President Reagan.

Madsen v. Women's Health Center, 512 U.S. 1277 (1994).

Maracek, J. (1991, January 10). *Psycho-social aspects of adolescent pregnancy and abortion*. Paper presented at the Congressional staff briefing on Teenagers and Abortion: The Impact of Parental Consent and Notification, Washington, DC.

Medical and psychological impact of abortion: Hearing before the Subcommittee on Human Resources and Intergovernmental Relations of the House Committee on Government Operations, 101st Cong., 1st Sess. (1989).

Melton, G. B., & Russo, N. F. (1987). Adolescent abortion: Psychological perspectives on public policy. *American Psychologist, 42*, 69–72.

National Organization for Women, Inc. v. Scheidler, 510 U.S. 249 (1994).

O'Keeffe, J. E., & Jones, J. M. (1990, Fall). Easing restrictions on minors' abortion rights. *Issues in Science and Technology*, pp. 17–23.

Roe v. Wade, 410 U.S. 113 (1973).

Rovner, J. (1991, July 27). House NIH vote overturns ban on fetal tissue research. *Congressional Quarterly*, pp. 2077–2079.

Rust v. Sullivan, 500 U.S. 173 (1991).

Schneider, W. (1995, February 18). Reopening the debate over abortion. *National Journal*, p. 462.

Steiner, G. Y. (Ed.). (1983). *The abortion dispute and the American system*. Washington, DC: Brookings Institution.

Tribe, L. W. (1990). *Abortion: The clash of absolutes*. New York: W. W. Norton & Co.

Victor, K. (1987, October 10). Not praying together. *National Journal*, pp. 2546–2551.

Webster v. Reproductive Health Services, 492 U.S. 490 (1989).

Wilmoth, G. H., Bussell, D., & Wilcox, B. L. (1991). Abortion and family policy: A mental health perspective. In E. Anderson & R. Huba (Eds.), *The reconstruction of family policy* (pp. 111–127). Westport, CT: Greenwood Press.

2

WHY IS ABORTION SUCH A CONTROVERSIAL ISSUE IN THE UNITED STATES?

NANCY FELIPE RUSSO AND JEAN E. DENIOUS

We are for *every* woman having exactly as many children as *she* wants, *when* she wants, *if* she wants. It's time the Bill of Rights applied to women.
—from the official statement of Jane,
legendary underground feminist abortion service (Kaplan, 1995)

We're in a war . . . until recently the casualties have only been on one side.
—Don Treshman, national director of Rescue America,
commenting on murders of abortion providers
(*New York Times*, Jan. 1, 1995, p. 26)

It seems fair to conclude that the majority does recognize abortion as *a troublesome, problematic, morally wrenching, wish it would go away, occasional necessity that I hope it never does but may someday face me, and in case it does I want the option (though I doubt I would want to exercise it) to decide what to do myself.*
—Barbara Craig and David O'Brien
(1993, p. 273, italics in the original)

A quarter of a century has passed since *Roe v. Wade* (1973) legalized abortion in the United States, and as these three very different quotations illustrate, that landmark ruling did little to settle the issue. Although over 70% of Americans believe abortion should be legal in some form, there is wide disagreement about the circumstances under which it should be permitted (Cook, Jelen, & Wilcox, 1992; Rubin, 1994). Despite the fact that tolerance, individualism, and freedom are core values of American culture (Williams, 1970), the public debate over legalizing abortion grows more impassioned and bitter with each passing year.

Why does legalized abortion continue to be controversial? There is

We thank Stephanie Wall and Angela Dumont for their assistance in collecting materials for this chapter and D. Allen Meyer for his helpful comments.

no simple answer. Efforts to restrict reproductive rights involve "a contest of meanings, a competition for how birth control should be understood," and these meanings vary over time (Gordon, 1990, p. 398). The movement to liberalize abortion laws that reached its legal peak with the passage of *Roe v. Wade* had advanced diverse reasons to justify legalizing abortion: to eliminate dangerous "back-alley" abortions, promote maternal health, reduce child abuse, alleviate poverty, slow population growth, and free up resources for addressing a host of other health and social problems (e.g., Calderone, 1960; Lader, 1973; Tietze & Lewit, 1969). Today, the public debate is dominated by two opposing perspectives: abortion as a right and means for attaining individual freedom, personal control, and social equality for women on the one hand, and abortion as a threat to morality and social cohesion on the other.

Although defining abortion as a moral issue plays a central role in contemporary debates, abortion involves complex issues and diverse values. As Cook et al. (1992) put it, abortion is a "mixed motive game" (p. 7), with players, including women, religious groups, and health professionals, holding a range of vested interests in its outcome—interests that change over time. In this chapter we examine some of those motives and interests. We explore various aspects of the sociopolitical context of abortion in the United States, beginning with the pro-life agenda that is designed to impede access to abortion. After considering the strategies and tactics that are used to advance that agenda and that intensify and shape the nature of the controversies surrounding abortion issues, we then consider interrelationships among feminist perspectives, women's roles, and attitudes toward abortion. We present research findings on relationships among abortion attitudes and attitudes toward other social issues and groups, including how they differ on the basis of religion, race, and class.[1] We consider how opinion poll research may have created distortions in the picture of public attitudes toward abortion and of the women who have abortions, and conclude with some thoughts and recommendations about where we go from here.

THE PRO-LIFE AGENDA: STRATEGIES AND TACTICS

The intensity of opposition to abortion is seen in the broad agenda of the pro-life forces. The complexity and comprehensiveness of this agenda has meant that access to abortion has been eroded on many fronts. Sophisticated, organized, and well-funded, this agenda is pursued on national and state levels, and encompasses political, legal, economic, and

---

[1]It is impossible to do justice to the complex history of abortion and other forms of birth control in the brief space available here. For excellent feminist historical analyses of these topics, see Gordon (1990) and Petchesky (1990).

psychological strategies. With public support insufficient for a constitutional amendment to ban abortion, electing pro-life legislators and appointing pro-life judges have been priorities—but only two of many in this multifaceted campaign. Some tactics seek direct legal limitations on service provision: restrictions on funds for family planning at home and abroad, bans on abortions in military hospitals, prohibitions against legalizing the drug RU486 in the United States, parental and spousal consent and notification requirements, mandated waiting periods, informed-consent scripts and "gag" rules that dictate what information can be given to patients, viability testing, record keeping and licensing requirements, hospitalization requirements, and guidelines on disposal of fetuses. Others try to limit public knowledge about abortion, including suppressing research on abortion techniques to lower the death rate of abortion, banning research using fetal tissue, prohibiting the Centers for Disease Control and Prevention from reporting death rates from childbirth and abortion in the same report, and funding "research" that can be used to "document" negative effects of abortion (including post-abortion emotional responses; Butler & Walbert, 1992; Devins & Watson, 1995a, 1995b, 1995c, Harrison & Gilbert, 1993; Lader, 1991, provide summaries of legislation, testimony, and research findings that reflect these tactics). Some antiabortion groups have begun establishing "fake abortion clinics" (Mertus, 1990). These organizations advertise services, attract women into their centers, and subject them to antiabortion "counseling." Training of physicians on how to do abortions has also diminished. In 1985, 25% of medical schools trained students on how to conduct first- and second-trimester abortions; by 1991, the figures had dropped to 12% and 7%, respectively (Blanchard, 1994).

Some legal strategies are to deter physicians from performing abortions by constructing abortion as a mental health threat. The idea is to hold physicans who perform abortions "fully liable for all the physical, psychological, and spiritual injuries they inflict on women" (Elliot Institute, 1997). By attributing previously existing psychological problems to the abortion experience, increasing the social stigma of abortion, and harassing women at clinic doors, abortion can be constructed as a mentally and physically damaging experience. Women with psychological problems can be offered "healing" and can be recruited to bring suits against abortion providers. For example, the web site for Priests for Life asks supporters to "encourage mothers who have been harmed by abortion to bring suits against the abortion industry" and provides telephone numbers of organizations that can help women bring suit. One of the listed organizations, Life Dynamics, is reported to have a nationwide network of 600 lawyers who are primed to file such suits (Farley, 1995). These activities are combined with attempts to pass laws that will go beyond usual malpractice liability and that will place civil liability on physicians for physical and psychological damages if they perform abortions (Reardon, 1996, 1997).

In April 1998, in deciding a lawsuit brought by the National Organization of Women and abortion clinics in Wisconsin and Delaware, a federal jury awarded damages against protesters for clinic vandalism and harassment. Because the case was brought under a federal racketeering law, the damages awarded to the clinics were tripled. The jury also found the Pro-Life League and Operation Rescue to be involved in the activity. This ruling opens the door for other suits for class-action damages, thus posing a financial threat to those pro-life groups that pursue a clinic harassment strategy. Its ultimate impact cannot be assessed until the appeal process is exhausted, however (Robinson, 1988).

Most pro-life supporters are nonviolent, pursuing their agenda by legal and political means. However, the fact of antiabortion clinic harassment and violence cannot be ignored. This harassment is often systematically organized; includes arson, death threats, kidnapping, and murder; and has distinct religious overtones. Blanchard and Prewitt (1993) described the wide range of tactics to foster "righteous" violence in the name of religion. In 1993, Florida physician David Gunn was murdered as he left his car to enter an abortion clinic, and in January 1997, the nation experienced its first bombing of an abortion clinic that involved a fatality (Reeves, 1997). Picketing outside clinics, tracing patients' identities, and invading their privacy; vandalizing and destroying facilities; and harassing doctors and their families at home or their children's schools are common tactics, and it is estimated that 83% of abortion patients have experienced some form of harassment (Forrest & Henshaw, 1987). (For a more in-depth discussion of the effects of picketing abotion clinics see Cozzarelli & Major, chap. 4, this volume). Joffe (1995) provided a moving (and chilling) description of the impact of such tactics on the lives of doctors who provide abortions. Every group has its extremists, and the systematic harassment and vandalism of abortion clinics is of concern to moderate pro-life forces as well as to pro-choice supporters. Indeed this extremism has even motivated representatives of different points of view to sit down and seek common ground in the debate, for example, by emphasizing family planning and prenatal care. Unfortunately, a vigorous and active portion of the pro-life leadership does not support use of modern methods of contraception (e.g., Eckel, 1997; Lewin, 1997), and this undermines such efforts to resolve controversies and find common ground.

Meanwhile, the controversy is intensified and emotions charged by sophisticated advertising campaigns associating abortions with gruesome images (e.g., decapitated or dismembered fetuses) and birth with images of bright-eyed, happy, well-loved children. Distribution of films such as "The Silent Scream" present a distorted view of fetal development and train viewers to attribute feeling and thinking to developing fetuses. Children are targeted by some of these campaigns, with activities ranging from demonstrations to art exhibitions that associate abortion with bloody, violent images.

Pro-life efforts have been effective in decreasing the availability of and access to abortion, particularly for women who are young or poor. Given the intensity, energy, and resources behind these efforts, pro-choice activities, which have focused on challenging restrictions to abortion services in court and electing pro-choice legislators, are low key in comparison. In the late 1980s, grassroots pro-choice activists responded to the pro-life intimidation and harassment by mobilizing Operation Respect, which sought to counter Operation Rescue with counseling and escorts for abortion clinics and to respond to pro-life chants with their own (Staggenborg, 1991; see also chapter 4 by Cozzarelli and Major in this volume). These efforts have been effective in diluting some of the impact caused to women crossing picket lines and enduring harassment when entering clinics (Cozzarelli & Major, 1994).

Amazingly, despite the concentrated pro-life campaign, public attitudes toward legalization show little change over time (Wetstein, 1996). Perhaps the fact that an estimated one in five adult women has had an abortion and can compare personal experience with the rhetoric has something to do with this attitude stability. Nonetheless, these activities set the context for public debates about abortion, intensify the controversial nature of the debate, and have a chilling effect on public discussions about abortion. In seeking to reduce controversy and find common ground, establishing "rules of engagement" will be an important first step in the process.

FEMINIST PERSPECTIVES, WOMEN'S ROLES, AND ATTITUDES TOWARD ABORTION

A woman is a woman because she can bear children. . . . To put it bluntly, an abortion amounts to a mutilation of the woman's body and to a denial of her nature. (Janet E. Smith, cited in Cunningham & Forsythe, 1992, p. 111)

The issue is whether you *trust women* to make choices of life and death significance. (Margaret Cerullo, 1990, p. 90)

Feminism means different things to different people, and people who identify with the label *feminist* are a diverse group (see Donovan, 1992). By definition, feminists recognize that women experience gender-based inequalities and share the goal of eliminating them. However, feminists differ in their definitions, ideologies, frameworks, and analyses of the conditions of women as well as in their view of what constitutes political, economic, and social inequality (Donavan, 1992; Hull, Scott, & Smith, 1982; Moraga & Anzaldúa, 1981). Given that feminists differ in their definition of feminism, it is not surprising that they differ in attitudes toward reproductive issues.

Here we take a broad view of feminism and use the definition of historian Linda Gordon, who defined *feminist* as "sharing in an impulse to increase the power of women and autonomy of women in their families, communities and/or society" (p. xvii). Abortion has been a divisive issue, even among self-identified feminists, from the very beginnings of the U.S. women's movement. Although control over reproduction has been an enduring feminist goal, a feminist perspective does not necessarily mean support for legal abortion.

In the 19th century, the cause of "voluntary motherhood" was more widely endorsed among women than women's suffrage. In the social context of the time, women's moral qualities were glorified in a "cult of domesticity" that held a negative view of sexuality (Welter, 1978). Consequently, advocates for voluntary motherhood emphasized abstinence as a means of fertility control. Abortion was seen as degrading women and encouraging male promiscuity. The feminist stance against abortion at this time can be interpreted as defending women's social status.

A parallel view is found today among pro-life feminists who consider abortion as denying the special values and concerns women bring to their reproductive experiences, encouraging male irresponsibility, and abandoning women to "heartless individualism" (Ginsburg, 1989, p. 215). Currently, several antiabortion organizations explicitly identify themselves as pro-women movements. Feminists for Life, Women Exploited by Abortion, Victims of Choice, and Concerned Women for America were formed by and are largely composed of women (Blanchard, 1994). The conservative religious foundation that underlies most antiabortion movements appears to play a central role in these female-based organizations.

The women's movement that reemerged in the late 1960s emphasized autonomy and liberation, and included a reproductive rights component promoting women's control over their own bodies. Pro-choice feminists rose to prominence in the abortion reform movement, working to broaden its agenda and empowering women to give voice to their abortion experiences (Petchesky, 1990). The dangers of illegal abortion were graphically described as women began to relate their experiences with abortion, obtained and denied (Condit, 1990). Some, as in the case of Sherri Finkbine, a popular television personality who had taken thalidomide during pregnancy and was forced to fly to Sweden to obtain an abortion, received national attention. These stories were so powerful that in 1967 members of the clergy formed the Clergy Consultation Service, a national network of thousands of clergy acting as "gentle lawbreakers" by referring women to reputable abortion providers in Great Britain, Puerto Rico, and some parts of the United States (Tribe, 1990, p. 40).

In addition to supporting abortion rights, the feminist reproductive agenda included contraceptive safety; ending sterilization abuse; empowerment of women in dealing with health professionals; and condemnation of using poor, minority, and Third World women in experiments. Feminist goals for reproductive policies also expanded beyond personal autonomy and freedom to encompass social goals such as social equality (Gordon, 1990; Petchesky, 1990).

Feminists have emphasized the link between attitudes toward birth control and abortion and the centrality of childbearing to women's roles and identity, that is, the "motherhood mandate" (Russo, 1976). Despite the fact that the female sex has a special vested interest in controlling reproduction, national polls suggest similar attitudes toward legalization of abortion among women and men. However, women who are homemakers or over 65 years of age are less supportive of abortion than men, suggesting that women's childbearing views may reflect both resistance and accommodation to their gender roles (e.g., wife, mother; Clark & Clark, 1996; Cook et al., 1992). Some research has found significant, albeit low, correlations between positive abortion attitudes and egalitarian gender role attitudes among women but not among men (Sitaraman, 1994). Thus, comparing men's and women's overall abortion attitudes may mask important subgroup attitudinal differences.

The way the question is worded is important. Although there is little evidence of an overall gender difference in attitudes toward legal abortion (e.g., Betzig & Lombardo, 1991), men are more approving than women when asked about personal feelings or the morality of abortion (Moore & Stief, 1991; Wright & Rogers, 1987). This may reflect women's defense of their roles, men's greater sexual permissiveness, or a combination of both.

A classic study of women pro-life and pro-choice activists by Kristin Luker (1984) demonstrates the usefulness of examining women's attitudes toward abortion in the context of their gender role resistance and accommodation. Luker found that pro-life activists held traditional attitudes toward gender roles and female sexuality. She concluded that employed women and housewives had different vested interests in the abortion debate. If housewives believe maternity is a biological and social destiny, they may regard the pro-choice view that motherhood is but one option among many as devaluing their role and undermining their status. Conversely, employed women have a vested interest in timing and controlling their pregnancies in pursuing their careers.

The conservativism of many homemakers' abortion attitudes may reflect what Blanchard (1994) has called "encapsulation." To the extent that individuals are isolated from others possessing alternative viewpoints, they are more likely to join highly activist organizations and to exercise extreme methods of protest. The homemaker's central identity as wife and mother, and the constraints the homemaker role can place on opportunities for exposure to diverse perspectives, thus may combine to place her more staunchly on the far right side of the abortion debate.

Neither homemakers nor employed women should be stereotyped in terms of either attitudes toward abortion or the women's movement, however. In an in-depth analysis of 1992 National Election Study data, Cal and Janet Clark (1996) explored women's social and political attitudes on a variety of issues. They found that homemakers were more likely to view family values as important than other women (57% vs. 48% of all women); nonetheless, 39% of homemakers expressed pro-choice views. Even among women classified as "antifeminist," nearly 1 out of 3 held pro-choice attitudes. The proportion of homemakers who expressed liking for the women's movement did not differ from that of all women (49%).

Both pro-life and pro-choice feminists seek to protect and respect pregnancy and motherhood, and oppose discrimination and support women's social and economic advancement. The difference appears to be that pro-life feminists believe abortion devalues motherhood and threatens social codes linking sex with reproduction and requiring fathers to support women who bear their children (Cunningham & Forsythe, 1992; Ginsburg, 1989). They argue that pro-choice feminists are "out of touch" with women's priorities and do not reflect women's "feminine" values of "intimacy, nurturance, community, responsibility and care" (Cunningham & Forsythe, 1992, p. 109).

Pro-choice feminists view abortion as a means to counter the differential effects of pregnancy on women; to empower women to control timing, spacing, and size of their families; and to maintain control over their work, sexuality, and relationships with their partners and children. Women's ability to choose if and when to bear children is viewed as enhancing motherhood's value, whereas forced motherhood is considered degrading to women and harmful to families and society (Ginsburg, 1989; Petchesky, 1990; Russo, 1976, 1979). Pro-choice feminists argue that pro-life feminists are out of touch with women's social and economic realities and that men's view of women as sexual objects and failure to support their wives and children preceded legalization of abortion. They regard forcing a woman to bear an unwanted child as "punishment" for sexual intercourse to be cruel to the child and damaging to society and to families. Research on the impaired development of unwanted children and the linkage between unwantedness in pregnancy and child abuse are cited in support of this perspective (Russo, 1992). Women's vulnerability to unplanned pregnancy has a long history of being used to justify educational and employment discrimination against women (regardless of whether the women actually have children). As a result, pro-choice feminists conclude access to abortion is necessary for women's full social and political equality (Petchesky, 1990; Russo, 1976).[2]

Support for abortion among pro-choice feminists has been defensive at times, with abortion portrayed as a "necessary evil." But choosing to have an abortion can be a moral, positive, self-enhancing, and empowering experience (Freeman, 1977; Lunneborg, 1992). As Rosalind Petchesky (1990) eloquently observed, an ambivalent stance toward abortion

> oddly forgets the spirit of buoyancy infusing not only feminists but masses of women after *Roe v. Wade*. Suddenly the years of terror, of silently fearing pregnancy, of sneaking off to possible sterility or death, and of sex ridden with shame were . . . going to end. This buoyancy was there . . . because abortion—easily available, cheap, administered under safe, hygienic conditions early in a pregnancy and in an ambience free of stigma and guilt—*is* a component (not just a condition) of women's liberation (p. 390).

From this perspective, legal and safe abortion is a "necessary good," a "positive benefit that society has an obligation to provide" (p. 391).

CONTROLLING FEMALE SEXUALITY

The anger of anti-abortionists seems to rise in direct proportion to the degree to which women can in good faith have abortions guilt-free. . . . The ire of the anti-abortionists cannot be understood outside the context of a larger sexual and cultural reaction to feminist gains.
—Lynn S. Chancer (1990, p. 118)

Petchesky (1990) emphasized the role of ideology surrounding both motherhood and sexuality in constructing abortion as evil, pointing out that one of the things that makes abortion "awful" is "the assumption that sex for pleasure is 'wrong' (for women) and that women who indulge in it have to pay a price" (pp. 390–391). Indeed, historical events have caused attitudes toward female sexuality and motherhood to be inextricably intertwined, particularly among Catholics.

During the age of conservative Victorian principles, abortions became damning evidence of illicit sexual behavior (Petchesky, 1990). The idea that sex could be separated from reproduction, essential for public acceptance of birth control, was considered immoral. Public acceptance of birth control required a major change in sexual values that has not uniformly occurred throughout society. Today, in addition to conservative ideas about

---

[2]The argument that access to abortion is critical for women's advancement assumes contraceptive technology is unavailable or inadequate for controlling women's fertility with certainty. This assumption is unlikely to become invalid any time soon. Nonetheless, it should be remembered that discussions of abortion attitudes are bound by sociocultural context. The state of contraceptive technology, which is bound by time and place, is a critical element in that context.

appropriate roles for women, religious and sexual values proscribing teenage sexual activity, extramarital sex, and homosexuality continue to be linked to abortion attitudes. People with more permissive sexual attitudes are more supportive of abortion (Wetstein, 1996). Insofar as abortion enables women to avoid consequences of illicit sexual activity, abortion debates are debates about "proper" sexual behavior (Cook et al., 1992).

Women are slightly more likely than men to consider family values important. This tendency is stronger among people with less than a high school education and a low family income (Clark & Clark, 1996). This finding is reversed among people who feel positive toward feminists or who have a college education, however. Among pro-life women, antagonism toward abortion appears more linked to traditional attitudes toward sexuality and reproduction rather than to disapproval of women's economic and political equality (Luker, 1984). This view has deep roots and is linked to religious ideology.

RELIGIOUS IDEOLOGY

The contraceptive mentality rejects a child as a gift from God.
—Judie Brown, American Life League (quoted in Eckel, 1997, p. B5)

Religious ideology with respect to abortion has many dimensions, reflecting the historical evolution of religious institutions: the location of authority and power in male–female relationships, conceptions of sexuality, the role of conscience in controlling fertility, the nature of personhood, and the relationship of morality to law (Simmons, 1992). In tracing the history of birth control, Linda Gordon (1990) suggested that when agricultural societies arose, individual restrictions on family size threatened community survival and led to ideologies banning birth control. Because enforcing social norms is easier when individuals internalize them, religious ideologies played a key role in controlling female sexuality and convincing people of the immorality of birth control. In Judeo-Christian traditions, which are most relevant to the U.S. context at this point, female sexuality became portrayed as an irresistible source of human suffering and evil. Writings of early church fathers are permeated with a view of sex as a source of weakness and corruption for men (Payne, 1989). As Gordon (1990) pointed out, such views served "to suppress women's resistance and discontent by instilling in them an immobilizing guilt and self-hatred, and by justifying men's enjoyment of their privileges" (p. 9).

Jesus argued for universal equality of all human beings and was extraordinarily pro-woman, particularly for his time. However, evolution of the Christian religion, which reflected values of the larger patriarchal social context and the drive to proselytize new members, proceeded in other directions. When extreme antisex and antiwoman ideologies of Christianity threatened to drive women from the Church, this conflict was ameliorated by offering women redemption of their sexual nature by sanctifying procreation. In the 13th century, Thomas Aquinas codified the view that sexual intercourse, an inherently sinful act, was appropriate only in marriage and, even then, justified only by the intent to procreate. As Gordon (1990) concluded, "Thus the connection between sex hatred and women hatred led to a lasting Christian emphasis on motherhood as women's destiny" (p. 9). A legacy of this history is found in survey data suggesting abortion attitudes become less favorable when women's desire for abortion is seen as rejection of motherhood (Rossi, 1967; Schur, 1965).

Today, the opposition of the Catholic Church to abortion remains rooted in its historical view of sexual intercourse as inevitably sinful and morally unjustifiable unless open to the possibility of conception. The Church views abortion as violating natural law—the right to life of innocent persons—and therefore concludes it should be banned by civil law as well. Since 1975, the National Council of Catholic Bishops has been one of the most powerful abortion opponents in the United States (Simmons, 1992). Blanchard (1994) reported that in 1990, with support of the Vatican, the NCCB hired the public relations giant Hill & Knowlton to conduct a five million dollar public relations campaign against legal abortion. The Catholic Church is also the driving force behind other major antiabortion organizations, such as the National Right to Life Committee, a group that boasts a membership and annual budget in the millions (Blanchard, 1994).

American Catholics have strong pro-choice voices, however. According to a 1987 poll, 85% of Catholics surveyed believed that a woman could both have an abortion and be a good Catholic (Simmons, 1992). Catholics for a Free Choice, as well as a number of prominent Roman Catholic theologians, have emphasized the centrality of personal conscience in moral decision making, arguing that historical teachings differ in their view of the moral status of the fetus and objecting to placing a higher moral status on a zygote than a woman. They emphasize pluralism as the norm for Catholics and stress the Catholic moral principle that applies when moral obligations are ambiguous: Dissent is permissible when reasonable and cogent reasons for the dissenting position are supported by a sufficient number of theologians and experts. In the case of abortion, they argue, individual conscience and not extrinsic authority should be the forum for decision making. They also point to the important role that separation of church and state has played in preserving religious liberty for Catholics and argue personal convictions against abortion should not be promoted as a political agenda (Simmons, 1992).

Many pro-life religious groups, not only the Catholic Church, have used abortion as an organizing issue to recruit new members, some of whom have little history of political activity. Preexisting social and religious networks have been key recruiting grounds for pro-life organizations (Cook et al., 1992). Even if individuals might be receptive to developing some consensus on abortion, religious organizations are ongoing institutional structures with a vested interest in perpetuating pro-life activism around religious values.

Pro-choice religious groups have also organized in support of abortion. The Religious Coalition for Abortion Rights represents about 30 national Christian, Jewish, and other religious groups holding diverse views about the morality of abortion. These groups are united in their position that (a) abortion is a "moral and theological concern;" (b) "an abortion decision should be the result of thoughtful consideration, based on one's conscience and religious beliefs;" (c) "there are some instances in which abortion may be a moral alternative to a problem pregnancy;" and (d) "in our pluralistic society, no one religious viewpoint on the beginning of human life should be imposed on all Americans by secular law" (Jenkins, 1990, p. 151). For these groups, belief in reproductive freedom is intimately related to belief in religious freedom.

It should not be surprising that religiosity continues to play an important role in explaining variation in abortion attitudes for both men and women (Adebayo, 1990; Esposito & Basow, 1995; Krishnan, 1991; Szafran & Clagett, 1988). Wetstein (1996) examined the relationship of attitudes toward premarital sex, opposition to teenage sex, frequency of church attendance, strength of religious affiliation, city size, age, education, and occupational prestige to support for abortion. These variables were found to represent five factors, labeled as religious/moral (church attendance, strength of affiliation), sexual liberalism (premarital sex, teen sex, and age), socioeconomic (income, education), and city size. All were found to be significantly related to abortion attitude. A LISREL analysis found that the religious/moral factor had the strongest relationship to abortion attitude (β = .32). The socioeconomic factor (β = .30) was close behind, followed by sexual liberalism (β = .21). The model, which uses eight indicators representing four latent factors, explained 43% of the variance in abortion attitudes measured in the study. Gender role attitudes were not included in the model, however, and how linkages among attitudes might differ among religious groups was not explored.

There are also large differences in abortion attitudes among religious groups, and both pro-choice and pro-life proponents can be found within any particular religious group (Adebayo, 1990; Hollis & Morris, 1992; Krishnan, 1991; Simmons, 1992). Despite the vehement opposition of the Catholic Church toward abortion, nearly 1 of 3 abortion patients (32%) is Catholic—491,120 women in 1987. More than 1 out of 6 (16%) identified as a "born again" Christian (Henshaw, Koonin, & Smith, 1991).

Jews are most supportive of abortion, with the life of the woman taking precedence over the fetus. The fetus is viewed as "part of its mother," and not a person until it has an independent existence. People are morally obligated to procreate, however, and casual abortion is morally repugnant (Simmons, 1992). Jews and mainline Protestant churches are more supportive than Catholics, Mormons, or Fundamentalist Christians (Cook et al., 1992; Wetstein, 1996).

A greater belief in the Bible is also associated with opposition to abortion. Protestant fundamentalists are more likely to oppose abortion than all other groups, including Catholics. People holding positive attitudes toward Fundamentalist Christians do not necessarily hold negative attitudes toward the women's movement, however. Clark and Clark (1996) found that 57% of women who had positive attitudes toward fundamentalists also held positive attitudes toward the women's movement, and 26% of such women were also pro-choice.

Research by Sitaraman (1994) suggests even more complexity to the picture: Linkages among gender role, abortion, human life issues, and sexual and reproductive concerns may differ among religious groups. In her study, attitudes toward church attendance, human life, abortion, sex, and reproduction were intercorrelated for both Catholics and non-Catholics. Only among non-Catholics, however, were liberal gender role and political orientation attitudes also related to all of these factors. In other words, egalitarian gender role attitudes were independent of conservative views on abortion, sex, and contraception among Catholics, but not non-Catholics.

CLASS AND RACE

Uneducated women, poor women, and women of color have a major stake in the abortion debate, as they are at higher risk for unintended pregnancies and have higher rates of abortion compared with other women. In 1987, after controlling for age, the abortion rate for poor women (family incomes under $11,000 per year) was more than three times that of women with higher family incomes (over $25,000 per year). Nonwhite women were 17% of the population, and 31% of abortion patients. Hispanic women (who may be of any race) were 8% of the population, and 13% of abortion patients (Henshaw & Silverman, 1988).

Class and race issues historically have played a role in restrictive abortion legislation. The 19th century was a time of societal upheaval, with an explosive growth in industry and technology associated with a decline in birth rates. This decline primarily was due to increasing rates of abortion among married women (Sitaraman, 1994). Worry over the fact that immigrant women were having larger families than their upper-class counterparts spawned a patently racist and classist eugenics movement. Belief in eugenics and the desire to encourage childbearing among the upper

"Yankee" classes fueled efforts to restrict abortion during this period (Petchesky, 1990). In 1905, no less a personage than President Theodore Roosevelt joined the cause, condemning smaller families as decadent and "criminal against the race." (cited in Gordon, 1990, p. 133). In the context of seeking to increase population, these concerns translated into restrictive family planning and abortion laws and policies.

Opposition to birth control around the turn of the 19th century thus went beyond viewing birth control as sinful and motherhood as a social duty. It reflected fear that immigrants would soon outnumber "Yankee stock" and, hence, a perceived need for a steadily growing population of large stable families. Linda Gordon (1990) eloquently described how these multiple sources of opposition mutually supported each other:

> Sin and small families weakened social cohesiveness and moral fiber, which encouraged and enabled women to stray from their proper sphere—home and children. Women's wanderings weakened the family, which in turn led women to stray further, in a vicious cycle of social degeneration. The Yankee upper classes, who believed themselves destined for political and economic leadership, saw this degeneration as weakening their position vis-à-vis those who continued to reproduce in larger numbers. The situation was culturally and morally fatal because, proportionally, the most valuable sectors of the citizenry were shrinking and the least valuable expanding. (pp. 134–135)

The relationship of birth control and abortion to racial, ethnic, and class issues continues to be complex. To some, the ability to control fertility is seen as a means to empower minority women, a path out of poverty, a mechanism for eliminating unwanted childbearing, and a means to enhance the health of women and children in high-risk populations. To others, controlling reproduction potentially undermines minority groups' political power; it is seen as devaluing motherhood and as functioning as a tool of genocide. Fertility norms and sexual practices vary across class and ethnic group and, in a climate of intolerance, can be a particularly strong source of intergroup friction (Fried, 1990).

Differences in abortion attitudes between Blacks and Whites have been the most studied, although results have been inconsistent (Combs & Welch, 1982; Hall & Ferree, 1986; Lynxwiler & Gay, 1994; Wilcox, 1990, 1992). Blacks are more religious than Whites, are more likely to be poor, and have lower education, attributes associated with increased opposition to abortion (Clark & Clark, 1996; Cook et al., 1992; Wetstein, 1996). However, recent research suggests that when socioeconomic status and religiosity are controlled, Blacks are slightly more supportive of abortion than Whites (Cook et al., 1992). Further, gender interacts with race: When income, education, and religious affiliation are controlled, Black women are more likely to support abortion than White women. The reverse is true for men: Black men are less likely to support abortion than comparable

White men (Wilcox, 1990). For a more complete discussion of these issues, see chapter 5 by Dugger in this volume.

THE ROLE OF GOVERNMENT

The American belief in separation of church and state has militated against explicitly and directly incorporating religious views on women's roles and family issues into national legislation, although they obviously influence governmental laws and policies indirectly. Tension resulting from this separation has been eased by the related idea of separation of private and public spheres. Emphasized by John Locke, this idea has guided the structure of the United States Constitution and society. But this distinction has not been universally accepted, creating conflict over the definition of appropriate boundaries. Conservatives, in particular, have chafed at their inability to enforce religious moral values in private domains. Similarly, some feminists have denounced the concept of separate spheres, albeit for different reasons (i.e., because it promotes inequalities between men and women). Unfortunately, whereas blurring the boundaries between public and private spheres may increase opportunities to promote women's rights in the family, it also opens the door for public debate and control over other family issues such as contraception and abortion. Two developments in American society have been important in moving abortion from a private to a public domain: changing conceptions of prenatal life and the changing role of the medical profession.

CONCEPTIONS OF PRENATAL LIFE

It is . . . the erasing of our personhood together with . . . the elevation of a fetus to the status of a "person" . . . that makes the antichoice campaign work.

—Sheila Ruth (1995, p. 227)

Abortion clinics are a world of death camps, contract killers and mass murder.
—New York Times description of National Pro-Life campaign statement (*New York Times*, Jan. 1, 1995, p. 26)

Issues regarding legalization of abortion in the United States get played out in a sociopolitical context where large proportions of Americans express "traditional family values" combined with a high value on individual autonomy and tolerance of others *as long as no one is being harmed*. As Cook et al. (1992) pointed out, in this context the construction of the embryo as a person who is being harmed by abortion becomes pivotal in making abortion a public rather than a private issue.

To what extent has there been agreement on the personhood of the embryo and fetus? The answer to this question has been controversial throughout the history of Western civilization, even among ancient Greeks. Although Plato and Aristotle approved of abortion in some circumstances, Pythagoreans considered the embryo a person from conception (Luker, 1984). Canon law defined the period of "ensoulment" at 40 or 80 days after conception, depending on whether the embryo was male or female, respectively. It wasn't until 1869, when Pope Pius IX rejected this view, that the Roman Catholic Church officially recognized the embryo as a person from the moment of conception.

> There is little doubt that the status of women is intimately related to prenatal technologies. Technology is never neutral—it both reflects and shapes social values . . . Because these technologies focus on the role of women as mothers, it may lead to diminution of other roles.
> —Merrick and Blank, 1993 (p. 16)

Changes in medical technology and scientific understanding of prenatal development have played an important role in changing conceptions of the embryo and fetus. Before attempts to criminalize abortion emerged in the 19th century, both English and American common law had defined quickening—the point at which the mother becomes aware of movement of the fetus—as the point beyond which abortion was considered a criminal act (Lader, 1991). Because the mother was the only reliable witness to the event, this meant that abortion was available very late in pregnancy. Abortions were performed mostly on poor, unmarried women and were conducted privately and quietly (Sitaraman, 1994). During this period, although abortion was controversial, abortifacients, including natural herbs and poisons, were widely marketed (Luker, 1984). Sufficient numbers of people found advertisements for abortion products unacceptable so that thinly disguised subterfuge and euphemisms were used to market them. For example, "French renovating pills" were billed as "a blessing to mothers," with the warning that pregnant women should avoid them because "they invariably produce a miscarriage" (Cook et al., 1992, p. 7).

In 1973, in *Roe v. Wade*, the Supreme Court ruled that the Constitutional right of privacy grounded in the Fourteenth Amendment is sufficiently broad to encompass a woman's decision to terminate her pregnancy. The Court held that a woman's right to an abortion may be counterbalanced by the state's interest in protecting maternal health and potential human life, interests that increase throughout the pregnancy as the fetus develops. At the point that the fetus reaches *viability*, that is, its brain and respiratory system have matured enough to enable it to survive outside the uterus, the State may exercise its interest in protecting potential life, and regulation and prohibition of abortion is permitted except when it would endanger the life or health of the woman. This occurs some time between 24 and 28 weeks after conception.

Beliefs in the beginning of human life are a major contributor to abortion attitudes. Lack of consensus about the moral status of the fetus means that fetal characteristics play a highly visible role in abortion debates, and beliefs about them have been found to play a role in women's postabortion well-being (Conklin & O'Connor, 1995). Increased participation in religious services and being female are independently associated with viewing human life as beginning closer to conception (Sitaraman, 1994).

Revolutionary developments in reproductive technology (e.g., genetic tests, in vitro fertilization, prenatal diagnosis and therapy) began snowballing in the late 1960s, just about the time pro-choice movements gathered momentum. Such progress in prenatal medicine facilitates social perception of the fetus as a separate individual. In particular, some methods of diagnosis, such as fetal monitoring and fetoscopy, allow for direct observation of the fetus. Visualization is an especially powerful tool for reconstructing people's notions of prenatal life.

> The pictures—a baby-like fetus, a smiling fetus, a fetus that sucks its thumb. Butchered fetuses—bloody mounds of human tissue, hacked arms, mangled legs, crushed skull. Without these compelling and brutal photographs the American abortion controversy probably would not continue.
>
> —Celeste Michelle Condit (1990, p. 79)

Disseminating highly magnified pictures of the developing fetus used as evidence for personhood has become a highly effective persuasion strategy. These pictures have been extremely controversial as they typically portray third-trimester fetuses and are not representative of the vast majority of abortions. More than 9 out of 10 abortions are performed at less than 13 weeks gestation—when the fetus is less than 2 inches long and weighs less than 1/2 ounce. About half of abortions are performed at 8 weeks or less, before a fetus is even formed, and more than 99% of abortions are performed before 21 weeks of gestation (Henshaw, 1990). Less than 1% (6%) are performed at 22 weeks or later, with such late abortions typically occurring only when continuing the pregnancy threatens the life of the mother or a serious, debilitating defect in the fetus is discovered (Henshaw et al., 1991).

In pro-life constructions of prenatal development, the implication is that the fetus is formed early in pregnancy, with the major difference between a 12-week and 24-week fetus being one of size. When pro-life advocates are taught to portray fetal development, they are instructed to establish the continuity of development by beginning with a picture of a baby and working backward (Condit, 1990). Have you had the experience of viewing an ambiguous figure and not seeing anything but a blur, but after looking at a clearer rendition of the picture, the ambiguous picture becomes unambiguous? If so, you can appreciate the power of this perceptual learning technique in enabling the individual to "see" the fetus as a baby.

The fetus is portrayed as able to feel pain, an idea that can be very disturbing to women contemplating abortion (Noonan, 1986). This inaccurate view is encouraged by language describing prenatal stages as they were conceptualized in the 19th century: zygote, embryo, and fetus. But today's science has discovered that the label *fetus* encompasses profound differences in the developing organism, particularly in the brain and nervous system.

It is not until 21 to 23 weeks after the woman's last menstrual period that rudimentary connections emerge between the higher centers of the developing fetal brain and the rest of the fetal body. These centers are located in the neocortex, the most recently evolved part of the brain, which contains human consciousness, thinking, problem solving, and language. Before the neocortex develops and is connected with the rest of the developing fetal body, the idea that a fetus can think or feel pain has no basis in biological fact. It takes at least 32 weeks after the woman's last menstrual period for the neocortex to begin to look and function like that of a newborn. At that point, continuous electrical activity and periodic fluctuations suggestive of the normal sleep—wake cycle are found. It is only at this point, which is after the point of fetal viability, that the major difference between a fetus and a newborn becomes one of size (Flowers, 1990).

The complex character of prenatal neural development is not communicated as easily in the popular media as a fetal picture. Evolving concepts of the fetus necessarily imply altering perceptions of the pregnant woman. With advances in fetal surgery, more cases will pit the interests of the fetus and the pregnant woman against each other (Merrick & Blank, 1993). The ever-increasing advancement and sophistication of reproductive technologies also means there remains an imbalance between doctors and patients in knowledge and, therefore, power with regard to reproductive control and rights. Although women have come a long way from the days in which many possessed little understanding of their own basic physiology (Kaplan, 1995), the medical community has been resistant to anything that will diminish the role and status of physicians.

THE ROLE OF THE HEALTH PROFESSIONS

The emergence of medicine as a profession in the 19th century contributed to defining abortion as a public issue and therefore subject to regulation. Characterizing abortion as a health issue moved it into the medical domain, and the medical profession was the first organized group to take up arms against abortion. Its goal was to control the practice rather than eliminate it, however (Petchesky, 1990). Emphasizing the need to protect women's health, the first statutes restricting abortion were designed to control certain dangerous poisons commonly used in abortifacients. Other laws emphasized the need to protect women from the dangers of the surgical procedure used at the time, especially by "irregular" (nonphysician) personnel (Mohr, 1978). Interestingly, religious authorities did not assume a role in legislative activities during this period, perhaps because defining abortion as a health issue gave them little standing in the debate.

Today, pharmaceutical and medical technology have undermined health arguments against abortion. Risk of death from abortion is lower than from childbirth—indeed lower than receiving a penicillin shot (Henshaw, 1990). Nonetheless, concerns about women's physical and mental health continue to be used as arguments for restrictive abortion laws. Such arguments give psychological knowledge and expertise a key role in abortion debates (Adler et al., 1990, 1992). Indeed, characterizing abortion as destructive to women's mental health has been a major linchpin supporting a rash of state legislation mandating informed-consent scripts that warn women of physical and mental health dangers of abortion. This continues despite the fact that every scientific review of the literature has concluded that, for the majority of women, freely chosen legal abortion is not found to have severe or lasting negative psychological effects, especially when the abortion is conducted during the first trimester of pregnancy (Adler et al., 1990, 1992; Schwartz, 1986; Russo, 1992).

As the medical profession has evolved in U.S. society, so too has its relationship to abortion issues. Kurt Back (1986–1987) argued that professions provided an outlet for tensions created by the shifting division of public and private spheres. In essence, professions have evolved as semi-autonomous social units that serve both public and private functions. This enables them to mediate between the state and the individual, operating as a public sector toward the individual (regulating access to abortion) and a private sector toward the larger society (maintaining women's privacy). The status of the professions and women's relationship to them thus plays a key role in availability and access of abortion.

Physicians' desire for professional status during the 19th century meant medicine was initially on the side of restrictive abortion laws. By taking a public position against abortion, physicians distinguished themselves from other health practitioners. Their claim to scientific knowledge of prenatal life made traditional assumptions about pregnancy seem outdated. Pregnancy became viewed as a continuous process, and the use of quickening to distinguish between acceptable and criminal abortions was questioned.

In addition to giving physicians a cause for advancing their professional status, restrictions on abortion had the advantage of eliminating competition from druggists and midwives. Using scientific expertise to consolidate its claims, in 1857 the American Medical Association commissioned an investigation into abortion rates, emphasizing its dangerousness and promoting a vocabulary describing abortion in provocative terms (e.g., "antenatal infanticide"; Gordon, 1990, p. 59). By the end of the Civil War, most states had outlawed abortion, and this situation persisted well into the 20th century.

As the medical profession gained influence and respect for its authority in health-related decisions, abortion became a medical decision, to be determined between a woman and her physician. This arrangement, which persisted throughout the early part of the 20th century, served the State's objectives while protecting women's privacy. Luker (1994) called the medical establishment's dominance over childbearing and abortion, which lasted from about 1850 to 1950, the "century of silence." Under this system, if a woman had money she had access to abortion for practically any reason, but the decision was the physician's, not the woman's.

Although reproductive rights movements for "birth control" and "planned parenthood" developed in the first half of the 20th century, it wasn't until the 1960s that legal abortion began to become a reality. The post-war baby boom and growing awareness of the danger of illegal abortion fueled a movement in support of abortion rights that included family planners, physicians, legal scholars, and feminists (Sitaraman, 1994). National Organization for Women and the National Association for Repeal of Abortion Laws in the late 1960s provided two strong national voices for pro-choice activism. Whereas lawyers and lobbyists worked for reform of abortion laws on the state and federal levels, secret underground networks worked to save women from the dangers of illegal abortion (Bart, 1981). Jane, the most renowned of such organizations, was founded in 1969 and provided counseling sessions and safe abortions to an estimated 11,000 women in the 4-year period preceding *Roe v. Wade* (Kaplan, 1995).

Feminist efforts to renegotiate the relationship between women and the medical profession and to redefine abortion as a woman's right had not anticipated political consequences for availability and accessibility of abortion, however. Moving abortion decisions from the private world of personal health to the public world of individual rights meant that a broad spectrum of interests and groups had a stake in defining issues and shaping their outcomes. The decline in respect for authority of the professions has meant that health, education, and family issues—including euthanasia, the right to have or refuse medical treatment, and relations between the sexes—have moved into the public domain, becoming open to popular debate and state intervention. In this context, the broad relationship between the individual and the state is subject to renegotiation, with all the potential opportunities and dangers that implies (Luker, 1984).

DISTORTIONS IN THE PICTURE OF PUBLIC ATTITUDES TOWARD ABORTION

With erosion of the constitutional protections of *Roe v. Wade*, public opinion can play an increasingly important role in directing and shaping legislative debates on abortion issues. The way public attitudes are measured shapes how abortion is understood. What's wrong with this picture?

The most widely used national poll data come from the General Social Surveys (GSS) conducted by the National Opinion Research Council. The GSS has included items assessing abortion attitudes nearly every year since its inception in 1972. These items have been incorporated into other polls and national surveys. They include the following:

Do you think it should be possible for a pregnant woman to obtain a legal abortion

1. if the woman's own health is seriously endangered by the pregnancy?
2. if she became pregnant as a result of rape?
3. if there is a strong chance of serious defect in the baby?
4. if the family has a low income and cannot afford any more children?
5. if she is unmarried and does not want to marry the man?
6. if she is married and does not want any more children?

Public support for abortion depends on the reasons for having one. There is strong support for legal abortion for the first three, more severe, reasons—76% of people surveyed from 1987 to 1991 supported abortion for all three reasons, whereas only 7% opposed abortion for all three reasons. There is deep division on the last three reasons, however; 47% opposed abortion in all three cases, whereas 37% supported it in all three cases (Cook et al., 1992).

A similar picture is obtained from Illinois Policy Survey (IPS) data. From 1990 to 1992, that survey annually asked a state sample of more than 800 people a more general question: "Regardless of how you personally feel about abortion, do you think it should be legal in all cases, legal in some cases, or not legal in any case?" For those 3 years, 37% to 39% of respondents said abortion should be legal in all cases, whereas from 11% to 14% said it should not be legal in any case. The largest group, from 45% to 49%, said it should be legal in some circumstances (Wetstein, 1996). Thus, although the public does not support a total ban on abortion, for the largest proportion of people—described as the "muddled middle"—approval depends on the women's reasons for seeking an abortion, which depend on her circumstances (Wetstein, 1996, p. 60).

Such poll findings arguably play an important role in shaping the public's perceptions of why women seek abortions and creating norms for what's considered an appropriate reason for doing so. In addition, they are likely to influence the conditions politicians will accept as legally permissible for obtaining an abortion. Unfortunately, items used in national opinion surveys, whether the GSS or others, generate a limited, simplistic image of women's reasons for abortion that neglects critical aspects of women's circumstances having profound implications for the women, their families, and society.

DISTORTION OF THE REALITIES OF WOMEN'S LIVES

Items typically used to measure abortion attitudes do not focus on the realities experienced by the majority of women seeking abortions. In general, they either ask about a limited number of reasons (e.g., the GSS) or they are pitched at a general level (e.g, IPS). In either instance, there is no consideration or communication of the important and multiple responsibilities women must juggle when thinking about having a child and no appreciation for the fact that women seeking abortions are in diverse life stages, with highly varied responsibilities and economic circumstances (Russo, Horn, & Schwartz, 1992; Torres & Forrest, 1988).

How do women's realities differ from the picture implied by the polls? For one thing, women typically have more than one reason for seeking an abortion (Torres & Forrest, 1988). The impression that a woman has simply one reason for abortion is grossly misleading. Second, abortion is constructed as a direct rebellion against traditional expectations that women should seek to be wives and mothers. In the highly influential GSS, the last two questions divide women into two categories—unmarried and wives and mothers—a text that facilitates constructing a stereotype of abortion patients as "selfishly" desiring to avoid family responsibilities.

But the reality is, marriage and motherhood do not go hand in hand. In 1987, among adult abortion patients (age 18 and over), 44% of unmarried women (i.e., never married, separated, or divorced) were mothers; for married women, 88% were mothers. Even a significant proportion (9%) of unmarried minors (17 years of age or younger) were already mothers (Russo et al., 1992).

Contrary to the picture of using abortion to eschew responsibilities of motherhood, Russo and Zierk (1992) found a small but significant correlation between number of children born and number of abortions obtained. About two out of three married abortion patients surveyed already had at least two children. Further, the majority of abortion patients said they intend to have more children (Russo et al., 1992).

A woman's ability to time, space, and limit her childbearing has important social, economic, and health implications, regardless of her marital status (see Russo, 1992, for a review). In the GSS, a married woman's general desire to limit family size is recognized as a reason for seeking abortion (Question 6) as is a poor family's inability to afford more children

(Question 5). The important benefits of enabling people to control family size beyond economic reasons are not recognized, however (Russo, 1992). Timing and spacing issues are ignored for all women, and it is assumed that unmarried women are childless.

Yet one of the most underrecognized contributions of abortion to the health and well-being of women and their families is its role in enabling women to lengthen their childbearing intervals. Longitudinal research has found that close child-spacing intervals are predictive of child abuse (Altemeier et al., 1984). Further, avoiding birth intervals of less than 2 years reduces the risk of low birth weight and neonatal death an estimated 5% to 10% (Miller, 1991). In 1987, 25% of adult mothers obtaining abortions had a youngest child under 2 years of age; 12% had a youngest child less than a year old. The sources of stress in these women's lives were not often accompanied by high levels of coping resources: 71% of these mothers were unmarried, and 39% had family incomes below the poverty level (Russo, Horn, & Tromp, 1993).

Another distortion of the reality of abortion for women occurs when surveys such as the GSS ask individuals to indicate the reasons or circumstances under which they feel legal abortion is acceptable. Although some smaller studies have focused on personal opinions about abortion (e.g., Esposito & Basow, 1995; Westfall, Kallail, & Walling, 1991), most national studies have emphasized attitudes toward legalization (Cook et al., 1992; Wetstein, 1996).

Framing measures of abortion attitudes in a legal context may create a knowledge base that helps politicians know whether their vote for legalizing abortion will be supported. But it also creates a demand to consider abortion in terms of rights, pitting a woman's right to choose abortion against the right of the fetus to be born. Examining stories women tell about their experiences with unplanned and unwanted pregnancy and abortion yields quite a different picture (Bonavoglia, 1991; Claire, 1995; Maloy & Patterson, 1992; Miller, 1993). Constructing the decision as a contest of rights is almost irrelevant to what women think about when faced with a pregnancy, which is how having a child will change their lives and whether they can meet their responsibilities—to the future child; to their current and future children; and to others who depend on them at home, at work, and in their communities (Russo et al., 1992; Torres & Forrest, 1988).

Framing the issue in a legal context has other implications. Responses to legally oriented questions reflect a balancing of several values, including separation of church and state, that are not specific to abortion. Indeed, one 1989 poll found that 78% of respondents agreed with the statement, "I personally feel that abortion is morally wrong, but I also feel that whether or not to have an abortion is a decision that has to be made by every woman for herself" (Craig & O'Brien, 1993). Such complex views are not easily picked up by polls that don't simultaneously consider a balance between moral and legal considerations. Though people may articulate the specific legal terms under which they consider abortion acceptable, those attitudes do not communicate how personally relevant and significant the issue is to the respondent. Two individuals citing similar opinions with regard to legal restrictions may have very different ideologies and personal experiences as a basis for those opinions. In fact, a person who disapproves of abortion may believe that making abortion illegal is undesirable (Scott, 1989).

A legal context promotes legal rhetoric, a rhetoric that is characteristically partisan and exaggerated, and focuses on the merits of one's own position and takes an uncompromising stand. As Mary Ann Glendon (1991) pointed out, "In its simple American form, the language of rights is the language of no compromise. The winner takes all, and the loser has to get out of town" (p. 9). Thus, framing the issue of abortion in terms of rights may undermine willingness to compromise and tolerate opposing views and abide by the rules of the democratic process.

OTHER METHODOLOGICAL ISSUES

Item context can have a profound effect on level of support (or opposition) expressed for abortion (Mellers & Cooke, 1996; Schuman, Kalton, & Ludwig, 1983). Even subtle differences in wording (e.g., "do you approve" vs. "do you oppose" vs. "would you support") can affect survey response. Although adequate evaluation of the impact of survey wording in abortion attitude studies has yet to be undertaken, research in other areas has documented powerful contextual effects (Huber, Payne, & Puto, 1982; Mellers & Cooke, 1996; Parducci, 1968, 1974; Strack, Schwarz, & Gschneidinger, 1985). Consider the following questions:

> "Should abortion be legal as it is now, or legal only in cases of rape, incest, or to save the life of the mother, or should it not be permitted at all?"
> "Do you think abortions should be legal under any circumstances, legal under certain circumstances, or illegal in all circumstances?"

These questions appeared on two independent abortion opinion polls conducted about the same time in 1989, using comparable representative samples. Nine percent of the respondents to the first poll said abortion should not be permitted at all. In contrast, 19% of respondents to the second poll said abortion should be illegal in all circumstances. The fact that the respondents evaluated different sets of alternatives before expressing their opinion led to very different pictures of the strength of the opposition (Craig & O'Brien, 1993).

Clearly, the current picture of abortion attitudes reflects the nature, number, order and direction of items used to measure them. Problems stemming from the fact that survey items are arbitrary (i.e., they don't fully and accurately portray women's reasons for abortion) are compounded when the items are used to construct an attitude scale (e.g., Cook et al., 1992). The proportion of the population depicted as pro-life or pro-choice, which becomes defined by the proportion of items approved, can be manipulated by selection and wording of the items. For example, adding more items of a "severe" nature (e.g., "because she has a severely disabled 10-month-old child that she must care for?") could create a more positive picture of support for abortion. More items of a "trivial" nature in the scale (e.g., "Do you think it should be possible for a pregnant woman to obtain a legal abortion because she feels ugly and unattractive when pregnant?") could create a more negative picture of abortion. Items constructed to pit women's choice against women's worth might even induce pro-choice feminist activists to express disapproval of abortion (e.g., "because she has found out the fetus is female and wants only male children?"). Effects of the larger context need to be considered as well: When respondents are asked if they support a woman's having a legal abortion "for any reason," what reasons come to mind? Insofar as pro-life propaganda leads to trivial reasons being available and accessible in memory, respondents may be more likely to withhold support.

Given the power of contrast and anchoring-and-adjustment effects on judgments, the fact that there are no truly trivial reasons included in the items may affect responses as well. Schuman, Presser, and Ludwig (1981) compared support for the GSS item "married and does not want any more children" (Question 6) when presented before or after "chance of serious defect in the baby" (Question 3). When the item was presented first, support was higher than when it was presented later (the order in which it usually appears on the GSS). Those authors speculated that, having supported a specific reason like fetal defect, the respondents were relieved of supporting the more general item. However, it may also be that responding three times in a row to severe reasons (health, rape, fetal defect), may make the other reasons presented seem inconsequential due to the processes of anchoring and adjustment.

Given the fact that national polls of abortion attitudes may shape views of the public and policy makers, and the wording of such polls can affect responses, manipulation of polls is of concern. Conduct of polls is governed by The Code of Disclosure, which mandates that reports of results include the population surveyed, sample size and method of drawing it, exact question wording, interview date, interview nature (e.g., telephone or mail survey), and identification of the poll's sponsor (Craig & O'Brien, 1993). This helps (but does not guarantee) the identification of purposely biased polls so that they can be refuted.

Although it may seem that difficulties in measuring public attitudes make these methodological problems intractable, Sitaraman (1994) demonstrated that alternative models that present women as having multiple reasons for abortion and communicate diversity in motivations and circumstances are possible. Using a factorial survey design, Sitaraman examined the characteristics of the situations affecting moral acceptance of abortion in a sample of 217 predominately White, middle-class respondents who had completed a telephone interview. This design involved experimentally varying a hypothetical description of a situation along 10 dimensions (independent variables): life course position (age, marital status, parity), personal circumstance (women's health and economic status), reasons for abortion (rape by stranger, fetal deformity, harmful pregnancy, desire to limit family size, financial problems, unmarried status, desire to remain childless, father's refusal to marry woman, incestuous rape by brother, and pregnancy from extramarital relationship), length of gestation (months pregnant), and relational context (quality of couple's relationship, parental approval/disapproval, partner's approval/disapproval). A computer generated random combinations of levels of the independent variables to produce vignettes describing the particular situation represented by that combination. Thus, opinion on abortion could be placed in the context of a complex weave of beliefs and attitudes related to gender roles and reproduction, sexuality, and human life.

Each respondent received only a limited number of the thousands of vignettes that were produced. In analyzing the impact of the situational dimensions, each vignette was the unit of analysis, not the individual respondent. Twenty vignettes were presented in random order, for a total of 4,340 unique vignettes used in the study. For the dependent variable, the respondents were given a 9-point scale (1 = *strongly approve* and 9 = *strongly disapprove*) and asked to circle "the number below that best expresses your opinion of this woman's decision to have an abortion."

Regression analyses revealed that when women were in their 40s, in very poor health, pregnant as a result of rape, with a defective fetus, or in a health-threatening situation, approval for abortion significantly increased. If women had a high income or were beyond the 4th month of gestation, approval significantly decreased. Financial problems, desire to limit family size, or remain childless produced slight decreases in approval, whereas pregnancy from a premarital or extramarital relationship produced slightly higher approval ratings. In examining effect of partner/parent's views, approval was highest when the partner approved in combination with parents disapproving, lowest when both partner and parents disapproved. Reasons for abortion explained the most variance in approval ratings (9%). That is, knowing the reason given for seeking an abortion predicted more variance in abortion attitudes toward the abortion than any of the other factors listed (e.g., partner approval).

The fact that all of these factors only explained 13% of the variance suggests that abortion attitudes are highly responsive to nuances of context. The range of factors influencing approval, including other reasons for seeking abortion, has yet to be fully identified. Further, the use of the word *approve* probably underestimates the number of people who would support a woman's decision to have an abortion in the particular circumstances. *Approve* is an active verb—had they been asked if they would *object* or *protest*, the resulting picture might different substantially. Nonetheless, finding differences in level of approval is a good indicator of relative support for a woman's decision across circumstances. In any case, alternative models to current approaches are possible and a concerted effort is needed to develop them.

Failing to distinguish between abortions performed at differing gestational ages continues to be a major problem. An "abortion" before implantation, at 8 weeks, and at 19 weeks of pregnancy are three very different experiences. In fact, some people suggest that new reproductive technology, including RU-486, may so radically change the assumptions made about the abortion context that the debates will become obsolete (Baulieu & Rosenblum, 1991; Lader, 1991; Tribe, 1990).

We consider this hope a bit optimistic. It is true that a pill enabling a woman to safely and completely terminate her pregnancy without having to go to a hospital or clinic would make many arguments and laws irrelevant (Tribe, 1990). However, the abortion debate does not hinge solely on fetal personhood, although that is indeed a critical issue. Even a "morning after" pill that works before implantation (i.e., before the woman is "officially" pregnant) still engenders objections rooted in traditional ideologies regarding female sexuality and gender roles. Promoting the notion that women will be encouraged to have unprotected sex and avoid the consequences of their shameful actions by popping a pill feeds into conservative ideas about women and sexuality and is likely to make a significant proportion of the public uncomfortable with this solution. When national leaders like Representative Dick Armey (R-Texas) proclaim women who seek abortion are "self-indulgent" and "damned careless" (quoted in Ivins, 1995, p. F5), it is obvious that a vivid and negative portrayal of women will be used to play on the public's discomfort with the idea of abortion as easy and accessible. Further, the drug must be taken early in pregnancy, and many women—particularly those who are young, uneducated, or ambivalent about the pregnancy—may not be able to readily obtain and use it properly. Nonetheless, for many women, access to such a drug would revolutionize the abortion context, making current knowledge irrelevant to their experience.

Although we have focused our methodological lens on characteristics of questions used in national polls, the validity of the results also depends on the size and representativeness of the sample, proper conduct on the part of the interviewer, and appropriate analysis of the results. We must consider size of the subsample as well as the overall sample when interpreting poll results—large differences may be meaningless if comparisons involve small subsamples (e.g., as when race and religious comparisons are being made). Craig and O'Brien (1993) demonstrated this point. They present responses to a 1989 Gallup poll that asked respondents if they opposed overturning *Roe v. Wade*, showing 58% of Whites and 55% of non-Whites were opposed. For the large subsample of Whites ($n = 1075$), the allowance for error is plus or minus 4 points. For the smaller subsample of non-Whites ($n = 166$), that allowance is plus or minus 11 points. In this context, the 3-point difference between the two groups becomes meaningless (p. 148).

WHERE DO WE GO FROM HERE?

What can we learn from this picture of the history and status of support for abortion in the United States? First, understanding the strategies and tactics used to express opposition to abortion is an initial step toward understanding the complex web of barriers to abortion access that is being constructed across the United States. Further, although abortion is an age-old practice, it has always been controversial for one reason or another. Meanings and purposes of reproductive control are socially and politically constructed, and express changing values and balances of political power between different groups in society. Even a brief survey of abortion's place in Western history reveals a multiplicity of views, motives, and vested interests participating in the abortion debate that go far beyond the question of embryonic personhood. Abortion appears to be at the intersection of multiple concerns, including values of tolerance, privacy, and individualism; gender role norms and the meaning of motherhood; control of female sexuality; the meaning of prenatal life; and the relationship of religion and the professions to the state. Abortion's relationship to sexuality, with its religious overtones and significance for societal survival, make it a particularly emotional and controversial issue when moved to the public sphere. Religious organizations, the status of the professions, economic conditions, and the state of medical technology all contribute to the sociopolitical context in which the meaning of abortion becomes constructed.

In this context, women become divided from one another on an issue affecting all women: control of whether and when they want to bear a child. Given that women's ability to control fertility is used to justify gender discrimination, even women who don't have children have a stake in making motherhood truly voluntary. All women also have a stake in the values placed on women's contributions, at home, at work, and in their communities. Can women find common ground when so many forces are working to divide them across lines of race, ethnicity, class, and religion? Unfortunately, national studies of abortion attitudes have overemphasized legal issues, and the resulting national knowledge base is not constructed to help answer that question.

The issue of abortion does not stand alone in a separate ideological space. Looking at related attitudes and issues may provide a fresh perspective for dealing with abortion issues. It's clear that pro-choice and pro-life individuals think about abortion in very different terms and link the issues to premises and values in different ways. Even among individuals identified as pro-choice or pro-life there is diversity in ways of thinking and evaluating abortion. We need to know more about those underlying beliefs and values and about the ongoing situational supports that harden people's positions and undermine meaningful dialogue.

We also need to be more clear about what the knowledge is for: to evoke negative images of abortion patients, identify points of common ground, or influence policy makers to support or oppose restrictive abortion policies? The biggest gap in our knowledge is what the attitudes mean for behaviors—deciding to give birth or have an abortion, writing letters to support a particular policy, donating money, voting, volunteering for escort or picket duty, throwing firebombs, writing book chapters? Surveys can link attitudes to behavioral intentions, but it will take methodologies that go beyond verbal report and that study other behaviors for us to learn what these attitudes mean for predicting a range of actions.

The "muddled middle" should play a critical role in redefining the grounds for the abortion debate. That middle does not want abortion to be legally prohibited but also doesn't want the abortion decision to be taken lightly. In this context, qualitative research that enables women to tell their stories—their motivations, circumstances, and experiences with abortion and its alternatives—becomes an important part of our knowledge base. Given the chilling, silencing effects of pro-life harassment and intimidation, providing support and outlets for women's stories can be an important contribution as well.

Perhaps seizing the ground and reframing the debate in terms of how to support a woman's pregnancy decision making such that she can act morally and responsibly in the context of her religious beliefs and values will be a positive step toward building bridges among pro-choice and pro-life feminists who already share so many concerns. Toward that end, psychological knowledge that goes beyond what is possible to obtain by public opinion polls is needed if a full understanding of the dynamics of the beliefs, values, attitudes, and emotions around abortion (and the related issues of sexuality and women's roles) and its relationship to behavior is to be achieved.

REFERENCES

Adebayo, A. (1990). Male attitudes toward abortion: An analysis of urban survey data. *Social Indicators Research, 22,* 213–228.

Adler, N. E., David, H. P., Major, B., Roth, S., Russo, N. F., & Wyatt, G. E. (1990). Psychological responses after abortion. *Science, 248,* 41–44.

Adler, N. F., David, H. P., Major, B. N., Roth, S. H., Russo, N. F., & Wyatt, G. E. (1992). Psychological factors in abortion: A review. *American Psychologist, 47,* 1194–1204.

Altemeier, W. A., O'Connor, S., Vietze, P., Sandler, H., & Sherrod, K. (1984). Prediction of child abuse: A prospective study of feasibility. *Child Abuse and Neglect 8,* 393–400.

Back, K. (1986–1987). Why is abortion a public issue? The role of professional control. *Politics and Society, 15(2),* 197–206.

Bart, P. B. (1981). Seizing the means of reproduction: An illegal feminist abortion collective. In H. Roberts (Ed.), *Women, health and reproduction.* New York: Routledge & Kegan Paul.

Baulieu, E., with Rosenblum, M. (1991). *The abortion pill: RU-486, a woman's choice* (pp. 109–128). New York: Simon & Schuster.

Betzig, L., & Lombardo, L. H. (1991). Who's pro-choice and why? *Ethology and Sociobiology, 13,* 49–71.

Blanchard, D. A. (1994). *The rise of the religious right: From polite to fiery protest.* New York: Twayne.

Blanchard, D. A., & Prewitt, T. J. (1993). *Religious violence and abortion: The Gideon Project.* Gainesville: University Press Florida.

Bonavoglia, A. (Ed.). (1991). *The choices we made.* New York: Random House.

Butler, J. D., & Walbert, D. F. (Eds.). (1992). *Abortion, medicine, and the law* (rev. ed.). New York: Facts on File.

Calderone, M. (1960). Illegal abortion as a public health problem. *American Journal of Public Health, 50,* 948.

Cerullo, M. (1990). Hidden history: An illegal abortion in 1968. In M. G. Fried (Ed.), *From abortion to reproductive freedom: Transforming a movement* (pp. 87–90). Boston, MA: South End Press.

Chancer, L. S. (1990). Abortion without apology. In M. G. Fried (Ed.), *From abortion to reproductive freedom: Transforming a movement* (pp. 113–120). Boston, MA: South End Press.

Claire, M. (1995). *The abortion dilemma: Personal views on a public issue.* New York: Plenum Press.

Clark, C., & Clark, J. (1996). Whither the gender gap? Converging and conflicting attitudes among women. In L. Lovelace (Ed.), *Women in politics: Outsiders or insiders?* (pp. 78–99). Upper Saddle River, NJ: Prentice Hall.

Combs, M. W., & Welch, S. (1982). Blacks, whites, and attitudes toward abortion. *Public Opinion Quarterly, 46,* 510–520.

Condit, C. M. (1990). *Decoding abortion rhetoric: Communicating social change*. Chicago: University of Illinois Press.

Conklin, M. P., & O'Connor, B. (1995). Beliefs about the fetus as a moderator of postabortion psychological well being. *Journal of Social and Clinical Psychology, 14*, 76–95.

Cook, E. A., Jelen, T. G., & Wilcox, C. (1992). *Between two absolutes: Public opinion and the politics of abortion*. Boulder, CO: Westview Press.

Cozzarelli, C., & Major, B. (1994). The effects of anti-abortion demonstrators and pro-choice escorts on women's psychological responses to abortion. *Journal of Social and Clinical Psychology, 13*, 404–427.

Craig, B. H., & O'Brien, D. M. (1993). *Abortion and American politics*. Chatham, NJ: Chatham House.

Cunningham, P. C., & Forsythe, C. D. (1992). Is abortion the "First Right" for women?: Some consequences of legal abortion. In J. D. Butler & D. F. Walbert (Eds.), *Abortion, medicine, and the law* (pp. 100–158). New York: Facts on File.

Devins, N., & Watson, W. L. (Eds.). (1995a). *Federal abortion politics: A documentary history. Volume I: Congressional action (Parts 1 & 2)*. New York: Garland.

Devins, N., & Watson, W. L. (Eds.). (1995b). *Federal abortion politics: A documentary history. Volume II: Executive initiatives (Parts 1 & 2)*. New York: Garland.

Devins, N., & Watson, W. L. (Eds.). (1995c). *Federal abortion politics: A documentary history. Volume III: Judicial nominations (Parts 1 & 2)*. New York: Garland.

Donovan, J. (1992). *Feminist theory: The intellectual traditions of American feminism* (2nd ed.). New York: Continuum.

Eckel, S. (1997, October 9). Pro-life forces rebuff bid to reduce abortion. *Arizona Republic*, p. B5.

Elliot Institute. (n. d.). Let Us Show You How We Will STOP ABORTION. Advertising flyer, Elliot Institute, P.O. Box 7348, Springfield, IL.

Esposito, C. L., & Basow, S. A. (1995). College students' attitudes toward abortion: The role of knowledge and demographic variables. *Journal of Applied Social Psychology, 25*, 1996–2017.

Farley, C. (1995, March 13). Malpractice as a weapon. *Time, 145*(10), p. 65.

Flowers, M. J. (1990). Coming into being: The prenatal development of humans. In J. D. Butler & D. F. Walbert (Eds.), *Abortion, medicine, and the law* (4th ed., pp. 437–452). New York: Facts on File.

Forrest, J. D., & Henshaw, S. K. (1987). The harassment of U.S. abortion providers. *Family Planning Perspectives, 19*(1), 9–13.

Freeman, E. W. (1977). Influence of personality attributes on abortion experiences. *American Journal of Orthopsychiatry, 47*(3), 503–513.

Fried, M. G. (1990). *From abortion to reproductive freedom: Transforming a movement*. Boston, MA: South End Press.

Ginsburg, F. D. (1989). *Contested lives: The abortion debate in an American community*. Berkeley: University of California Press/Goodman, Ellen.

Glendon, M. A. (1991). *Rights talk: The impoverishment of political discourse.* New York: Free Press.

Gordon, L. (1990). *Woman's body, woman's right: Birth control in America.* New York: Penguin Books.

Hall, E. J., & Ferree, M. M. (1986). Race differences in abortion attitudes. *Public Opinion Quarterly, 50,* 193–207.

Harrison, M., & Gilbert, S. (Eds.). (1993). *Abortion decisions of the United States Supreme Court.* Beverly Hills, CA: Excellent Books.

Henshaw, S. (1990). Induced abortion: A world review, 1990. *Family Planning Perspectives, 22*(2), 76–89.

Henshaw, S. K., Koonin, L. M., & Smith, J. C. (1991). Characteristics of U.S. women having abortions. *Family Planning Perspectives, 23,* 75–81.

Henshaw, S. K., & Silverman, J. (1988). The characteristics and prior contraceptive use of U.S. abortion patients. *Family Planning Perspectives, 20*(4), 158–168.

Hollis, H. M., & Morris, T. M. (1992). Attitudes toward abortion in female undergraduates. *College Student Journal, 26,* 70–74.

Huber, J. J., Payne, W., & Puto, C. (1982). Adding asymmetrically dominated alternatives: Violations of regularity and the similarity hypothesis. *Journal of Consumer Research, 9,* 90–98.

Hull, G. T., Scott, P. B., & Smith, B. (Eds.). (1982). *All the women are white, all the blacks are men, but some of us are brave: Black women's studies.* Old Westbury, NY: The Feminist Press.

Ivins, M. (1995, February 5). Lack of civility plagues politicians. *The Arizona Republic* [Editorial/Opinions section], p. F5.

Jenkins, S. (1990). Abortion rights, poor women, and religious diversity. In M. G. Fried (Ed.), *From abortion to reproductive freedom: Transforming a movement* (pp. 151–156). Boston, MA: South End Press.

Joffe, C. (1995). *Doctors of conscience: The struggle to provide abortion before and after Roe v. Wade.* Boston, MA: Beacon Press.

Kaplan, L. (1995). *The story of Jane: The legendary underground feminist abortion service.* New York: Pantheon.

Krishnan, V. (1991). Abortion in Canada: Religious and ideological dimensions of women's attitudes. *Social Biology, 38,* 249–257.

Lader, L. (1973). *Abortion II: Making the revolution.* Boston, MA: Beacon Press.

Lader, L. (1991). *RU-486: The pill that could end the abortion wars and why American women don't have it.* Reading, MA: Addison-Wesley.

Lewin, T. (1997, December 21). New techniques blur line between abortion, contraception: But foes say moral issues are the same. *The Arizona Republic,* p. A5.

Luker, K. (1984). *Abortion and politics of motherhood.* Berkeley: University of California Press.

Lunneborg, P. (1992). *Abortion: A positive decision.* Westport, CT: Greenwood Press.

Lynxwiler, J., & Gay, D. (1994). Reconsidering race differences in abortion attitudes. *Social Science Quarterly, 75,* 67–84.

Maloy, K., & Patterson, M. J. (1992). *Birth or abortion? Private struggles in a political world.* New York: Plenum Press.

Mellers, B. A., & Cooke, A. D. J. (1996). The role of task and context in preference measurement. *Psychological Science, 7,* 76–82.

Merrick, J. C., & Blank, R. H. (Eds.). (1993). *The politics of pregnancy: Policy dilemmas in the maternal-fetal relationship.* New York: Harrington Park Press.

Mertus, J. A. (1990). Fake abortion clinics: The threat to reproductive self-determination. *Women and Health, 16,* 95–113.

Miller, J. E. (1991). Birth intervals and perinatal health: An investigation of three hypotheses. *Family Planning Perspectives, 23*(2), 62–70.

Miller, P. G. (1993). *The worst of times: Illegal abortion—Survivors, practitioners, coroners, cops, and children of women who died talk about its horror.* New York: Harper Collins.

Mohr, J. (1978). *Abortion in America: The origins and evolution of national policy, 1800–1900.* Oxford, England: Oxford University Press.

Moore, K. A., & Stief, T. M. (1991). Changes in marriage and fertility behavior. *Youth and Society, 22,* 362–386.

Moraga, C., & Anzaldúa, G. (Eds.). (1981). *This bridge called my back: Writings by radical women of color.* New York: Kitchen Table: Women of Color Press.

Noonan, J. T. (1986). The experience of pain in the unborn. In J. D. Butler & D. F. Walbert (Eds.), *Abortion, medicine, and the law* (3rd ed., pp. 360–369). New York: Facts on File.

Parducci, A. (1968). The relativism of absolute judgment. *Scientific American, 219,* 84–90.

Parducci, A. (1974). Contextual effects: A range–frequency analysis. In E. C. Carterette & M. P. Friedman (Eds.), *Handbook of perception* (Vol. 2, pp. 127–141). New York: Academic Press.

Payne, R. (1989). *Fathers of the Eastern church.* New York: Dorset Press.

Petchesky, R. (1990). *Abortion and a woman's choice: The state, sexuality and conditions of reproductive freedom* (rev. ed.). Longman, NY: Northeastern University Press.

Reardon, D. (1996). *Making abortion rare: A healing strategy for a divided nation.* Springfield, IL: Acorn Books.

Reardon, D. (1997, May). *Predictive factors of post-abortion adjustment: Clinical, legal, and ethical implications.* Paper presented at the annual meeting of the American Psychiatric Association, San Diego, CA.

Reeves, J. (1998, January 30). Abortion clinic blast is 1st to be deadly. *Arizona Republic,* pp. A1, A11.

Robinson, M. (1998, April 21). Abortion foes lose key case. *The Arizona Republic,* pp. A1, A13.

Roe v. Wade, 410 U.S. 113 (1973).

Rossi, A. S. (1967). Public views on abortion. In A. F. Guttmacher (Ed.), *The case for legalized abortion now*. Berkeley, CA: Diablo Press.

Rubin, E. A. (1994). *The abortion controversy: A documentary history*. Westport, CT: Greenwood Press.

Russo, N. F. (1976). The motherhood mandate. *Journal of Social Issues, 32*, 143–154.

Russo, N. F. (Ed.). (1979). *The motherhood mandate* [Special issue, *Psychology of Women Quarterly*]. New York: Human Sciences Press.

Russo, N. F. (1992). Psychological aspects of unwanted pregnancy and its resolution. In J. D. Butler & D. F. Walbert (Eds.), *Abortion, medicine, and the law* (4th ed., pp. 593–626). New York: Facts on File.

Russo, N. F., Horn, J. D., & Schwartz, R. (1992). U.S. abortion in context: Selected characteristics and motivations of women seeking abortions. *Journal of Social Issues, 48*, 183–202.

Russo, N. F., Horn, J., & Tromp, S. (1993). Childspacing intervals and abortion among blacks and whites: A brief report. *Women & Health, 20*(3), 43–52.

Russo, N. F., & Zierk, K. L. (1992). Abortion, childbearing, and women's well-being. *Professional psychology: Research and Practice, 23*, 269–280.

Ruth, S. (1995). *Issues in feminism*. (3rd ed.). Mountain View, CA: Mayfield.

Schuman, H., Kalton, G., & Ludwig, J. (1983). Context and contiguity in survey questionnaires. *Public Opinion Quarterly, 47*, 112–115.

Schuman, H., Presser, S., & Ludwig, J. (1981). Context effects on survey responses to questions about abortion. *Public Opinion Quarterly, 45*(2), 216–222.

Schur, E. M. (1965). *Crimes without victims: Deviant behavior and public policy—abortion, homosexuality, drug addiction*. Englewood Cliffs, NJ: Prentice-Hall.

Schwartz, R. A. (1986). Abortion on request: The psychiatric implications. In J. D. Butler & D. F. Walbert (Eds.), *Abortion, medicine, and the law* (pp. 323–340). New York: Facts on File.

Scott, J. (1989). Conflicting beliefs about abortion: Legal approval and moral doubts. *Social Psychology Quarterly, 52*, 319–326.

Simmons, P. D. (1992). Religious approaches to abortion. In J. D. Butler & D. F. Walbert. *Abortion, medicine, and the law* (pp. 712–728). New York: Facts on File.

Sitaraman, B. (1994). *The middleground: The American public and the abortion debate*. New York: Garland Publishing, Inc.

Staggenborg, S. (1991). *The prochoice movement*. New York: Oxford University Press.

Strack, F., Schwarz, N., & Gschneidinger, E. (1985). Happiness and reminiscing: The role of time perspective, affect, and mode of thinking. *Journal of Personality and Social Psychology, 6*, 1460–1469.

Szafran, R. F., & Clagett, A. F. (1988). Variable predictors of attitudes toward the legalization of abortion. *Social Indicators Research, 20*, 271–290.

Thompson, J. J. (1971). A defense of abortion. *Philosophy and Public Affairs 1*, 44–66.

Tietze, C., & Lewit, S. (1969). Abortion. *Scientific American, 220*, 21–27.

Torres, A., & Forrest, J. D. (1988). Why do women have abortions? *Family Planning Perspectives, 20*(4), 169–176.

Tribe, L. H. (1990). *Abortion: The clash of absolutes.* New York: Norton.

Walzer, S. (1994). The role of gender in determining abortion attitudes. *Social Science Quarterly, 75*, 686–693.

Warren, M. A. (1979). On the moral and legal status of the unborn. In S. Bishop & M. Weinzweig (Eds.), *Philosophy and women* (pp. 216–266). Belmont, CA: Wadsworth.

Welch, M. R., Leege, D. C., & Cavendish, J. C. (1995). Attitudes toward abortion among U.S. Catholics: Another case of symbolic politics? *Social Science Quarterly, 76*, 142–157.

Welter, B. (1978). The cult of true womanhood: 1820–1860. In M. Gordon (Ed.). *The American family in socio-historical perspective* (2nd ed., pp. 313–333). New York: St. Martin's Press.

Westfall, J. M., Kallail, K. J., & Walling, A. D. (1991). Abortion attitudes and practices of family and general practice physicians. *The Journal of Family Practice, 33*, 47–51.

Wetstein, M. E. (1996). *Abortion rates in the United States: The influence of opinion and policy.* Albany: State University of New York Press.

Wilcox, C. (1990). Race differences in abortion attitudes: Some additional evidence. *Public Opinion Quarterly, 54*, 248–255.

Wilcox, C. (1992). Race, region, and abortion attitudes. *Sociological Analysis, 53*, 97–105.

Williams, R. M., Jr. (1970). *American society* (3rd ed.). New York: Alfred A. Knopf.

Wright, L. S., & Rogers, R. R. (1987). Variables related to pro-choice attitudes among undergraduates. *Adolescence, 22*, 517–524.

3

BARRIERS TO ACCESS TO ABORTION SERVICES

STANLEY K. HENSHAW

In recent years reproductive health care providers and advocates for women's health have become alarmed by the apparent decline in the number of physicians willing to perform abortions and the consequent decrease in the availability of abortion services in the United States (Grimes, 1991). Although abortion services still are readily available to those in large urban areas who are able to pay, access to services may be curtailed for many women because of barriers such as distance from the nearest provider, cost of the procedure, and harassment. Using data from the Alan Guttmacher Institute's (AGI) 1993 Abortion Provider Survey, in this chapter we examine two major issues: (a) the declining number of abortion providers, which negatively impacts service availability, and (b) the multitude of other barriers that can hinder access to abortion services.

THE DATA SET

The data reported in this chapter primarily were obtained from the 1993 Abortion Provider Survey of AGI. The most complete data on the availability of abortion services come from periodic surveys conducted by AGI of all known abortion providers in the United States. These surveys ask questions about the number of abortions provided and contain questions that vary from survey to survey about provider characteristics and conditions of service. The surveys are the only national source of information on the number and type of abortion providers and their geographic distribution. In addition, for most states and for the United States as a whole, they are the most complete sources of information on the number of abortions performed.

The 1993 Abortion Provider Survey is the 11th survey of all known abortion providers in the United States. Its methodology is described in more detail by Henshaw and Van Vort (1994). In February 1993, questionnaires were mailed to a total of 3,156 potential providers, including all hospitals, clinics, and physicians' offices thought to have provided abortions during 1991 and 1992. The mailing list included all facilities that indicated in an earlier 1989 AGI survey that they performed abortions and was updated with names of possible new providers obtained from known providers, advocacy groups, the telephone yellow pages, newspaper articles, and a commercial mailing list. If a response was not received within 3 weeks of the mailing, we sent as many as three follow-up mailings. For facilities that still did not respond, health department data were used in states that provided such information for individual facilities. The remaining nonresponding facilities or individuals were contacted by telephone. Of the 3,156 facilities surveyed, we received 1,606 completed questionnaires, interviewed 831 providers by telephone, and used health department data for 328 providers. Thus, data were available for 84% of the facilities surveyed. Of 391 facilities for which data were not available, 211 did not respond to requests and 174 closed, moved, or could not be located. However, it was possible to estimate the number of abortions performed for 206 of these providers from community sources or data provided for earlier years.

Two versions of the survey questionnaire were used: one for hospitals and one for clinics and other nonhospital facilities. In addition to requesting information about the number of abortions provided, the questionnaire for nonhospital providers included questions about the proportion of patients who travel 50 to 100 miles or more than 100 miles for abortion services, the maximum gestation age at which abortions are provided, the days of the week services are offered, whether abortions can be performed during a patient's first visit, costs of abortion, and any problems affecting the facility's ability to offer abortion services. Providers also were asked about the frequency of harassment by antiabortion activists during 1992. Because the additional topics covered in the hospital questionnaire were confined to gestation limits and antiabortion harassment, most of the information on barriers to services in this chapter pertains only to nonhospital providers. Hospitals performed only 7% of all abortions in 1992. Therefore, these data describe the services offered to most women who had an abortion during that year. One limitation of the data is that not all providers gave information on all questionnaire items. For instance, of the 1,525 nonhospital abortion providers, 73% provided information on gestation limits, 60% on costs, and 55% to 61% on other items.

We divided nonhospital facilities into three groups: abortion clinics, nonspecialized clinics, and physicians' offices. An abortion clinic was defined as a clinic where at least 50% of a provider's patient visits in 1992 were for abortion services or, if no information was provided about proportion of visits for abortion services, the facility provided 1,000 or more abortions during 1992. Because response rates were higher for nonhospital facilities and facilities with larger caseloads than for hospitals and small facilities, results were weighted to reflect the correct national proportions according to facility type and caseload.

THE DECLINE IN ABORTION RATES

After remaining at around 1,600,000 abortions per year from 1980 through 1990, the total number of abortions in the United States appears to have begun to decline. Table 1 shows the numbers of reported abortions from 1973 to 1992. Approximately 1,529,000 abortions were performed in 1992, marking the first time since 1979 that fewer than 1,550,000 abortions were reported.

In 1992, the abortion rate was 25.9 abortions per 1,000 women aged 15 to 44 in the population, and the ratio was 27.5 per 100 live births plus abortions. An abortion ratio of 27.5 per 100 means that about 27.5% of pregnancies (excluding miscarriages) were terminated by abortion; when the estimated number of pregnancies ending in miscarriage are included, the percentage is 23.5%. Both the abortion rate and ratio have gradually, though irregularly, declined since approximately 1981 and have now reached their lowest levels since 1976. They are nevertheless higher than those in any Western European country with accurate statistics, although much lower than those in most of Eastern Europe and in some developing countries (Henshaw, 1990).

The largest numbers of abortions are performed in the most populous states, California (304,000 abortions in 1992), New York (195,000), and Texas (97,000). These states plus Florida and Illinois account for almost half (49%) of all the country's abortions. At the other end of the spectrum is Wyoming, the state with the fewest abortions; only 460 were performed there in 1992.

TABLE 1
Number of Reported Abortions, by Metropolitan Status; Rate of
Abortions per 1,000 Women Aged 15–44; and Ratio of Abortions
per 100 Pregnancies Ending in Abortions or Live Births:
United States (1973–1992)

Year	Abortions (in thousands)			Rate	Ratio[b]
	Total	Metro[a]	Nonmetro		
1973	744.6	720.2	24.4	16.3	19.3
1974	898.6	860.7	37.9	19.3	22.0
1975	1,034.2	985.7	48.5	21.7	24.9
1976	1,179.3	1,123.3	56.0	24.2	26.5
1977	1,316.7	1,258.0	58.7	26.4	28.6
1978	1,409.6	1,345.2	64.4	27.7	29.2
1979	1,497.7	1,430.9	66.8	28.8	29.6
1980	1,553.9	1,507.7	46.2	29.3	30.0
1981	1,577.3	1,538.3	39.0	29.3	30.1
1982	1,573.9	1,537.3	36.6	28.8	30.0
1983	1,573.0*	—	—	28.5*	30.4*
1984	1,577.2	1,543.9	33.3	28.1	29.7
1985	1,588.6	1,556.4	32.2	28.0	29.7
1986	1,574.0	—	—	27.4*	29.4*
1987	1,559.1	1,532.0	27.1	26.9	28.8
1988	1,590.8	1,563.4	27.4	27.3	28.6
1989	1,566.9*	—	—	26.8*	27.5*
1990	1,608.6*	—	—	27.4*	28.0*
1991	1,556.5	1,531.0	25.5	26.3	27.4
1992	1,528.9	1,506.1	22.8	25.9	27.5

Note. Asterisks indicate that data are estimated by interpolation of numbers of abortions; dashes
indicate data were unavailable.
[a]For 1973 to 1979, metropolitan status is defined according to criteria published by the Office of
Management and Budget (OMB), October 1975. For 1980 to 1988, definitions by the OMB based
on the 1980 census are used. For 1991 to 1992, OMB's June 30, 1990, definitions are used.
[b]For each year, the ratio is based on births occurring during the 12-month period starting in July of
that year (to match times of conception for pregnancies ending in births with those for pregnancies
ending in abortions).

Abortion rates vary widely among the states.[1] New York and Hawaii
have the highest rates at 46 abortions per 1,000 female residents 15 to 44,
and rates are also above 40 in California and Nevada. The rate for the
District of Columbia (DC), 138, is higher than that of any state; relatively
high rates are characteristic of central cities generally, and the rate includes
large numbers of women from outside the District who seek abortion services in DC. The census divisions with the highest rates per 1,000 are on
the East and West Coasts: Pacific (39), Middle Atlantic (35), South At-

[1]Abortion rates by state of occurrence should be interpreted cautiously because they do not
always reflect the extent of use of abortion by residents, who may travel to other states for
services. For example, in 1987, the number of Wyoming residents who had abortions in other
states was greater than the number of residents who had abortions in the state, and in Indiana,
South Dakota, and West Virginia, the abortion rate of state residents was more than 35%
higher than the rate based on the abortions occurring in the state (Henshaw, Koonin, &
Smith, 1987).

lantic (26), and New England (25). The lowest rates are found in Wyoming (4 per 1,000), South Dakota (7), Idaho (7), West Virginia (8), and Utah (9). All of these states except Utah are largely rural with no large metropolitan areas.

Factors that can cause wide variation in abortion rates by state of occurrence include the proportion of the population that is non-White, Hispanic, or unmarried (characteristics associated with higher abortion rates); the degree of urbanization (large cities tend to have higher rates); the extent of subsidies for abortion services for low-income women; and the availability of abortion services.

Between 1988 and 1992, abortion rates decreased in 36 states and DC, as well as in the country as a whole. The largest declines occurred in the West North Central states, where the number of abortions decreased by 15%, and in one of that region's states, Missouri, by 29%. Other states with declines of more than 25% were North Dakota (28%) and Utah (27%). In North Dakota, two physicians stopped performing abortions, leaving only one provider. In Michigan and DC, where funding of Medicaid abortions stopped at the end of 1988, declines in abortion rates between 1988 and 1991 were greater than the overall U.S. decline. The abortion rate increased in only one census division (Middle Atlantic),[2] and only five states (Mississippi, South Dakota, Arkansas, Kansas, and Montana) experienced rate increases of more than 10%. In summary, the 1992 Abortion Survey data show a trend toward lower abortion rates on both a national and a state-by-state level.

Reasons for Decreasing Abortions

The latest data indicate that abortion levels, whether measured by the rate per 1,000 women of reproductive age or the ratio of abortions to pregnancies, have decreased slowly but persistently since the early 1980s. Why are abortion rates declining at this particular time? The changing age distribution of women of reproductive age could be affecting the abortion rate. Women of the "baby boom" generation, now in their 30s and 40s, have fewer abortions as they age. However, when 1988 age-specific abortion rates are applied to 1992 population estimates, the difference between number of abortions expected in 1992 and the actual number in 1988 amounts to about one sixth of the actual decline of 62,000 abortions. Thus, the changing age distribution appears to account for only a small part, about one sixth, of the actual decline in the number of abortions in 1992 (Henshaw & Van Vort, 1994). Moreover, the abortion ratio should be affected even less by the changing age distribution, because birthrates as well as abortion rates decline after age 30.

---

[2]The rise of 2% was entirely the result of a 7% increase in New York.

Other reasons for the decline in abortion rates may include the following: decreases in the number of unintended pregnancies, less accepting attitudes toward abortion, or greater acceptance of childbirth outside of marriage. Although there is little evidence to support these first two explanations (Henshaw & Van Vort, 1994), the soaring birth rate of unmarried women—which was 30 per 1,000 unmarried women of reproductive age in 1981, 39 per 1,000 in 1988, and 45 per 1,000 in 1991 (National Center for Health Statistics, 1983; National Center for Health Statistics, 1990, 1993)—suggests that nonmarital childbearing is increasingly considered acceptable. Further, between 1981 and 1988 the proportion of pregnancies ending in abortion declined by 14% for unmarried women, as compared with 5% for married women (Henshaw & Van Vort, 1992).

It is unlikely, however, that any of these factors can entirely explain the decline in abortion rates. One important explanation is that this decline is due to decreasing availability of abortion services, which, in turn, restricts women's ability to freely choose among pregnancy resolution options. The evidence presented below suggests that a declining number of abortion providers and changes in geographic concentration and types of providers may be influencing declines in the abortion rate.

Availability of Abortion Services

One measure of the availability of abortion services is the proportion of counties that have abortion providers and the proportion of women who live in a county with a provider. The presence of a small provider, however, may not represent true availability of services because small providers often do not want a large abortion caseload, they usually do not advertise, and hence women may have difficulty finding out about and obtaining services from them. In 1992, 84% of all U.S. counties had no identified abortion provider, and 92% had none that performed 400 or more abortions. Thirty percent of women of reproductive age lived in the counties that had no provider and 41% lived in counties with no large provider. The number of counties with a provider declined from 714 in 1978 to 495 in 1992, a decrease of 31%.

In 1992, abortion services were provided by 2,380 facilities in the United States, a decline of 202 since 1988. The number of abortion providers declined by 18%, from a high of 2,908 in 1982. The loss of providers accelerated in the most recent survey period, from an average of 33 lost per year from 1985 to 1988, to an average of 51 per year from 1988 to 1992. Moreover, the loss in the latest period was greater than appears in these figures because in 1992 providers omitted from past surveys were identified through additional sampling procedures (Henshaw & Van Vort, 1994).

Wide state differences also are evident when other indicators of the availability of abortion services are examined. Of the country's 320 metropolitan areas,[3] 91 had no identified abortion provider and another 14 had providers who together performed fewer than 50 abortions in 1992; thus, 33% of metropolitan areas were underserved. These numbers have increased since 1988, when 70 metropolitan areas had no provider and 20 had providers who performed fewer than 50 abortions. The states with the most underserved metropolitan areas were Texas, with 13, and Indiana, Pennsylvania, and Wisconsin, each with 7. In 22 states, no more than 5 counties had a facility that reported at least 1 abortion in 1992, and in only 11 states did as many as half the counties have any abortion services. In 8 states, fewer than one third of women lived in a county with a provider. Several states experienced a distinct loss of providers since 1988. The greatest numerical losses occurred in California (which had a net loss of 54 providers), New York (16), Texas (12), North Carolina (11), and Florida (10). Large proportionate changes took place in several states in the middle of the country, including Indiana, Iowa, Kansas, Missouri, and Tennessee, which lost 20% to 40% of their providers. Since 1988, North Dakota has lost 2 of its 3 providers and joined South Dakota in having only one facility where women can find abortion services.

The scarcity of providers was much greater in nonmetropolitan than in metropolitan counties. Ninety-four percent of nonmetropolitan counties had no abortion services, and 85% of nonmetropolitan women lived in unserved counties. In 1992, only 23,000 abortions took place in nonmetropolitan counties, and this number has fallen sharply over time from 67,000 in 1979. Even among metropolitan counties, however, half had no services in 1992.

Types of Providers

Relatively few abortions were performed in hospitals in 1992. Table 2 presents the number and percentage of abortion providers and abortions for 1992. The 855 hospital providers accounted for 110,000 abortions, or 7% of the total. The proportion of abortions performed in hospitals has fallen steadily since 1973, when it was more than half (Henshaw & Van Vort, 1992). This decline in the number of hospital abortions has occurred because fewer abortions are performed at each hospital and fewer hospitals offer abortion services.

In 1992, only 16% of the country's short-term, general hospitals provided abortion services, down from 19% in 1988. Hospitals that offer abortion services tend to provide few abortions. Hospitals that allow abortions to be performed only when a woman's life or health is threatened by the

[3]The Office of Management and Budget defines a metropolitan area as a county containing a central city with a population of 50,000 or more along with any contiguous counties with close economic ties to the central county.

TABLE 2
Number and Percentage Distribution of Abortion Providers and Abortions, by Type of Facility, According to Caseload (1992)

Caseload[a]	Total		Hospitals		Abortion clinics		Other clinics		Physicians' offices	
	n	%	n	%	n	%	n	%	n	%
Providers	2,380	100	855	36	441	19	448	19	636	27
<30	699	29	439	18	0	0	45	2	215	9
30–390	926	39	351	15	13	1	141	6	421	18
400–990	282	12	45	2	68	3	169	7	na	na
1,000–4,990	428	18	18	1	318	13	92	4	na	na
≥5,000	45	2	2	++	42	2	1	++	na	na
Abortions	1,528,930	100	109,950	7	1,057,500	69	307,020	20	54,460	4
<30	6,480	++	3,390	++	0	0	510	++	2,580	++
30–390	111,970	7	35,170	2	2,740	++	22,180	1	51,880	3
400–990	183,970	12	26,640	2	49,610	3	107,720	7	na	na
1,000–4,990	877,430	57	30,840	2	679,980	44	166,610	11	na	na
≥5,000	349,080	23	13,910	1	325,170	21	10,000	1	na	na

Note. na = not applicable. Percentages may not add to 100 because of rounding.
[a] Caseloads are rounded to nearest 10.
+ Physicians' offices reporting 400 or more abortions a year are classified as clinics (either abortion clinics or "other clinics").
++ Fewer than 0.5%.

continuation of her pregnancy are counted as abortion providers even if only one abortion was performed. A majority (51%) of the hospitals that reported providing abortions performed fewer than 30 each; these facilities together accounted for only 3,000 of the procedures. Only 20 hospitals performed 1,000 or more. In 1992, only 10.8% of hospital abortions, or 0.8% of all abortions, were performed as inpatient procedures.

Most abortions are performed in the country's 441 abortion clinics, defined as nonhospital facilities in which half or more of patient visits are for abortion services. The largest of these clinics (those that reported 5,000 or more abortions in 1992) together provided 325,000 abortions, or 21% of all abortions performed during the year. Of all abortions, the proportion performed in abortion clinics had increased from 60% in 1985 to 64% in 1988 and 69% in 1992.

The category called "nonspecialized clinics" includes group practices with clinic names, surgical centers, health maintenance organizations, and other facilities with clinic names. In addition, physicians' offices were included as "other clinics" if they provided 400 or more abortions in 1992 and did not qualify as abortion clinics. There were as many of these facilities as there were abortion clinics, but they accounted for only 20% of all abortions.

The category of physicians' offices is made up of solo practitioners or group practitioners who performed fewer than 400 abortions per year. Together this group provided 4% of all reported abortions. Despite the underestimation that may occur because of the difficulty in identifying physicians who perform only a few abortions in their offices, it is clear that this group accounts for only a small percentage of all abortions.

The decline in the number of abortion providers since 1977 is substantial among both metropolitan and nonmetropolitan hospitals. In the most recent 4-year interval for which survey data are provided, 1988 to 1992, the total number of hospital providers fell by 185 (or 18%). The percentage drop was greatest among hospitals in nonmetropolitan counties where the number of providers fell from 427 in 1977 to 96 in 1992 (a 78% decrease), as compared with a 38% decline in metropolitan hospitals. The number of clinics and physicians' offices providing abortion services in nonmetropolitan areas also fell, from 145 in 1978 to 100 in 1992, although these types of facilities have held steady in metropolitan areas at slightly more than 1,400 since 1987.

IMPEDIMENTS TO SERVICE ACCESS

The decline in service availability negatively impacts women's ability to gain access to needed abortion services. At the same time, characteristics of the facilities that remain, together with the social context of women's lives, hinder access to services for women who choose to terminate a pregnancy. The extreme variation in abortion rates of state residents suggests that barriers to services affect the abortion rate. Abortion is semiurgent care because risk of complications increases with gestation. It becomes impossible if delayed too long, and most women who have chosen to terminate their pregnancies want to do so as early in gestation as possible. Yet, women seeking surgical abortion must cope with numerous barriers that are not typical of other types of semiurgent care. Although the impact of many of these barriers is impossible to quantify, with the present data set we can examine information on the percentage of women who travel long distances to obtain abortion services, the availability of services during the second trimester of pregnancy, the need to make more than one trip to the abortion facility, the amount that providers charge for abortion services, and the antiabortion harassment of abortion providers and their patients.

Distance

According to the estimates of abortion providers, 8% of women having abortions in nonhospital facilities travel more than 100 miles for abortion services, and an additional 16% travel 50 to 100 miles. The need to travel is greatest in the East South Central census division (Alabama, Kentucky, Mississippi, and Tennessee), where an estimated 15% of women having abortions in nonhospital facilities lived more than 100 miles from the provider and about 31% lived 50 to 100 miles away. Sixty-one percent of the women in this census division lived in a county with no abortion provider. Distances traveled were also higher in the other noncoastal census divisions except East North Central.

Where travel distances are shortest—in the Pacific and Mid-Atlantic census divisions—15% and 17%, respectively, of patients traveled 50 miles or more. The Mid-Atlantic states are dominated by large urban areas well supplied with abortion clinics, as is California, which dominates the Pacific census division. However, even in these states, 15% and 6%, respectively, of women lived in counties with no abortion provider.

The larger the facility, the higher the proportion of patients who traveled long distances for services. Among those providers reporting 1,000 or more abortions in 1992, 25% of patients traveled at least 50 miles, as compared with only 5% of patients of the smallest providers (fewer than 30 abortions in 1992). Women who need or prefer to go to a distant facility are probably more likely to go to large providers, which advertise more widely and are less expensive on average than are small providers.

Women may travel long distances not because their area lacks an abortion provider, but because they desire anonymity or are minors who want to avoid state parental involvement requirements (Cartoff & Klerman, 1986). If mandatory waiting periods are adopted by more states, travel to states without such restrictions will probably increase (Althaus & Henshaw, 1994). Other women may choose a distant provider to take advantage of lower fees or services such as general anesthesia that may not be available from small local providers.

Gestation Limits

Even if a woman seeking abortion services has located an abortion provider and secured transportation, there is a possibility that services will not be available to her from that provider if her pregnancy has passed the earliest gestational stages. The later in pregnancy an abortion is performed, the more complex the procedure and the greater the risk of complications. The maximum gestation age at which providers will perform abortions varies widely, depending on physicians' skills, preferences, and other factors. At 8 weeks from the start of the last menstrual period, 98% of facilities will provide services. Table 3 presents the percentage of abortion facilities performing procedures at 8 to 24 weeks of gestation for 1993. Many physicians, hospitals, and nonspecialized clinics provide services only during the first 12 weeks, often considered the dividing point between the first and second trimester of pregnancy. Abortion clinics are far more likely to

TABLE 3
Percentage of Abortion Facilities Performing Procedures at 8 to 24
Weeks of Gestation, by Type of Facility (1993)

Weeks of gestation	All[a] (N = 1,492)	Hospitals (n = 386)	Abortion clinics (n = 377)	Nonspecialized clinics (n = 326)	Physicians' offices (n = 403)
8	98	99	100	99	96
9	92	93	99	95	85
10	90	92	99	93	81
11	81	86	97	89	60
12	79	84	97	85	54
13	48	52	84	49	17
14	44	50	78	43	13
15	34	46	61	26	6
16	32	45	57	24	4
17	28	43	46	18	3
18	26	42	41	15	3
19	23	38	35	13	2
20	22	38	31	11	1
21	13	20	21	7	1
22	12	19	20	6	1
23	8	12	14	4	+
24	7	10	12	3	+

[a]Standardized to the actual percentage distribution of abortion providers to account for differences in response rates by type of provider.
+Less than 0.5%.

provide second-trimester abortions than other facilities. For instance, although only 17% of physicians provide abortions in their offices at 13 weeks of gestation and about half of hospitals and nonspecialty clinics provide such services, 84% of abortion clinics perform abortions at 13 weeks of gestation. Fewer than half (48%) of facilities overall provide services at 13 weeks, and the proportion declines rapidly beyond that point to 22% at 20 weeks and 7% at 24 weeks. Although abortions after 26 weeks of gestation are unrestricted in many states, they are rarely performed. Only three providers are known to perform abortions during the third trimester, and they accept patients past 26 weeks only under certain conditions such as known fetal abnormalities and severe medical complications (Kolata, 1992).

The larger a facility's abortion caseload, the later its maximum gestation limit is likely to be. For example, 57% of abortion clinics that performed 2,000 or more abortions in 1992 offered services at 17 weeks, compared with only 35% of those that reported fewer than 1,000 abortions.

Between the 1989 and 1993 surveys, the proportion of facilities that offered services in the second trimester increased, continuing a trend from earlier years. The increase was greatest at the highest gestations (Henshaw, 1995).[4]

Appointment Availability

How soon a woman is able to have an abortion depends not only on how long it takes her to locate a provider and on the provider's gestation limits, but also is affected by how often the facility is open and how long it takes to get an appointment. Nonhospital facilities were asked, "What is the average interval between the first telephone or walk-in contact with a woman and the procedure?" Most facilities reported short average periods between first contact and the abortion procedure. A period of 1 to 3 days was estimated by 33% of the facilities, 4 days by 17%, 5 to 6 days by 17%, 7 days by 18%, and more than 7 days by 14%.

Abortion clinics report much less time between first contact and the procedure than do other facilities. Periods of 1 week or more were indicated by 17% of abortion clinics, as compared with 43% of nonspecialized clinics and 35% of physicians' offices. Similarly, periods of 1 week or more were reported by 25% of clinics with 1992 abortion caseloads of 400 or more,

---

[4]In addition to maximum gestation limits, most providers set a minimum gestation before which they will not perform an abortion. This is because studies have found a higher rate of complications in very early procedures and because the small size of the embryo makes it difficult to be sure that the pregnancy has been ended. The most common requirement is 6 weeks since the last menstrual period, which is used by 43% of nonhospital facilities. Patients who come before the minimum are asked to return after enough time has elapsed. Later gestations are required by some facilities: 19% require 7 weeks and 5% 8 weeks, while 19% set their minimums at 5 weeks and 7% at 4 weeks.

as compared with 38% of smaller facilities. The period between first contact and the pregnancy termination is longer now than in 1981, when a survey of providers of 400 or more abortions indicated that only 11% typically needed 7 or more days (Henshaw, 1982), as compared with 25% in 1993.

A certain amount of delay is inevitable if facilities perform abortions only a few days a week, as is the case with many smaller providers. For example, a woman seeking services from a provider that performs abortions only 1 day a week might have to wait up to 6 days for an appointment if the facility always has appointment slots available, and longer if all the appointments are taken. Of all nonhospital providers, 11% perform abortions on only 1 day per week and 15% on only 2 days. Only a minority—38%—perform abortions 5 or more days each week. Physicians with small abortion practices are most likely to perform abortions any day of the week (51%), whereas nonspecialized clinics are most likely to offer the procedure on only 1 or 2 days (41%). Evidently the facilities most likely to perform abortions on only 1 or 2 days a week are those that are large enough to have specialized abortion sessions but small enough to need only one or two such sessions a week.

Once an appointment has been made, a woman is usually able to have her pregnancy terminated in one trip to the facility unless state laws require two visits (Althaus & Henshaw, 1994). Sixty percent of nonhospital providers said it is their usual procedure to perform first-trimester abortions on the woman's first visit, and all but 14% will provide services on one visit under some circumstances, for instance, if the woman would have to travel a long distance for a second visit (24%), if a delay would move her beyond maximum gestation limits or into a higher cost category (20%), or if she had already received counseling or preliminary evaluation from another source (19%).

The availability of abortion services during the first visit is highly dependent on the abortion caseload of the provider. Clinics where 2,000 or more abortions a year are performed almost all (91%) routinely provide services in one visit, whereas only 25% of facilities with the smallest caseloads do so. Because most women go to facilities with large caseloads, 86% of women having nonhospital abortions are able to obtain services in one visit if they choose to do so.

Costs

Although exact data are unavailable, abortion providers report that a large majority of abortions are paid for by the patients themselves rather than by insurance. There are several reasons for this self-payment. About one third of women have no employer-based insurance, and although some of the remaining third are covered by Medicaid, in most states Medicaid rarely pays for abortions. One third of insurance plans do not cover abortions or cover it only for certain medical indications (AGI, 1994). Women with insurance that covers abortion may not have met their deductible requirements, or they may not use their insurance because of concerns that confidentiality might be jeopardized by benefits statements sent to their homes, the need for someone else's signature, or reports sent to the employer. Therefore, cost can be a significant barrier for many women, particularly those who have low incomes, lack health insurance that covers abortion services, and desire to keep the abortion confidential. Cost may be a barrier for many adolescents who desire to conceal the abortion from family or friends.

The average nonhospital facility charged $341 for an abortion at 10 weeks with local anesthesia in 1992; the median fee was $298 and the range was $140 to $1,700. Clinics performing at least 400 abortions per year reported the lowest average charges ($287–$296), followed by facilities reporting 30 to 390 abortions ($391) and those performing even fewer ($463). Table 4 presents costs for nonhospital abortions, by weeks of gestation and facility caseload, for procedures at 10, 16, and 20 weeks. Because

TABLE 4
Charges for Nonhospital Abortion, by Weeks of Gestation and Facility Caseload for Procedures at 10, 16, and 20 Weeks, According to Type of Facility

Weeks of gestation and caseload[a]	Total	Abortion clinics	Non-specialized clinics	Physicians' offices
10 weeks				
<30	$463 (87)	na (0)	$404 (10)	$471 (77)
30–390	391 (299)	297 (13)	417 (67)	389 (219)
400–990	296 (174)	295 (60)	296 (114)	na
1,000–4,990	293 (335)	285 (251)	314 (84)	na
≥5,000	287 (19)	289 (18)	(1)[+]	na
Mean charge[b]	341 (914)	288 (342)	335 (276)	410 (296)
Median	298 (914)	276 (342)	297 (276)	353 (296)
Range	140–1,700	140–1,350	170–1,000	180–1,700
Mean amount paid[+]	296 (1,020)	289 (740)	310 (250)	365 (30)
16 weeks				
Mean charge[b]	$604 (304)	$577 (200)	$639 (76)	$700 (28)
Median	550 (304)	546 (200)	570 (76)	599 (28)
Range	275–2,500	275–1,900	300–2,500	350–2,500
20 weeks				
Mean charge[a]	$1,067 (159)	$1,014 (115)	$1,220 (36)	(8)[++]
Median	946 (159)	935 (115)	990 (36)	(8)[++]
Range	350–3,015	600–3,015	350–3,015	[++]

Note. na = not applicable.
[a]Caseloads are rounded to the nearest 10.
[b]Averaged over the number of facilities (shown in parentheses).
[+]Averaged over the number of abortions (shown in parentheses in thousands).
[++]Too few cases to report statistics.

most women go to the larger clinics with lower fees, the average patient paid about $296, excluding, of course, her other expenses such as travel and time missed from work and additional medical services that might be needed.

The average amount paid in 1993, $296, reflected an 18% increase from the average amount paid in 1989. This increase is much less than the 35% increase in the consumer price index for medical care over the same period and is about the same as the 17% rise in the consumer price index for all items. Prices increase sharply with gestation after about 12 weeks. At 16 weeks, the average charge was $604 and at 20 weeks it was $1,067 for nonhospital providers.

Charges in abortion clinics, which averaged $288 at 10 weeks, were distinctly lower than charges at other clinics ($335) or physicians' offices ($410), but the differences largely disappear when the volume of services is taken into account. At 16 and 20 weeks as well, the mean and median charges of physicians operating in their offices were higher than those of nonspecialized clinics, which in turn were higher than those of abortion clinics, but the differences may be attributable to variations in the volume of services. If one controls for number of abortions performed, the cost differential disappears.

Although no data were collected in 1993 on charges for abortion services in hospitals, the average hospital charged $1,757 for a first-trimester outpatient abortion in 1991 (Henshaw, 1991). These charges, which included the fees of the hospital, surgeon, and, where required, anesthesiologist, were about six times that of the average nonhospital facility. Because nonhospital facility charges have risen more slowly than the consumer price index for medical care, the average charge for a hospital abortion today is probably at least six times that of a nonhospital abortion in 1993 (Henshaw, 1995).

For women who seek abortions with general anesthesia, costs may be significantly higher. Relatively few nonhospital providers offer general anesthesia—only 33% of abortion clinics, 17% of other clinics, and 17% of physicians' offices. Sixty-three percent of facilities that offer general anesthesia charge extra for it. The extra charge varies according to provider type, averaging $114 at abortion clinics, $136 in other clinics, and $306 in physicians' offices.

Harassment

Another barrier facing many women seeking abortion services is harassment by antiabortion protestors, which also affects the ability of facilities to offer services. Providers were asked to indicate the number of times they had experienced various types of harassment during 1992. In all, 55% of nonhospital providers reported at least one type of harassment during

1992. Harassment was strongly associated with the abortion caseload; 86% of facilities that performed 400 or more abortions in 1992 reported some harassment, compared with only 29% of smaller providers. Harassment varied by region of the country, the Midwest reporting the highest level and the West the lowest. In the Midwest, 48% of the larger clinics (nonhospital providers of 400 or more abortions during 1992) experienced 4 or more types of harassment, compared with 22% of those in the West. The experience of larger providers is shown in Table 5. Picketing, the most common type of harassment, was reported by 83% of the larger providers (those performing 400 or more abortions in 1992). Demonstrations resulting in arrests were reported by 34% of these clinics, almost the same number that reported blockades (30%). When nonhospital providers were asked for a list of problems that had affected their ability to provide abortion services

TABLE 5
Percentage Distribution of Nonhospital Facilities Performing 400 or More Abortions in 1992, by Number of Incidents of Harassment Experienced and Percentage Experiencing any Incident by Year, According to Type of Harassment

Type	No. of incidents in 1992					Incidents		
	None	1–4	5–19	≥20	Total	1985	1988	1992
Picketing ($n = 514$)	17	11	10	62	100	80	81	83
Picketing with physical contact or blocking of patients ($n = 491$)	50	27	10	13	100	47	46	50
Vandalism ($n = 492$)	58	32	8	2	100	28	34	42
Demonstrations resulting in arrests ($n = 494$)	66	27	5	2	100	—	38	34
Stalking staff or patients ($n = 487$)	70	17	7	6	100	—	—	30
Blockades ($n = 489$)	70	23	5	2	100	—	—	30
Picketing homes of staff members ($n = 491$)	72	19	5	4	100	16	17	28
Tracing of patients' license plates ($n = 464$)	76	11	7	6	100	16	—	24
Bomb threats ($n = 490$)	76	21	2	1	100	48	36	24
Chemical attacks ($n = 490$)	88	12	0	0	100	—	—	12

Note. 1988 and 1992 percentages are weighted to adjust for nonresponses; ns are unweighted. Dashes indicate that question was not asked.

during the previous 12 months, 30% cited conditions directly associated with harassment as their most important problem, and an additional 11% mentioned physician shortage and other staffing problems that may have been indirectly related to harassment. More detailed information on harassment and its effect on women seeking abortion is provided by Cozzerelli and Majors (chap. 4, this volume).

RECOMMENDATIONS AND CONCLUSION

The latest data indicate that abortion levels, whether measured by the rate per 1,000 women of reproductive age or the ratio of abortions to pregnancies, have decreased slowly but persistently since the early 1980s (30.0 per 100 pregnancies in 1982 vs. 25.9 per 100 pregnancies in 1992). The cause of most of the decline is not clear, but one important reason appears to be the decreasing availability of abortion providers. The declining number of providers suggests that services are becoming more difficult to obtain, especially for women living in nonmetropolitan areas, in smaller cities, and in the Midwest.

Decreases in the numbers of providers have been especially steep for hospitals. The most important reason for this change is the relatively high cost of hospital abortion services (Henshaw, 1991). Changes in hospital policies in response to pressure from antiabortion elements may also be a factor. Even where nonhospital services are available, however, the presence of hospital abortion services is vitally important to the minority of women whose health status requires overnight postoperative observation or emergency equipment that only a hospital can provide. Abortion services in hospitals also are important as backup for clinics and for training residents in obstetrics and gynecology in performing abortions. On February 14, 1995, The Accreditation Committee for Graduate Medical Education released a policy change that requires residents in obstetrics and gynecology to learn abortion procedures during their hospital training. If hospitals do not provide the service, it is unclear where residents will be trained.

The reduction in the number of providers has been accompanied by increasing concentration of services in specialized abortion clinics, where 69% of abortions are now performed. Thus, abortion services are becoming even more isolated from the mainstream of medical care, making the physicians who provide them vulnerable to stigmatization within both the medical profession and the general community. Although abortion services that are organizationally separate from other medical care may offer a number of benefits including greater confidentiality, lower cost, and expertise that result from high volume, services should also be available in the same facilities as other gynecological care. Coordinated and comprehensive health care for women demands that abortion be treated like any other semiurgent care.

Unlike other kinds of semiurgent medical and surgical care, however, women seeking abortions must cope with numerous barriers, ranging from having to travel great distances to a provider to having to pass through lines of demonstrators. This chapter presents information on some of the key barriers to women's access but is not meant to cover all difficulties women face in obtaining abortions or that providers face in making services available. Wilcox, Robbenolt, and O'Keeffe discuss legislative barriers to abortion in chapter 1 of this volume, and as previously mentioned, Cozzerelli and Major examine the impact of harassment on women seeking abortions in chapter 4. Therefore, these issues are only briefly mentioned here.

In some ways and for some women, the abortion service system provides efficient and, judging from the low mortality and morbidity rates, high-quality care. Women who live in large urban areas and have the necessary financial resources can usually obtain abortion services in a single visit without a long wait for an appointment.

Many women who have unintended pregnancies, however, have low incomes and no health insurance that covers abortion services. For these women, the average charge of $296 for first-trimester nonhospital abortion services may be a significant barrier. Women living at the poverty level or in limited financial circumstances also are disproportionately likely to be ethnic minorities. Although the poverty rate for the total United States in 1993 was 15.1%, 33.1% of African Americans and 30.6% of Hispanics lived below the poverty level (U.S. Bureau of the Census, 1995, Table 744).

Nonfinancial obstacles affect some women of all income levels, although those with few financial resources may have the most difficulty overcoming them. Distance from a provider is often a problem, especially for women who need second-trimester services. Evidence of an increasing provider shortage may be seen in the increase over the past 10 years in the average time between a woman's first contact with a provider and the day the abortion is performed. Fourteen percent of nonhospital providers cite an average delay of more than 1 week.[5]

Harassment of women and providers, always a problem, has become more widespread. The increase in the proportion of clinics subject to frequent picketing suggests that more people than ever are engaged in the most common antiabortion activity. It is in this context of gradually es-

---

[5]These data were collected before a 24-hour waiting period was in effect in any state except Mississippi. As of April, 1996, 24-hour mandatory delay laws were being enforced in eight states—Louisiana, Mississippi, Nebraska, North Dakota, Ohio, Pennsylvania, South Dakota, and Utah—an 8-hour-delay law was in effect in Kansas and a 1-hour-delay law was in effect in South Carolina.

calating violence that the fatal shootings of two physicians and a clinic escort should be viewed.

Legislation and government regulation have created additional barriers for both women and providers. The exclusion of abortion from Medicaid coverage in most states is perhaps the most severe legislative restriction now in effect (National Abortion and Reproductive Rights Action League Foundation, 1998). Laws requiring two clinic visits would cause delay for most women, often of more than 1 day. At present, services are commonly provided in one clinic visit, and almost all women who travel long distances for abortion services or have other reasons to need immediate care can have their pregnancies terminated in a single visit (National Center for Health Statistics, 1993). Because a majority of providers do not perform abortions every day of the week, the need for two visits can easily cause a delay of more than 1 day.

Many of the difficulties in accessing and providing abortion services would disappear if abortion were integrated with other health care for women, but this cannot happen as long as opposition to abortion is widespread. Alternatively, availability of medical methods of early abortion, such as mifepristone in combination with a prostaglandin, has the potential to change both the numbers and types of abortion providers and to reduce some of the barriers. For example, early gestational limits might be dropped and an emphasis placed on women's coming to a provider as early in pregnancy as possible. If abortion services become available in more locations, distances and waiting times for services would be reduced.

Medical abortion, however, will not solve all the problems of access. The method can be used only at very early gestations, surgical backup facilities are needed, charges are likely to be at least as high for surgical abortion, two or more physician visits will be required, and antiabortion harassment will still be possible in many cases. Legal restrictions on abortion will remain, regardless of changes in abortion technology.

As new contraceptive technologies become available and women learn to be more effective contraceptors, the abortion rates in the United States should decrease. Until this happens, it is essential that those working on women's health issues devote special effort to making high-quality abortion services available to all women who wish to terminate an unwanted pregnancy, especially rural residents, teenagers, women with few economic resources, and women of color, who because of their disadvantaged status in American society, have difficulties accessing services.

REFERENCES

Alan Guttmacher Institute. (1994). *Uneven and unequal: Insurance coverage and reproductive health services.* New York: Author.

Althaus, F. A., & Henshaw, S. K. (1994). The effects of mandatory delay laws on abortion patients and providers. *Family Planning Perspectives, 26,* 228–231, 233.

Cartoof, V. G., & Klerman, L. V. (1986). Parental consent for abortion: Impact of the Massachusetts law. *American Journal of Public Health, 76,* 397–400.

Grimes, D. A. (1991). *Who will provide abortions?* Washington, DC: National Abortion Federation.

Henshaw, S. K. (1982). Freestanding abortion clinics: Services, structure, fees. *Family Planning Perspectives, 14,* 248–256.

Henshaw, S. K. (1990). Induced abortion: A world review. *Family Planning Perspectives, 22,* 76–79.

Henshaw, S. K. (1991). The accessibility of abortion services in the United States. *Family Planning Perspectives, 23,* 246–253.

Henshaw, S. K. (1995). Factors hindering access to abortion services. *Family Planning Perspectives, 27,* 54–59, 87.

Henshaw, S. K., Koonin, L. M., & Smith, J. C. (1987). Characteristics of U.S. women having abortions. *Family Planning Perspectives, 23,* 75–81.

Henshaw, S. K., & Van Vort, J. (1992). *Abortion factbook, 1992 edition: Reading, trends, and state and local data to 1988.* New York: The Alan Guttmacher Institute.

Henshaw, S. K., & Van Vort, J. (1994). Abortion services in the United States. *Family Planning Perspectives, 26,* 100–106, 112.

Kolata, G. (1992, Jan. 5). In late abortions, decisions are painful and options few. *The New York Times,* p. 1.

National Abortion and Reproductive Rights Action League Foundation. (1998). *A state-by-state review of abortion and reproductive rights.* Washington, DC: Author.

National Center for Health Statistics. (1983). Advance report of final natality statistics. *Monthly Vital Statistics Report* (Vol., 32, No. 9, Suppl., Table 15). Washington, DC: U.S. Government Printing Office.

National Center for Health Statistics. (1990). Advance report of final natality statistics, 1988. *Monthly Vital Statistics Report* (Vol. 39, No. 4, Supplement 1990, Table 18). Washington, DC: U.S. Government Printing Office.

National Center for Health Statistics. (1993). Advance report of final natality statistics, 1991. *Monthly Vital Statistics Report* (Vol. 42, No. 3, Suppl., Table 16). Washington, DC: U.S. Government Printing Office.

U.S. Bureau of the Census. (1995). *Statistical abstract of the United States: 1995.* (115th ed.). Washington, DC: U.S. Government Printing Office.

4

THE IMPACT OF ANTIABORTION ACTIVITIES ON WOMEN SEEKING ABORTIONS

CATHERINE COZZARELLI AND BRENDA MAJOR

In the minds of many Americans, the issue of abortion has become inextricably linked with images of fervent antiabortion or "pro-life" demonstrations. Indeed, through the media, we are treated to a steady diet of chanting picketers, blockaded clinics, and even murder. Such images serve continually to remind us that abortion is a divisive issue, one that engenders violent moral debate and deeply ambivalent feelings for many Americans. Nevertheless, despite the whirlwind of controversy that surrounds the availability of abortion, large numbers of American women continue to have abortions. According to the Alan Guttmacher Institute (AGI), 1,529,000 abortions were performed in 1992 (Henshaw & Van Vort, 1994). Thus, many women are having abortions in a historical context that includes national awareness of antiabortion sentiments and the possibility of personally encountering antiabortion demonstrators. It is therefore vitally

Preparation of this chapter was supported by National Institute of Mental Health Grant 5R01MH47989. We thank the staffs of Buffalo GYN Womenservices Clinic, Erie Medical Center, and Shalom Press. Without their help and goodwill, the data we have collected on antiabortion picketing could not have been gathered.

important to understand the impact of antiabortion activities on women seeking to obtain an abortion. Such impact could take many forms. A woman could decide not to have an abortion, knowing that her local clinic is likely to be picketed. Or, it may be difficult for a woman to locate a doctor still willing to perform abortions in these contentious times. If she does obtain an abortion, a woman may suffer negative postabortion psychological outcomes as a result of encounters with intense antiabortion demonstrations on her way into the abortion clinic. The purpose of this chapter is to explore some of the many pathways by which antiabortion activities can affect women seeking an abortion. Unfortunately, the empirical literature (especially in psychology) has had little to say about this issue. Thus, in many places, our analysis is, of necessity, speculative. However, in discussing the psychological effects of antiabortion activities on women who do obtain an abortion, we rely on conclusions drawn from data we have collected.

SCOPE OF PICKETING ACTIVITIES

What is the nature and scope of antiabortion activities currently directed against U.S. abortion providers, and have these activities changed from the 1970s to the present? Although precise estimates of these phenomena are difficult to obtain, the most complete documentation of antiabortion activities has been conducted by AGI and the National Abortion Federation (NAF). Both of these organizations receive their information directly from facilities that provide abortions. Data from both AGI and NAF (as cited in Blanchard, 1994) suggest that antiabortion activity is widespread and persistent and that the preferred modes of expressing antiabortion sentiments have changed somewhat over time.

The earliest antiabortion organizations were created in the 1960s in response to campaigns seeking to liberalize state abortion laws (Blanchard, 1994; Luker, 1984). The individuals involved in these organizations were typically professionals (e.g., physicians and social workers) who were personally involved in the abortion issue. Because of the need to maintain professional decorum, early expressions of antiabortion sentiment were typically peaceful, polite, and devoid of intensive activism. In the 1960s and 1970s, national antiabortion organizations (e.g., National Right to Life Committee and Committee on Family Life) began to arise. Initially, these organizations relied on lobbying, political pressure, and threatened boycotts in attempting to achieve their aims (Blanchard, 1994). Thus, for example, there were no bombings of abortion clinics prior to 1977. However, with the failure of such relatively peaceful tactics to secure major reversals in the trend toward liberalization of abortion laws, more radical organizations (e.g., Pro-Life Direct Action League and Pro-Life Action Network) began to surface in the late 1970s and early 1980s. These organizations initiated now commonplace activities such as the extensive picketing of abortion clinics and attempts to convince women trying to enter such clinics not to go through with their abortions.

In the early 1980s, major shifts toward increasing levels of violence in the expression of antiabortion sentiments took place. In its 1985 survey of all known abortion providers in the U.S., AGI included several questions designed to assess the extent to which facilities that provide abortions had been subjected to antiabortion activities. The results of this survey revealed that although no type of abortion provider was exempt from antiabortion activity, large, nonhospital facilities that provided more than 400 abortions per year (e.g., abortion clinics) were especially likely to be subjected to antiabortion harassment. Eighty-eight percent of these facilities reported that they had experienced at least one form of antiabortion activity in 1985 and 82% said they had been subjected to multiple forms of harassment (Forrest & Henshaw, 1987). Picketing was most commonly reported, but almost half of the large, nonhospital facilities that responded to this survey also reported experiencing a wide array of antiabortion activities including bomb threats, clinic blockades, jamming of telephone lines, invasion of the facility, and distribution of antiabortion literature. In addition, 19% of these facilities reported that their staff members had received death threats and 16% reported picketing of staff members' homes. Typically, most antiabortion activities were not experienced as single episodes but were part of on-going pressure directed at either the facility or its staff.

Data collected by NAF corroborate the results of the AGI survey and point to the early to mid-1980s as a peak in some forms of violent antiabortion activity. For example, according to NAF statistics (reported in Blanchard, 1994), the largest numbers of arsons and bombings were reported in 1984 and 1985 (30 and 22, respectively). These were also the years with the highest numbers of reported death threats. Blanchard has hypothesized that the peak of violence in the mid-1980s was a byproduct of increased frustration resulting from unrealized hopes that a Reagan presidency would ensure legal victories for the antiabortion movement.

In the late 1980s, bombings and arson became less frequent (see Blanchard, 1994; Henshaw, 1991), but other forms of antiabortion activism increased. The year 1987 saw the formation of Operation Rescue and the initiation of large-scale clinic blockades. In 1987, two clinic blockades were reported to NAF, whereas in 1988, the number rose to 182. In response to the initiation of clinic blockades by Operation Rescue and other groups, AGI added an item to the 1988 survey of abortion providers to assess whether providers had experienced antiabortion demonstrations with resulting arrests. Thirty-eight percent of the large abortion facilities responding to the survey reported such demonstrations.

According to the results of the most recent AGI survey (Henshaw, 1995; Henshaw & Van Vort, 1994), 86% of large, nonhospital abortion facilities were subjected to antiabortion activities in 1992. This percentage is almost identical to those obtained in earlier surveys. Picketing remained the most commonly reported form of such activities; 83% of larger providers reported being picketed, in many cases, quite regularly. In addition, from 1988 to 1992, the proportion of large providers that experienced vandalism, tracing of patients' license plates, and picketing at the homes of staff members increased. Some providers also experienced two relatively new forms of harassment: stalking of clinic staff or patients (30% of facilities) and chemical attacks, usually involving butyric acid (12%). Butyric acid is a foul-smelling chemical that when sprayed into clinics has the effect of forcing a temporary suspension of activities and, in some cases, causing illness. Eighty such chemical attacks were reported in 1992. Finally, the number of demonstrations with attendant arrests decreased slightly from 1988 to 1992, as did reports of bomb threats (48% of clinics in 1985 to 24% in 1992).

Thus, in the early 1990s, antiabortion activism was common and affected a large proportion of women seeking to obtain abortions. In addition to vandalism, picketing, chemical attacks, and stalkings, in the early 1990s several individuals who were affiliated with the provision of abortion services were shot or killed. Blanchard (1994) hypothesized that the 1993 murder of Dr. David Gunn and the shooting of Dr. George Tiller reflected rising frustration among antiabortion activists in response to the election of William J. Clinton as U.S. president. President Clinton made it clear that he opposed severe restrictions on abortion and early in his term reversed some of the limitations on abortion that had been imposed during the Reagan presidency.

In 1994, President Clinton signed into law legislation that makes it a federal crime to use force or the threat of force to intimidate either clinic workers or women entering abortion clinics (see Wilcox, Robbennolt, & O'Keeffe, chap. 1, this volume). Although there have been some reports that this legislation has decreased the intensity of antiabortion protests (e.g., Serrano, 1996), future research will be needed to support or refute these claims.

WHO IS LIKELY TO TAKE PART IN ANTIABORTION ACTIVITIES?

First, it must be noted that antiabortion activists have always been a diverse group, and not everyone joins antiabortion organizations for similar reasons. Some join on the basis of a personal philosophy of life that is incompatible with abortion, whereas others become active because abortion is one manifestation of a general pro-life position that also includes concern about issues such as the death penalty (Blanchard, 1994). Some women join the antiabortion movement because they had an abortion that they later regretted or because they experienced other negative reproduction-related events. For example, in her study of antiabortion activists, Luker (1984) found that one third of those she interviewed decided to become active in the antiabortion movement because of a problem related to parenthood such as an inability to conceive, a miscarriage, a newborn lost to congenital disease, or an older child lost to illness. In many cases, these individuals had already held antiabortion attitudes, but the experience of these reproduction-related losses transformed the abstract into the deeply personal and galvanized them into action.

Although the reasons for joining antiabortion organizations are varied, researchers have noted some trends in the types of individuals most likely to become involved with such groups. As was mentioned, the earliest antiabortion activists were predominantly professionals who objected to the liberalization of abortion laws. As such liberalization came to pass, however, concern about the abortion issue spread to nonprofessionals (e.g., housewives and blue collar workers) who actively sought out and joined antiabortion organizations. These individuals were often operating from a basis of personal religious beliefs and strongly objected to the logic that embryos did not yet represent fully developed persons with constitutionally protected rights. The organizations they joined were primarily Catholic (Blanchard, 1994). Beginning in the 1980s, however, Protestant evangelicals began to become active in larger numbers, and the tenor of the antiabortion movement shifted toward the overarching conservative views of the New Right (Guth, Smidt, Kellstedt, & Green, 1993).

Historically, one of the strongest motivations for joining activist antiabortion organizations has been a belief in cultural fundamentalism, a central feature of many fundamentalist religious orientations (Blanchard, 1994). *Cultural fundamentalism* is defined as a strong desire to return to a more "traditional" culture, in which men are dominant and women subservient, and in which sexual liberation and deviant lifestyles are strongly rejected. The majority of the antiabortion activists interviewed by Luker (1984) felt that men and women naturally excel in different spheres and that women's talents are best suited for a focus on husband, home, and children. Given these beliefs, it is not surprising that the women in Luker's antiabortion sample were less educated, less likely to work in the paid labor force, more likely to be housewives, less likely to be divorced, and more likely to be or have been married and to have children than the women in her pro-choice sample (see also Guth et al., 1993).

Although the various fundamentalist sects differ in the precise nature of their religious beliefs, all of these groups share, to some extent, an ideology that reflects core tenets of cultural fundamentalism: a dislike of ambiguity, a strong belief in the rights of the individual, patriotic American-ism, the acceptance and endorsement of paternalism, a fervent belief in Capitalism, anti-intellectualism, and a commitment to the traditional fam-ily structure (Blanchard, 1994; Petchesky, 1984). Although the connec-tions between some of these ideologies may not be readily apparent, Pet-chesky (1984) argued that antiabortion attitudes and conservative views on social policy are cut from the same cloth. From her perspective, the efforts of the New Right to dismantle social welfare (including funding for abortion, welfare, busing, Medicaid, Occupational Safety and Health Ad-ministration, etc.) are primarily targeted at women, minorities, and the poor, and are intended both to maintain the established power structure and to punish women who try to function outside the bounds of the tra-ditional family. Thus, in a general sense, the common perceptions that many antiabortion activists are antagonistic toward women's liberation and a woman's right to control her reproductive history are compatible with cultural fundamentalist beliefs (see also Cook, Jelen, & Wilcox, 1992; Himmelstein, 1986).[1]

THE EFFECTS OF ANTIABORTION ACTIVITIES ON PROVIDERS

Antiabortion activities might indirectly impact women seeking abor-tions by making it less likely that these women will be able to obtain an abortion, even though it is their legal right to do so. Such a scenario could result from the effects of antiabortion activities on the number of physi-cians who are willing to provide abortions, the increasing difficulty abortion clinics might encounter in attempting to hire competent medical and counseling staff, and the rising cost of providing abortions in the face of threats to the security of abortion clinics and staff. Do antiabortion activ-ities have such effects? Little research has examined this issue directly. The 1993 AGI survey included a question asking providers to list, in order of importance, the factors that had most affected their ability to provide abor-tions in the previous 12 months. Abortion providers who responded to this item saw antiabortion harassment as the single most important factor af-fecting their ability to provide services (Henshaw, 1995). Overall, 30% cited conditions directly associated with antiabortion activities as their most pressing problem: Commonly mentioned activities included picketing (8%), demonstrations and blockades (5%), and vandalism and other direct action (8%). In addition, 11% mentioned problems that might be indi-

---

[1]One very extreme expression of cultural fundamentalism is reflected in the tenets of Christian Reconstructionism (to which Randall Terry of Operation Rescue subscribes). Christian Reconstructionists endorse replacing our currently democratic society with one based on the bible. In a society run by "God's laws," the church would wield ultimate power over nearly every aspect of daily life, and the punishment for many forms of morally "deviant" behavior would be death (Blanchard, 1994).

rectly related to antiabortion activities, such as difficulty in securing physicians or other clinic staff.

Other, more indirect evidence suggests that antiabortion activities might make it more difficult for facilities to provide abortions by increasing the cost of keeping clinics open in the face of escalating antiabortion protests. For example, during 1982 to 1985, bombings and fires at abortion clinics resulted in more than $2 million worth of damage (Donovan, 1985) and almost certainly translated into increased costs for the affected clinics. Similarly, according to Forrest and Henshaw (1987), large, nonhospital facilities that experienced antiabortion activity (beyond picketing) in 1985 were also more likely to experience a host of service-related problems. For example, experiencing harassment was significantly related to higher security costs, higher legal costs, increased security personnel, difficulty in hiring staff, and the revocation of fire or casualty insurance. In particular, providers that reported increased difficulty in hiring staff were more likely to have experienced clinic blockades, loud demonstrations, bomb threats, mass scheduling of no-show appointments, and tracing of license plates.

The large-scale demonstrations and clinic blockades organized by groups such as Operation Rescue beginning in the late 1980s resulted in increased costs not only for the affected clinics but also for the communities in which these activities occurred. For example, in the summer of 1991, Operation Rescue orchestrated a 46-day protest in Wichita, Kansas, that drew over 25,000 individuals against abortion from across the country. Three abortion clinics were closed down for a week and more than 3,000 arrests were made (Hull, 1991). The six weeks of activity cost taxpayers a total of $846,447 (Forero & Linstedt, 1992). In April 1992, Operation Rescue began a similar campaign to stop abortions by blockading clinics in Buffalo, New York. Unlike the earlier demonstration in Wichita, the blockades in Buffalo were unsuccessful: The clinics remained open and women seeking abortions were able to keep their appointments. Even so, 615 people were arrested, and police officials estimated that the demonstrations cost the financially struggling Erie County more than $500,000 in overtime police pay and other costs (Wallin, 1992).

The above-mentioned statistics imply that it has become financially more costly to provide abortions, and common sense would suggest that increases in violent antiabortion activities such as stalkings and murder could have a dampening effect on the number of physicians and facilities that are willing to provide abortions. Even if not exposed to extreme forms of antiabortion violence, clinic personnel may simply tire of dealing with persistent, low-level harassment. Consonant with these suggestions, the number of facilities providing abortions nationally has been decreasing at a rate of about 65 facilities per year since 1988 (Henshaw & Van Vort, 1994). The overall number of providers dropped 8% between 1988 and 1992 and 18% between 1982 and 1992. In addition, the number of women who obtained abortions in 1992 was the lowest since 1979 (Henshaw & Van Vort, 1994). It is difficult, however, to determine the precise magnitude of the impact of antiabortion activities on these numbers. Most likely, these decreases reflect the combination of antiabortion activities and other barriers to obtaining an abortion (e.g., the refusal of many states to allow Medicaid to pay for an abortion, the passage of laws requiring minors to obtain parental consent, and mandated waiting periods). A precise estimate of the extent to which antiabortion activities have resulted in fewer abortions being performed would, at a minimum, require information from providers who cease conducting abortions. It is likely that reliable information of this type would be difficult to obtain.

THE DIRECT EFFECTS OF ANTIABORTION ACTIVITIES ON WOMEN SEEKING ABORTIONS

Effects on the Decision to Abort

It is possible that antiabortion activities may persuade some women not to have an abortion. This is certainly the hope and in many cases the claim of individuals who are actively opposed to abortion (e.g., Reardon, 1987; Scheidler, 1985). Whether this claim is true is extremely difficult to evaluate, as most women decide whether to seek an abortion in the privacy of their own homes. Nevertheless, it is possible that awareness of the arguments and activities of antiabortion activists may result in some women deciding not to obtain an abortion but rather to carry their pregnancies to term. Alternatively, the activities of antiabortion activists may have the effect of making the abortion decision more difficult or prolonged for some women. Given that a more difficult or conflicted decision about whether to obtain an abortion leads to poorer postabortion adjustment (Major & Cozzarelli, 1992), such a delay could have potentially negative consequences for women who eventually decide to abort.

It is also possible that some women change their minds about obtaining an abortion after confronting demonstrators outside an abortion clinic. An empirical study by Cozzarelli and Major (1994), however, suggests that this response is rare. In this study, objective coders stationed outside a Buffalo abortion clinic reported that nearly all of the women observed approaching the clinic were confronted by antiabortion demonstrators. Despite this, not a single woman (out of approximately 400) was observed to turn back after being approached by these demonstrators. Whether this finding is generalizeable to other settings is difficult to assess, but it does suggest that antiabortion demonstrators may not have a strong influence over a woman's abortion decision by the time she arrives at an abortion clinic.

The Psychological Effects of Antiabortion Demonstrators

Although most women may decide to go through with an abortion after encountering antiabortion demonstrators as they enter a picketed clinic, it is quite possible that contact with these activists might have an impact on their preabortion affective state, postabortion adjustment, or both. Next, we discuss several aspects of this issue. Throughout this discussion, we refer to data we collected several years ago as part of an investigation of the psychological effects of antiabortion demonstration on women obtaining an abortion.

Some of the analyses we conducted on these data also were presented in Cozzarelli and Major (1994). However, we present the results of additional analyses that have not been previously published. To facilitate a smoother discussion of these data, we first present a brief description of the methodology of this study. The results of various analyses are described where they are relevant to the discussion.

The data for this study were collected in 1990 at a large, private abortion clinic in Buffalo, New York, where approximately 30 first-trimester suction abortions are performed each week. On each day the study was conducted, a research assistant stationed outside the clinic rated several aspects of antiabortion demonstrator and pro-choice escort activity for each 15-minute interval in which she was present. Specifically, these "coders" provided a count of the number of antiabortion demonstrators outside the clinic and rated the intensity of their activity. (Intensity was operationalized as the average of scores on two 7-point scales, one reflecting the general activity level of the demonstrators and the other, demonstrators' level of verbal aggressiveness.) The coders also counted the number of pro-choice escorts that were present and rated the escorts' general activity level (on a 7-point scale).

In addition, all English speaking women seeking a first-trimester abortion at the clinic were asked to participate in our study; 88% agreed to do so. After excluding women who did not complete our questionnaires (typically because they were judged ineligible for a first-trimester abortion by the clinic staff), our final sample was 291 women. This group was predominantly young (M = 23.3 years), Catholic (45%) or Protestant (44%), White (66%), single (75%), had obtained at least a high school diploma (71%), and had no prior abortions (59%). Participants were asked whether they had seen antiabortion demonstrators and, if they had, whether these demonstrators had spoken to them or tried to block their access to the clinic (using a yes–no response format). Women were also asked the degree to which they had been upset by the demonstrators (on a scale ranging from 1 [*they did not upset me at all*] to 5 [*they upset me a great deal*]). Thirty minutes after her abortion and just before she left the clinic, each woman's level of depression was assessed using the SCL-90 Depression subscale

(Derogatis, 1983), a well-known and frequently used measure of state depression. Finally, the receptionist at the clinic recorded each woman's time of arrival; thus, we were able to link each participant in our study with a coder's objective report of demonstrator activity during the 15-minute period when she arrived.

Women's Preabortion Responses to Antiabortion Demonstration

To date, very few empirical studies have included questions asking women entering abortion clinics whether they were approached by antiabortion demonstrators or how they felt about this contact. The few studies that have included such questions, however, suggest that a large number of women do encounter protesters and that for the majority of these women, such contact is perceived as negative. In this study, objective coders stationed outside an abortion clinic reported that 96% of the women who attempted to enter the clinic during the 3 months in which this study was being conducted encountered antiabortion demonstrators. The number of demonstrators present ranged from 0 to 43 (M = 11.55), and on average, their activity level was coded as moderate (M = 3.02, on a 7-point scale). In addition, 71% of the women participating in the study who encountered such demonstrators said the demonstrators spoke to them, and 54% reported that the demonstrators tried to stop them from entering the clinic. On average, women reported being moderately upset by the demonstrators (M = 2.68, where a 5 indicates the greatest degree of upset). Sixty-six percent of the women reported being upset to some degree, and 34% of the women said they were not at all upset by the demonstrators.[2]

We recently completed the data collection for a 2-year longitudinal study of the psychosocial predictors of adjustment to abortion (see Major, Richards, Cooper, Cozzarelli, & Zubek, 1998; Major, Zubek, Cooper, Cozzarelli, & Richards, 1997, for more information on these data). Although this study was designed to explore a wide range of issues, we included several items that addressed various aspects of antiabortion activities. Of 615 women who obtained an abortion at one of three facilities in Buffalo, New York, during a 6-month period in 1993, 537 (or 87.7%) reported that they had seen antiabortion demonstrators when they entered the clinic; 76.5% of these women said that the demonstrators had spoken to them, and 42.2% reported that the demonstrators had tried to keep them from entering the clinic. Women who reported having seen antiabortion demonstrators were also asked the extent to which the demonstrators had "made them feel like" each of 12 different descriptors of emotional states (e.g., mad, confused, happy, sad, or like they had done the wrong thing).

---

[2]We also found that being older, $r(254) = .11$, $p < .08$, White rather than Black, $r(255) = 1.25$, $p < .01$, and married rather than single, $r(252) = -.20$, $p < .01$, were related to being more upset by the antiabortion demonstrators.

Responses to these items could range from 1 (*not at all*) to 5 (*a great deal*). The results of a factor analysis of these items suggested that women's emotional responses fell into two broad categories that we labeled *guilt* (tense, afraid, guilty, did the wrong thing, confused, sad, ashamed [coefficient alpha equal to .91]) and *anger* (mad, angry, determined [coefficient alpha equal to .83]). Two items (happy and strong) did not load on either factor. Inspection of the mean scores on the two scales derived from the factor analysis, and the two remaining items revealed that, on average, women reported the highest level of anger (M = 2.63), followed by guilt (M = 2.00) and feelings of strength (M = 1.95). On average, women did not report feeling at all happy (M = 1.12) after encountering antiabortion picketers.

Finally, Nasman (1992) conducted a survey of 142 women obtaining an abortion and 51 friends or other individuals who accompanied these women to an abortion clinic in Dayton, Ohio. All women who entered the clinic were asked to participate in the study by a receptionist, and the women who agreed were demographically similar to the general population of women who obtained abortions at this facility. Seventy-five percent of Nasman's sample completed a series of items pertaining to antiabortion activities. Fifty-nine percent of these respondents reported that they had seen antiabortion protesters outside the clinic, and 47% said they had asked the protesters to leave them alone; 62% specified that the protesters had failed to respect that request. Seventy-five percent of respondents said the demonstrators in some way made direct contact with them (e.g., by speaking directly to them, handing them literature, etc.). In addition, 81% said the protesters should mind their own business, 82% said the protesters were invading their privacy, and 35% said the protesters wished to challenge their religious freedom. However, not all women felt that the motivations or actions of the protesters were completely negative. Fifteen percent of the women in this study felt that the protesters were trying to help women, 12% believed the protesters were sincerely respectful and concerned about their life, and 1% said they were sincerely interested in what the protesters had to say.

In sum, the combined results of these studies suggest that women most frequently respond to antiabortion demonstrators with feelings of anger or the conviction that protesters are intruding on a private matter. Responses indicative of upset or other negative affective responses such as guilt, confusion, and anxiety appear to be only slightly less common. A minority of women believed the demonstrators had their interests at heart or were guided by positive motivations, but very few reported being happy in response to encounters with these activists. Of course, the extent to which these patterns can confidently be said to generalize across large numbers of women cannot be determined until more data have been collected. Thus, these conclusions must be considered tentative.

The Effects of Antiabortion Activities on Women's Postabortion Adjustment

Does exposure to antiabortion demonstrators have a detrimental effect on women's postabortion adjustment? Anecdotal evidence suggests that this may indeed be the case. For example, on the basis of observations at abortion clinics, Hern (1991) asserted that some women show obvious signs of physical distress (including sweating, palpitations, anger, crying, or hyperventilation) after encountering antiabortion demonstrators. Our own observations made during the process of collecting data at abortion clinics are consistent with Hern's. It is plausible to hypothesize that women who are more agitated prior to their abortions may be at increased risk for problems both during and after the abortion procedure.

There are also theoretical reasons to predict that antiabortion demonstrators may have a negative impact on women's postabortion adjustment. Specifically, the encounters that many women have with demonstrators are consistent with the social psychological definition of negative social interactions (interactions that are affectively unpleasant, conflictive, interfering or hostile; Ruehlman & Karoly, 1991). Research has suggested that negative social interactions may serve as direct sources of stress and can result in depression, anxiety, physical symptoms, and reduced quality of life (e.g., Fiore, Becker, & Coppel, 1983; Rook 1984; Ruehlman & Wolchik, 1988). In addition, the combination of high life stress and negative social interactions is thought to strain an individual's coping abilities and precipitate even greater distress than would negative social interactions alone (Coyne, Wortman, & Lehman, 1988; Rook, 1984; Shinn, Lehman, & Wong, 1984).

To our knowledge, our 1994 study represents the only empirical investigation designed to explore the effects of exposure to antiabortion picketing on women's postabortion psychological adjustment. In that study we hypothesized that increased antiabortion activity would result in higher postabortion depression scores for women obtaining an abortion at a picketed clinic on the basis of the psychological literature indicating that conflictive social interactions can have negative psychological effects. We also anticipated that women's subjective reports of being more upset by the picketers would mediate the relationship between higher levels of antiabortion activity and higher postabortion depression.

The model we tested is depicted in Figure 1. As can be seen by inspecting this figure, a set of objective and subjective indicators of antiabortion demonstrator and pro-choice escort activity outside the clinic was entered as a block into the path model we tested. The objective indices included the coders' reports of the numbers of antiabortion demonstrators and pro-choice escorts who were present and their ratings of the intensity of antiabortion activity. Subjective indices included women's reports of

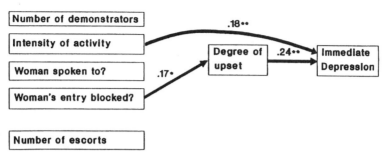

Figure 1. The impact of antiabortion activities and number of pro-choice escorts on women's postabortion depression. From "The Effects of Antiabortion Demonstrators and Pro-Choice Escorts on Women's Psychological Responses to Abortion," by C. Cozzarelli and B. Major, 1994, *Journal of Social and Clinical Psychology, 13,* p. 417. Copyright 1994 by Guilford Press. Reprinted with permission.
**$p < .01$. *$p < .05$.

whether they were spoken to or blocked by antiabortion demonstrators. The extent to which women reported being upset by the antiabortion demonstrators was entered into the model as a mediator variable. Results revealed that women who said the demonstrators had tried to block their entry to the clinic were more upset by the demonstrators than those who said their entry was not blocked. Being more upset by the demonstrators was, in turn, related to increased levels of depression 30 minutes after the abortion. Finally, the more intense the antiabortion activity outside the clinic when a woman tried to enter, the more depressed she was postabortion. In sum, exposure to intense antiabortion activity, perceived attempts to block entry to the clinic, and being upset by demonstrators were all linked to increased postabortion depression.

We also included measures of postabortion adjustment in our more recent longitudinal study. Although we are still in the process of analyzing whether various emotional responses to antiabortion demonstrators (e.g., anger vs. guilt) relate in similar ways to short-term postabortion adjustment (Cozzarelli, Karrasch, Fuegen, & Major, 1997), at this point, we do know how these variables are correlated. In this study, short-term adjustment was assessed at an average of 39 days postabortion with measures of distress (the SCL90-R; Derogatis, 1983), decision satisfaction (a composite of two items designed for this study), and positive well-being (Ryff's, 1989, 18-item Positive Well-Being scale). Experiencing guilt in response to the demonstrators was related to increased postabortion distress, $r(522) = .39$, $p < .01$; lower decision satisfaction, $r(504) = -.38$, $p < .01$; and lower positive well-being, $r(520) = -.25$, $p < .01$. Feelings of anger were also related to increased distress, $r(524) = .16$, $p < .01$, but were unrelated to decision satisfaction or positive well-being. Feeling happy in response to the demonstrators was not related to any of the adjustment variables, most likely because there was almost no variance on this item. Finally, feeling strong was related to increased decision satisfaction, $r(501) = .15$, $p < .01$, and positive well-being, $r(516) = .12$, $p < .01$.

Thus, the small amount of accumulated evidence suggests that encounters with antiabortion demonstrators can have a negative impact on women's postabortion adjustment. Women who encounter intense picketing or who perceive that demonstrators attempted to block their entry to an abortion clinic were more depressed after their abortions than women who did not encounter these circumstances. It also appears that a wide range of negative emotional responses to antiabortion demonstrators (e.g., upset, anger, guilt) is related to at least some degree of negative postabortion psychological outcomes, although some of these emotional responses are associated with more uniformly negative outcomes than others. For example, guilt in response to picketing on the day of an abortion was negatively related to all three of the postabortion adjustment measures assessed at 1 month postabortion in our most recent study. Anger, on the other hand, was only correlated with postabortion distress and was not related to lower levels of decision satisfaction or positive well-being. Thus, although a variety of emotional responses to antiabortion demonstration may relate to increased levels of postabortion distress, it is possible that experiencing guilt causes one to reevaluate an abortion decision, but becoming angry does not.

Finally, the fact that feeling strong in response to antiabortion demonstrators was related to more positive postabortion adjustment suggests that some emotional responses to these activists may actually have beneficial effects for the women who experience them. Another important agenda for future research will be to determine the characteristics that distinguish women who experience such relatively beneficial responses from those who respond more negatively. It is likely that a host of personal (e.g., preabortion levels of depression, self-esteem), social (e.g., degree of social support), and situational (e.g., the nature of the antiabortion activities that women encounter) variables are involved. Although published research to date has not explored these issues, we have conducted secondary analyses on the data collected for our 1994 study to explore the effects of personal conflict on responses to antiabortion picketing.

The Effects of High Personal Conflict on Responses to Antiabortion Demonstrators

In general, previous research has suggested that women who experience high levels of personal conflict in the context of an abortion are more likely to experience postabortion distress (or lesser satisfaction with their decision to abort) than those who experience low levels of preabortion conflict (see Adler et al., 1992; Lemkau, 1988; Major & Cozzarelli, 1992, for reviews). For example, Catholic and more religious women (in general) appear to be at increased risk for negative postabortion sequelae (Adler, 1975; Osofsky, Osofsky, & Rajan, 1973; Payne, Kravitz, Notman, & Anderson, 1976). In a study that compared emotionally distressed and emotionally nondistressed women who had had an abortion, Congleton and Calhoun (1993) found that the distressed group had significantly higher scores on religiosity and were more likely to belong to conservative churches than were the women in the nondistressed group. In addition, satisfaction with the decision to abort has been related to a generally favorable opinion of the abortion option or favorable prepregnancy attitudes toward abortion (e.g., Bracken, Klerman, & Bracken, 1978; Eisen & Zellman, 1984). Thus, women with personal religious or attitudinal conflict over their abortion decisions may find the abortion experience especially stressful. Because the combination of high stress and negative social interactions has been shown to be related to detrimental psychological effects, it is quite conceivable that exposure to active antiabortion demonstrators could exacerbate the effects of an already stressful situation for women high in personal conflict and increase their level of postabortion depression.

As mentioned earlier, we performed additional analyses on our data to explore this issue. In addition to the variables described earlier, women who participated in the study were asked to rate (a) the extent to which having this abortion conflicted with their personal religious beliefs (on a scale from 1 [not at all in conflict] to 5 [very much in conflict] and (b) their attitude toward abortion prior to this pregnancy (on a scale from 1 [definitely in favor of legalized abortion] to 5 [definitely against legalized abortion]. Means computed on these variables suggested that, on average, women experienced a moderate level of religious conflict (M = 2.61) and that prior to this pregnancy, most women held an opinion that was basically in favor of legalized abortion (M = 1.84). The higher the religious conflict a woman reported, $r(247) = .24$, $p < .01$, and the less favorable her prepregnancy attitude toward abortion, $r(249) = -.25$, $p < .01$, the more upset she reported being by the antiabortion demonstrators.

To explore whether personal conflict exacerbated the effects of antiabortion activities on postabortion depression, we looked at whether the number of demonstrators present or the intensity of their activities interacted with either religious conflict or prepregnancy attitude toward abortion in predicting postabortion distress. Results revealed that religious conflict did not interact with either picketing variable but that prior attitude toward abortion interacted with both. The overall nature of these two interactions was quite similar (see Figures 2 and 3). Women who held a prepregnancy attitude that was relatively favorable toward abortion had roughly the same low depression scores regardless of the number of picketers outside the clinic or the intensity of their activity. However, women who held more negative prepregnancy attitudes were more depressed over-

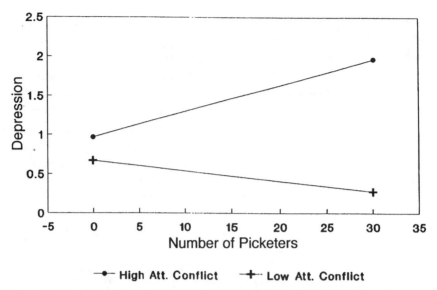

Figure 2. The interaction of attitudinal (Att.) conflict and the number of antiabortion demonstrators on women's postabortion depression.

all than those with more positive attitudes, and their depression levels increased as the number of picketers or the intensity of their activities increased.

The results of the above-mentioned analyses suggest that encounters with antiabortion demonstrators can have negative ramifications for

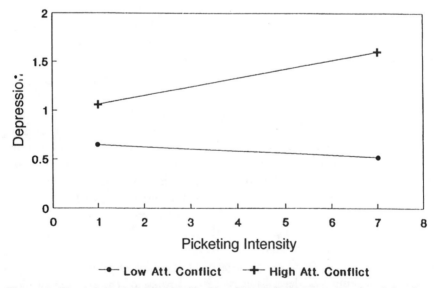

Figure 3. The interaction of attitudinal conflict and the intensity of antiabortion picketing on women's postabortion depression. Higher numbers equal higher depression.

women who experience relatively high levels of attitudinal conflict over having an abortion. Exactly how this occurs is unclear, but it is possible that the demonstrators serve to prime or remind these women of their own unfavorable attitudes toward abortion. Once primed, these negative attitudes may be especially prominent as determinants of women's emotional states.

Applied Issues

In a variety of ways, lawmakers and individuals have begun to engage in attempts to limit the activities or impact of antiabortion demonstrators (see Wilcox et al., chap. 1, this volume). Next, we discuss the potential effects both of injunctions aimed at curtailing antiabortion activities and of pro-choice escorts.

Injunctions

In response to the growing perception that antiabortion activities such as picketing, stalking, and blocking access to clinics represent forms of harassment, many communities are seeking injunctions mandating that a given distance be maintained between demonstrators and individuals entering abortion facilities or limiting certain types of antiabortion activities. For example, in response to continued violence directed against an abortion clinic in Boulder, Colorado, the City Council adopted an ordinance requiring demonstrators to remain at least 8 feet from anyone approaching a health care facility, unless that person agrees to let the demonstrator approach (Hern, 1991). In Buffalo, a court order in 1992 restricted antiabortion activities outside clinics where abortions are performed. Demonstrators were specifically barred from blocking or obstructing access to abortion facilities, demonstrating within 15 feet of all clinic entryways and parking lot entrances, using amplification devices, and harassing clinic patients or staff (Wallin, 1992). Most recently, the Supreme Court upheld the legality of a 36-foot buffer zone around an abortion clinic (Wilcox et al., chap. 1, this volume).

To our knowledge, no data exist that can address the issue of whether such injunctions are effective in reducing the potential distress resulting from unwanted interactions with antiabortion demonstrators. However, it seems likely that enforcing these injunctions would aid women in gaining unimpeded access to abortion clinics and may also serve to diffuse the perceived intensity of antiabortion activity. In light of the results of Cozzarelli and Major (1994), it seems likely this would have positive effects on women's postabortion adjustment.

In addition, it has been argued that distances of less than 10 or 12 feet are abnormally short when compared with the distance that Americans normally maintain while receiving messages from strangers. As cited in Hern (1991), being approached by a stranger at shorter distances, especially in a situation that is perceived as negatively toned, leads to perceptions of threat and heightened distress. Thus, forcing demonstrators to remain at distances of 12 feet or more may well lead to some reduction of distress for women entering clinics. However, even at distances of 12 feet, women entering abortion facilities would still be able to hear the content of antiabortion messages and be able to read inscriptions on antiabortion placards. Whether these kinds of messages have a negative effect on women is currently unknown and is a question worthy of future investigation. Finally, although there is also no data to address the issue, it is reasonable to speculate that doctors and clinic personnel would be more likely to continue providing abortions if they and their families were not subjected to antiabortion harassment.

Pro-Choice Escorts

Pro-choice escorts are volunteers whose function it is to ensure that women seeking to enter a picketed abortion clinic are able to do so. Unfortunately, there is little systematic empirical research on why individuals join pro-choice organizations or on the worldviews of those who volunteer to escort. However, Luker (1984) argued that the views of those who are active in the pro-choice movement are often diametrically opposed to those of antiabortion activists. For example, she argued that pro-choice individuals are likely to see abortion as an issue of self-determination for women. That is, control over reproduction is seen as a key factor in allowing women to reach their fullest potential. However, many of those in Luker's pro-choice sample were uncomfortable with the idea of using abortion as a routine form of birth control and would prefer to see women make use of more traditional forms of contraception. The pro-choice activists in Luker's study were also less likely to believe that men and women are fundamentally different, less likely to equate fulfillment for women solely with motherhood, and more likely to endorse the belief that it is acceptable to separate sex from reproduction, as compared with those in her antiabortion sample.

Traditionally, the escort role has been defined as a response to the activities of those who picket or block access to abortion clinics and, in this sense, is often thought of as defensive in nature, rather than proactive. As is the case with antiabortion activists, however, it is likely that pro-choice escorts vary in their personal beliefs and in the extent to which they are active or aggressive while escorting. It is also likely that women entering abortion clinics vary in terms of how they conceptualize the nature of an escort presence.

To our knowledge, with the exception of our 1994 study, there is no empirical evidence regarding how many women entering abortion clinics encounter pro-choice escorts or addressing how women feel about these individuals. In our study, the coders who were responsible for rating anti-abortion activities also counted the number of pro-choice escorts who were present outside the clinic and rated their overall activity level. We also asked the women who participated in our study whether they saw pro-choice escorts and if they did, how the escorts made them feel on a scale from 1 (*they made me feel much worse*) to 5 (*they made me feel much better*).

According to the coders, pro-choice escorts were present during 38.3% of the coding intervals (most often on Saturdays, when the largest numbers of antiabortion demonstrators were present). The number of escorts present ranged from 0 to 27, with an average of 3.51. In general, the escorts were described as moderately active (M = 2.74). Only 19% of the women in our study reported seeing escorts when they entered the clinic. On average, these women reported that the escorts made them feel better (M = 3.90). In addition, as the number of escorts increased, women were less likely to report that the antiabortion demonstrators had spoken to them, $r(224) = -.12$, $p < .04$, or tried to prevent them from entering the clinic, $r(224) = -.12$, $p < .05$, and as coder ratings of the intensity of escort activity increased, women were less likely to report that the antiabortion demonstrators had blocked their entry, $r(86) = -.23$, $p < .05$. Finally, as the number of antiabortion demonstrators increased, the extent to which women were likely to say that the escorts made them feel better increased as well, $r(50) = .27$, $p < .05$. In a similar vein, Nasman (1992) reported that 75% of the individuals in her study who encountered anti-abortion demonstrators reported receiving assistance from pro-choice escorts. All of those who received this service specified that they appreciated it.

These results suggest that women entering abortion clinics perceive the presence of pro-choice escorts in a positive manner. An equally intriguing issue concerns whether these escorts are able to buffer women against the negative psychological effects related to encountering antiabortion demonstrators. In our study, we found that the number of pro-choice escorts present when a woman entered an abortion clinic was not a significant predictor of her postabortion depression. This led us to speculate that the precise number of escorts present outside an abortion clinic may not matter as much as whether there are any escorts present versus none at all. That is, perhaps it is simply an escort presence, per se, that is critical for establishing a physical or psychological buffer. To test this possibility, we examined whether the number of antiabortion demonstrators present outside a clinic or the activity levels of the escorts interacted with the presence and absence of pro-choice escorts in predicting women's postabortion depression. We found that when no pro-choice escorts were present, as the number of antiabortion demonstrators increased, so did women's levels of immediate postabortion depression. However, when pro-choice escorts were present, increasing numbers of antiabortion demonstrators did not result in increased depression (see Figure 4). In contrast, the intensity of anti-abortion activity levels did not interact with the presence or absence of escorts.

The results of the various analyses that have been reviewed suggest that, overall, women entering abortion clinics perceive pro-choice escorts positively and that, to some extent, an escort presence can help reduce the psychological effects of large numbers of antiabortion demonstrators. How this occurs is still somewhat unclear, but it may be that escorts achieve this effect, in part, by preventing antiabortion activists from having personal contact with women entering an abortion clinic. Thus, escorts may serve to blunt or prevent the negative social interactions attributable to antiabortion demonstrators. In addition, the presence of pro-choice escorts may serve as symbolic support for a woman's decision to obtain an abortion. If this is the case, the number of escorts present or the exact nature of their activities may not matter as much as the simple fact that they are there. Thus, escorts may be perceived not just as an antidote to negative social interactions but also as a source of positive interactions or affirmation.

Our finding that pro-choice escorts were able to buffer women from the effects of large numbers of demonstrators, but not from the effects of intense antiabortion activities, is provocative. It is possible that adding escorts to a situation that is already perceived as intense by women entering

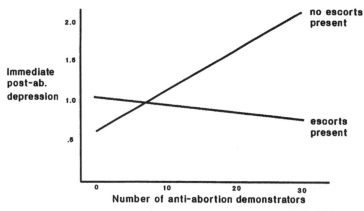

Figure 4. The interaction of presence/absence of pro-choice escorts and the number of antiabortion demonstrators on women's postabortion (post-ab.) depression. Higher numbers equal more demonstrators, greater activity, being spoken to, having one's entry blocked, being more upset, more escorts, and greater depression. From "The Effects of Antiabortion Demonstrations and Pro-Choice Escorts on Women's Psychological Response to Abortion, by C. Cozzarelli and B. Major, 1994, *Journal of Social and Clinical Psychology, 13,* p. 419. Copyright 1994 Guilford Press. Reprinted with permission.

an abortion clinic does not serve to lessen that perception, particularly if these individuals are also very active. Indeed, this is often likely to be the case, as it is presumably more difficult to ensure women's access to clinics that are surrounded by relatively large numbers of antiabortion demonstrators. In a practical sense, this suggests that escorts may be most effective when they are able to achieve the difficult combination of maintaining access to a picketed clinic without causing an escalation in the overall activity level confronting women as they attempt to enter that clinic.

DIRECTIONS FOR FUTURE RESEARCH

We have documented that antiabortion demonstrations are widespread and that they affect a majority of women entering clinics to obtain an abortion. We also reviewed evidence suggesting that encounters with antiabortion demonstrators can have a negative impact on women obtaining an abortion and that pro-choice escorts may, to some extent, be able to offset these negative effects. However, it is quite clear that, in a general sense, many of our conclusions must be considered tentative until they are confirmed by additional empirical data. In particular, theoretical models of the mechanisms by which antiabortion demonstrators affect women's postabortion adjustment are sorely lacking. It is quite possible that different mechanisms may be operating for different women. For some women, antiabortion demonstrators may have a negative impact by priming their own conflicts about abortion, whereas for others, negative effects may arise from the fact that encounters with these demonstrators serve to make the abortion experience that much more negative. It also remains to be seen whether encounters with antiabortion demonstrators have any long-term effects on women's postabortion adjustment. Although being blocked by demonstrators, encountering intense antiabortion activities, and feeling guilt after encountering demonstrators all seem to have negative effects on short-term postabortion adjustment, it is currently unknown whether such effects are likely to persist or to dissipate over time. To address this issue, we are in the process of examining whether exposure to antiabortion activities affects adjustment 2 years after an abortion.

In addition, there is almost a complete lack of data concerning how women feel about pro-choice escorts and about how various escort activities may impact women obtaining abortions. Future research would do well to address and more clearly delineate the conditions under which escorts have positive effects on women's health from those conditions where an escort presence or escort activities might exacerbate an already negative situation. Finally, the passage of federal laws restricting antiabortion activities requires that researchers obtain new estimates of the prevalence of antiabortion activities and new data concerning the percentage of women seeking abortions who are likely to encounter such demonstrators. Although fewer women may now be exposed to antiabortion demonstrators than was the case when we collected our data, these women may still suffer the negative effects we have described.

We are well aware that research on the impact of antiabortion and pro-choice activities on women's postabortion adjustment is difficult and costly to conduct, both in terms of time and money. However, given the large numbers of women who continue to obtain abortions and the likelihood that abortion clinics and clinic staff will continue to experience various forms of antiabortion activities, we believe that such research is of vital interest to both the scientific community and the American public.

REFERENCES

Adler, N. (1975). Emotional responses of women following therapeutic abortion. *American Journal of Orthopsychiatry, 45,* 446–454.

Adler, N. E., David, H. P., Major, B. N., Roth, S. H., Russo, N. F., & Wyatt, G. E. (1992). Psychological factors in abortion: A review. *American Psychologist, 47,* 1194–1204.

Blanchard, D. A. (1994). *The anti-abortion movement and the rise of the religious right: From polite to fiery protest.* New York: Twayne.

Bracken, M. B., Klerman, L. V., & Bracken, M. (1978). Coping with pregnancy resolution among never-married women. *Journal of Orthopsychiatry, 48,* 320–334.

Cook, E. A., Jelen, T. G., & Wilcox, C. (1991). *Between two absolutes: Public opinion and the politics of abortion.* Boulder, CO: Westview.

Congleton, G. K., & Calhoun, L. G. (1993). Post-abortion perceptions: A comparison of self-identified distressed and nondistressed populations. *The International Journal of Social Psychiatry, 39,* 255–265.

Coyne, J., Wortman, C., & Lehman, D. (1988). The other side of support: Emotional overinvolvement and miscarried helping. In B. Gottlieb (Ed.), *Marshalling social support* (pp. 305–330). Beverly Hills, CA: Sage.

Cozzarelli, C., Major, B., Karrasch, A., & Fuegen, K. (1997). *The impact of emotional responses to antiabortion picketers on short and long-term postabortion adjustment.* Manuscript in preparation.

Cozzarelli, C., & Major, B. (1994). The effects of anti-abortion demonstrators and pro-choice escorts on women's psychological responses to abortion. *Journal of Social and Clinical Psychology, 13,* 404–427.

Derogatis, L. R. (1983). *SCL-90-R Manual 1.* Baltimore: Johns Hopkins University Press.

Donovan, P. (1985). The holy war. *Family Planning Perspectives, 17,* 5–9.

Eisen, M., & Zellman, G. (1984). Factors predicting pregnancy resolution decision satisfaction of unmarried adolescents. *The Journal of Genetic Psychology, 145,* 231–239.

Fiore, J., Becker, J., & Coppel, D. B. (1983). Social network interactions: A buffer or a stress? *American Journal of Community Psychology, 11,* 423–439.

Forero, J., & Linstedt, S. (1992, April 23). Police union sees strain on precincts. *Buffalo Evening News,* p. A-14.

Forrest, J. D., & Henshaw, S. K. (1987). The harassment of U.S. abortion providers. *Family Planning Perspectives, 19,* 9–13.

Guth, J. L., Smidt, C. E., Kellstedt, L., & Green, J. C. (1993). The sources of antiabortion attitudes: The case of religious political activists. In M. L. Goggin (Ed.), *Understanding the new politics of abortion* (pp. 44–56). Newbury Park, CA: Sage.

Henshaw, S. K. (1991). The accessibility of abortion services in the United States. *Family Planning Perspectives, 23,* 246–252.

Henshaw, S. K. (1995). Factors hindering access to abortion services. *Family Planning Perspectives, 27,* 54–59.

Henshaw, S. K., & Van Vort, J. (1994). Abortion services in the United States, 1991 and 1992. *Family Planning Perspectives, 26,* 100–106.

Hern, W. M. (1991). Proxemics: The application of theory to conflict arising from antiabortion demonstrations. *Population and Environment: A Journal of Interdisciplinary Studies, 12,* 379–388.

Himmelstein, J. (1986). The social basis of anti-feminism. *Journal for the Scientific Study of Religion, 25,* 1–15.

Hull, J. D. (1991, Sept. 9). Whose side are you on? For weary Wichitans, the protests may be subsiding, but the healing has yet to begin. *Time,* p. 19.

Lemkau, J. P. (1988). Emotional sequelae of abortion: Implications for clinical practice. *Psychology of Women Quarterly, 12,* 461–472.

Luker, K. (1984). *Abortion and the politics of motherhood.* Berkeley: University of California Press.

Major, B., & Cozzarelli, C. (1992). Psychosocial predictors of adjustment to abortion. *Journal of Social Issues, 48,* 121–142.

Major, B., Richards, C., Cooper, M. L., Cozzarelli, C., & Zubek, J. (1998). Personal resilience, cognitive appraisals, and coping: An integrative model of adjustment to abortion. *Journal of Personality and Social Psychology, 74,* 735–752.

Major, B., Zubek, J. M., Cooper, M. L., Cozzarelli, C., & Richards, C. (1997). Mixed messages: Implications of social conflict and social support within close relationships for adjustment to a stressful life event. *Journal of Personality and Social Psychology, 72,* 1349–1363.

Nasman, V. T. (1992). . . . *And then the decision was mine.* Unpublished manuscript, Dayton, OH.

Osofsky, J. D., Osofsky, H. J., & Rajan, R. (1973). Psychological effects of abortion: With emphasis on the immediate reactions and follow-up. In H. J. Osofsky

& J. D. Osofsky (Eds.), *The abortion experience* (pp. 189–205). Hagerstown, MD: Harper & Row.

Payne, E., Kravitz, A., Notman, M., & Anderson, J. (1976). Outcome following therapeutic abortion. *Archives of General Psychiatry, 33,* 725–733.

Petchesky, R. P. (1984). *Abortion and woman's choice.* New York: Longman.

Reardon, D. (1987). *Aborted women: Silent no more.* Chicago: Loyola University Press.

Rook, K. S. (1984). The negative side of social interaction: Impact on psychological well-being. *Journal of Personality and Social Psychology, 46,* 1097–1108.

Ruehlman, L. S., & Karoly, P. (1991). With a little flak from my friends: Development and preliminary validation of the Test of Negative Social Exchange (TENSE). *Journal of Consulting and Clinical Psychology, 59,* 97–104.

Ruehlman, L. S., & Wolchik, S. A. (1988). Personal goals and interpersonal support and hindrance as factors in psychological distress and well-being. *Journal of Personality and Social Psychology, 55,* 293–301.

Ryff, C. D. (1989). Happiness is everything, or is it? Explorations on the meaning of psychological well-being. *Journal of Personality and Social Psychology, 57,* 839–852.

Scheidler, J. M. (1985). *Closed: 99 ways to stop abortion.* Westchester, IL: Crossway Books.

Serrano, R. A. (1996, Dec. 8). Law protecting abortion clinics thwarts protests. *LA Times,* pp. A1, A28.

Shinn, M., Lehman, S., & Wong, N. W. (1984). Social interactions and social support. *Journal of Social Issues, 40,* 55–76.

Wallin, C. (1992). *Report on Operation Rescue demonstrations in Buffalo, NY.* New York: New York Civil Liberties Union.

II

THE CULTURAL CONTEXT
OF ABORTION

5

BLACK WOMEN AND THE QUESTION OF ABORTION

KAREN DUGGER

Black women's relationship to abortion, both symbolically and in practice, cannot be apprehended outside the nexus of race, class, and gender relations of power in which it is situated. Black women's use of abortion, their attitudes toward abortion, and their relative absence from the mainstream reproductive rights movement must be considered in light of the existing social and economic realities they confront, as well as in the context of their historical and contemporary social location vis-à-vis reproductive technologies. Black women have higher rates of unintended pregnancies and three times the rate of abortion than White women do (Centers for Disease Control and Prevention [CDC], 1994). Yet, survey after survey consistently show that from the 1960s to the present Blacks tend to be less supportive of legalized abortion than Whites. How is this seeming contradiction to be reconciled? What is the basis of Black women's relative ideological opposition to legalized abortion in spite of apparent need? How do Black women construe the issue of "reproductive rights," and where does this issue fit in their political agenda? The present chapter addresses these questions.

Before exploring these issues, I want to caution against a universalistic interpretation of the phrase "black women." A universalistic understanding assumes Black women share some essential commonality or experience, such as racism, that provides a basis for unity among them. But, the impact of racism on the reproductive lives of Black women is not uniform. Class, for instance, is a significant factor, with poor Black women having fewer options and subjected to greater coercion than their middle-class sisters. A focus on comparisons between Black and White abortion attitudes and practices has resulted in a dearth of research on divisions within the Black community, perpetuating a totalizing image of Black women. But as the following analysis demonstrates, Black women are not a homogeneous grouping. Rather, they are divided by a variety of factors including class, sexuality, religiosity, ideology, and age, all of which influence their views on abortion. Although given little attention by the mainstream media, there have been and continues to be strong divisions within the Black community and among Black women over the abortion issue.

ATTITUDES TOWARD LEGALIZED ABORTION

Black–White differences in support for legalized abortion have been the subject of both a good deal of study and a good deal of controversy. Researchers have offered essentially six explanations for the racial disparity in abortion attitudes. These include (a) sociodemographic differences between Blacks and Whites, (b) cultural differences between Blacks and Whites, (c) the greater religious orthodoxy and fundamentalism of Blacks as compared with Whites, (d) race-specific generational differences, (e) race-specific life cycle differences, and (f) the theme of abortion and birth control as forms of Black genocide hypothesized as prevalent within Black communities.

The Demographic Hypothesis

The debate over the antecedents of racial differences in abortion attitudes began with a study by Combs and Welch (1982). Using data from the 1972–1980 General Social Survey (GSS), Combs and Welch found that the same demographic variables that are related to abortion support in the larger population—education, occupation, income, rural and southern residence, and various measures of religiosity—also predicted Black attitudes. Controlling for these demographic and religious variables they found that although a small but statistically significant difference remained, the racial gap was substantially reduced. On the basis of these findings Combs and Welch argued that the abortion attitudes of Blacks and Whites are converging and concluded that "patterns in attitudes toward abortion in the black community mirror those in the larger society, and thus seem to be shaped by the same forces as white attitudes" (p. 517). Thus, Combs and Welch posited a sociodemographic explanation for the racial gap in abortion attitudes, maintaining that as Blacks become more structurally assimilated into American society their attitudes will become indistinguishable from those of Whites.

The Cultural Differences Hypothesis

Challenging both conceptually and empirically the conclusions of Combs and Welch (1982) is research by Hall and Ferree (1986). Hall and Ferree conceptualized race not primarily in sociodemographic, but in cultural and political, terms. For them, race is viewed as producing different sets of experiences that inform how members of various racial groups interpret political and social realities. Consistent with much feminist research into the sources of opposing worldviews on abortion, Hall and Ferree maintain that abortion attitudes are largely a product of cultural understandings surrounding the meanings of family, sexuality, motherhood, and gender roles. Their analysis extended the GSS data set used by Combs and Welch through 1984 and included the same sociodemographic and religious variables. In addition, Hall and Ferree incorporated measures of attitudes toward premarital sex, family size, and gender roles. They found that although the inclusion of the latter variables substantially increased the amount of variance explained, it did not reduce racial differences in support for legal abortions.

Hall and Ferree's (1986) data also provide tentative support for their contention that cultural differences between Blacks and Whites may be at the crux of the differences in their abortion attitudes. Their results showed that attitudes toward premarital sex more strongly predicted the abortion attitudes of Whites than Blacks and that Blacks were more likely than Whites to recognize economic need as opposed to being a single woman as a legitimate reason for an abortion. They also found a race–age interaction, wherein older Whites but younger Blacks were more pro-choice. These findings suggest that the sex–gender belief system in which attitudes toward legalized abortion are embedded may be race specific.

My own research explored this possibility, namely, that Black women's abortion attitudes are not grounded in the same ideological configuration as that of White women (Dugger, 1991). For this purpose, I used data from the 1980 Virginia Slims American Women's Opinion Poll, which, unlike GSS data, offered a rich variety of measures of sex, family, and gender-role attitudes. Extant research on both abortion activists and the general public demonstrates that support or opposition to legalized abortion tends to be grounded in a matrix of interrelated beliefs regarding sex, family, and gender issues (Barnartt & Harris, 1982; Blake & Del Pinal, 1980; Conover & Gray, 1983; Gordon & Hunter, 1977; Granberg, 1978; Granberg & Granberg, 1980; Harding, 1981; Luker, 1984; Petchesky, 1984). Given this, attitudes toward abortion are often understood as indicative of a more general feminist or antifeminist orientation. However, the research on which such conclusions are based was conducted primarily with White women, whose experiences of motherhood, family, and work differ from those of Black women. Consequently, I suspected that the ideological correlates of Black women's abortion attitudes might likewise differ.

This suspicion was confirmed. Whereas sex, family, and gender-role beliefs were associated with both Black and White women's abortion attitudes, the strength and pattern of these associations were race specific. Attitudes toward sexual morality and family were substantially stronger predictors of White than Black women's perspectives on legalized abortion. In terms of gender-role attitudes, White women who believed that women's status should be enhanced and their roles changed were more likely to support legal abortions. These attitudes failed, however, to distinguish between Black supporters and opponents of abortion.

For Black women, the most important attitudinal determinant of their abortion attitudes was whether they believed women suffer from discrimination. In addition, education and the extent to which women were invested in the labor market more strongly predicted Black women's attitudes toward legal abortion than those of White women. Collectively, the predictor variables explained significantly less variance in Black women's abortion attitudes than was the case for White women. Thus, my results indicate that for Black women, legalized abortion is not a referendum on feminism. That is, abortion does not appear to hold the same symbolic or political significance for Black women that it does for White women. Rather, given the three variables that most strongly predicted Black women's stance on abortion (education, investment in the labor market, and a belief that women were discriminated against), I concluded that "for Black women abortion is more a practical consideration grounded in the realization of the consequences of unwanted pregnancies than it is a symbolic issue" (Dugger, 1991, p. 583).

Differences in Religiosity

Other researchers have explored different dimensions and added new spins to the controversy over racial differences in abortion attitudes. In a variety of publications, Wilcox (1990) has insisted on the importance of religion in structuring the abortion attitudes of Blacks. His 1990 study updated the research of Combs and Welch (1982) and Hall and Ferree (1986) by adding 4 more years of GSS data (1985–1988) and including additional measures of religiosity. He contended that the different conclusions reached by these two teams of researchers about whether the racial gap in abortion attitudes was declining or persisting was largely due to differences in the survey years each examined and the relatively weak measures of religiosity available during those years. Inclusion of the new religious variables increased the variance explained and eliminated racial differences, leading Wilcox (1990) to conclude that the racial gap in abortion support is "in part a function of the greater religiosity and doctrinal orthodoxy of the black population" (p. 254). Although Wilcox's findings supported the convergence hypothesis of Combs and Welch, his data did not support their explanation of this convergence. Rather, his data showed relative stability in the abortion attitudes of Blacks, but declining support among Whites. Hence, he concluded that "Blacks are not becoming more supportive over time as their socioeconomic position improves—whites are becoming less supportive as the political climate changes" (p. 254).

In two later articles, Wilcox (1992; Wilcox & Thomas, 1992) further pursued his claim that the greater religiosity of Blacks largely accounts for their less permissive stance on abortion. Both studies tested the hypothesis that various measures of religiosity would prove especially important in explaining the abortion attitudes of Blacks. Surprisingly, however, the results of the first study (Wilcox, 1992) were to the contrary. Religious variables had a larger impact on the abortion attitudes of Whites than they did on those of Blacks. Their inclusion in the regression equations increased the explained variance in White abortion attitudes by an average of 14%, but added only 0.5% to that of Blacks. Moreover, the combination of religious, demographic, and sexual morality variables collectively explained a substantially greater proportion of the variance for Whites than for Blacks. Such findings underscore the point that the sources of Black abortion attitudes are not well understood. Nonetheless, because controlling for the religious variables did erase the racial gap in abortion attitudes, Wilcox maintains that religiosity exerts a considerable force on Black support for legal abortions.

The second study drew on a sample of African American women residing in Washington, DC. In this instance, Wilcox and Thomas (1992) argued that religiosity combines with the influence of Black women's experience of a variety of reproductive abuses, both historically and in the present, to produce mixed feelings toward abortion. Their findings showed that religious involvement and doctrinal orthodoxy were strongly associated with Black women's opposition to legal abortion.

However, these same measures of religiosity were not predictive of Black women's attitudes toward gender equality. In fact, for Black women, greater religiosity, in some instances, led to greater support for feminist organizations and objectives. This finding runs counter to research showing that for White women, greater religiosity results in increased opposition to feminism. Wilcox and Thomas (1992) explained this discrepancy by pointing to the role of the Black church in advocating racial equality and collective action. Such messages of liberation and equality, they argued, spill over into the realm of gender politics, leading to increased support for feminism by Black women. The finding that religiosity is negatively related to opposition to abortion but positively associated with support for feminism is consistent with the claim that, for Black women, abortion is not necessarily symbolic of a broader feminist or antifeminist orientation.

Generational Versus Life Cycle Explanations

The finding by Hall and Ferree (1986) that the effect of age on support for abortion was race specific, with older Whites but younger Blacks being more pro-choice, prompted exploration of the meaning of this difference. To this end, Cook, Jelen, and Wilcox (1993) examined cohort differences among Blacks and Whites in their abortion attitudes. They constructed seven cohorts, ranging from those who reached age 18 before or during the Great Depression to those who came of age during the Reagan era. These researchers found that, for Whites, the youngest (i.e., the Reagan cohort) women were less supportive of legal abortion than those who came of age during the 1960s and 1970s. By contrast, among Blacks, the Reagan cohort was considerably more likely than older cohorts to be supportive of legalized abortion. A longitudinal trend analysis of the White sample revealed that the rank ordering of the cohorts over the time period from 1972 to 1988 remained constant. In other words, for each of the time periods examined, the younger Reagan cohort consistently showed less support for legal abortions than the 1960s and 1970s cohorts. The authors interpreted this finding as evidence of enduring generational differences and argued that "the process of generational replacement will greatly shift the average position of the black community on legal abortion" (Cook et al., 1993, p. 38). This conclusion, however, may be premature. Given the small size of the Black sample, no longitudinal trend analysis was performed. This leaves open the possibility that the cohort differences discovered among Blacks is a product of life-cycle rather than generational differences.

The hypothesis that stage in the life cycle critically structures the abortion attitudes of both Black and White women was explored by Lynxwiler and Gay (1994), who sought to adjudicate the controversy over whether the racial difference in abortion attitudes was persistent or declining. Lynxwiler and Gay reasoned that because the social and economic costs associated with an unintended pregnancy are most salient for childbearing women (those 44 and younger), such women are likely to take an instrumental approach to the abortion issue. Consequently, they argued that practical considerations may influence childbearing women's support for the legality of abortion and override "other value systems and definitions of its morality that they have internalized" (p. 70).

Lynxwiler and Gay (1994) expected and found no racial differences in support for legal abortion among women of childbearing age. With only a few exceptions, there were no mean differences in Black and White women's abortion attitudes from 1972 to 1988. Similarly, controlling for sociodemographic variables; religiosity; and sex, family, and gender-role attitudes over four time clusters from 1972 to 1978 they found no net difference in support for abortion between Black and White women of childbearing age. Differences did surface, however, with regard to other categories of Blacks and Whites. Older White women were the most pro-choice and older Black women the least, which, the authors posit, may explain Hall and Ferree's (1986) findings of persisting racial differences. On the other hand, Black men, whose abortion attitudes were less permissive than that of women of childbearing age, showed a trend toward convergence with the latter, a finding consistent with that of Combs and Welch (1982).

Although the effect of generational differences may be a contributing factor in the formation of Black and White women's abortion attitudes, Lynxwiler and Gay (1994) maintain that such differences are insufficient in accounting for the race-specific patterns they observed. Rather, they view the differential effect of life-cycle experiences as key. Drawing on analyses from prior research (Dugger, 1991; Gump, 1980; Luker, 1984; Plutzer, 1988; Walters, 1985), Lynxwiler and Gay (1994) endorsed the argument that abortion is more symbolic of the politics of gender for White women than for Black women. Because attitudes with high symbolic content tend to develop early in life and crystallize over the life course (Sears, 1975, 1988), White women's stance on abortion should intensify and stabilize over the life course. Such an explanation is consistent with their finding that older White women are the more pro-choice.

Lynxwiler and Gay's (1994) interpretation of the pattern of Black women's abortion support draws on my (Dugger, 1991) conclusion that abortion for Black women is largely a practical rather than a symbolic issue. Distinguishing between support for legal abortion and definitions of abortion as a moral issue, Lynxwiler and Gay posited that it is possible for women to support legalized abortion while viewing abortion itself as morally wrong. Given this logic they argued that

> as black women leave their childbearing years, the salience of an unwanted pregnancy will decline. In the absence of practical considerations on which their support for legal abortion is premised ... black women's definitions concerning the morality of abortion tend to become more salient. (p. 80)

Although taking no stand, the authors offered several speculations regarding factors that might shape Black women's moral perspective on abortion to produce a less permissive stance. These include greater acceptance of nonnuclear family forms and out-of-wedlock births, perceptions of abortion as placing self-aggrandizement above concerns for preserving the Black family and community, and the sentiment that abortion is a form of Black genocide.

Abortion as Black Genocide

Some researchers have speculated that the less permissive attitudes of Blacks toward legal abortion may in part be due to perceptions within Black communities that abortion is a form of race genocide (Petchesky, 1984; Wilcox, 1990; Wilcox & Thomas, 1992). Although there is no research to my knowledge that directly investigates this hypothesis, several researchers have documented the strong theme of birth control and abortion as forms of Black genocide in the culture of Black communities and among some political leaders during the 1960s and 1970s (Brown & Eisenberg, 1995; Littlewood, 1977; Sarvis & Rodman, 1974; Shapiro, 1985; Weisbord, 1975). At the Black Power conference in 1971, for example, participants endorsed the view of abortion as genocide (Schulder & Kennedy, 1971). Similarly, Littlewood (1977) pointed to the suspicion with which some Blacks viewed the placement of birth control clinics in Black neighborhoods and specifically described the attempt by the National Association for the Advancement of Colored People (NAACP) in Pittsburgh to close down one such clinic. Charles Willie (1970) maintained that

> Many people in the black community are deeply suspicious of any family planning program initiated by whites . . . The genocidal charge is neither absurd nor hollow . . . Neither is it limited to residents of the ghetto . . . Indeed my studies of black college students indicate that young educated blacks fear black genocide. (p. 257)

Blacks during this time were not, however, united on the abortion issue. Those associated with Black nationalist causes were most likely to view birth control and abortion as genocidal. Black women, on the other hand, were more likely than Black men to argue for the right to choice and to distinguish between population control and birth control (Littlewood, 1977; Weisbord, 1975).

The observation of Rodman, Sarvis, and Walker (1987) that the theme of Black genocide since the 1970s has receded into the background appears questionable. Following the legalization of Norplant in the 1990s, Turner (1993) acknowledged that rumors suggesting its coercive use on African American women in the inner city began to circulate in the Black community, recalling for some the theme of Black genocide from the 1970s. A survey of Black democratic activists during the 1992 Democratic Convention by *Emerge* magazine found that although the majority (50%) supported choice, a significant minority (almost 40%) believed that the hypothesis "abortion is genocide" was somewhat or largely true. Such perceptions, proposes Malveaux (1993), may account for the ambiguous stance of Blacks toward abortion, particularly the failure of Black political leaders to weigh in on the issue and the absence of any resolutions on legal abortions from major civil rights organizations such as the NAACP. Both Malveaux and Cary (1992) argued that the association of family planning and abortion with Black genocide must be understood in the context of U.S. race relations wherein the needs and humanity of Black Americans have historically been devalued. "Genocide," according to Malveaux,

> is often a code word for the many inequities related to race and reproductive rights—the use of Norplant ... forced on poor black women; the unavailability of basic health care for many low-income and working people in our community; the apparent disinterest of pro-choice activists in a broader range of social issues that affect the black community. (p. 34)

To place Black attitudes toward legal abortion in the larger context of U.S. race, class, and gender relations I turn to a discussion of the inequities to which Malveaux refers.

BLACK WOMEN AND REPRODUCTIVE TECHNOLOGIES

Evidence of the punitive and coercive manipulation of Black women's reproductive options is abundant (Brown & Eisenberg, 1995; Gordon, 1977; Hartmann, 1987; Solinger, 1992). From the beginning of the birth control movement to the present, Black women have been subjected to the repressive administration of reproductive technologies. The tarnished legacy of the birth control movement is reflected in the infamous assertion by Margaret Sanger, who in 1921 established the American Birth Control League (ABCL). In her advocacy for the legalization of birth control, Sanger and the ABCL opportunistically built alliances with leaders in the Eugenics movement and the population control establishment. Endorsing the view of racial progress through sterilization, Sanger proclaimed that the chief issue of birth control was "more children from the fit and less from the unfit" (cited in Hartmann, 1987, p. 97). The racist character of the ABCL can also be glimpsed from its proposal of the Negro Project. Designed in 1939, the Negro Project sought to hire Black ministers who were to travel through the South to enlist the support of Black doctors for birth control. According to Gordon (1977), the project proposal argued that

> the mass of negroes, particularly in the South, still breed carelessly and disastrously, with the result that the increase among Negroes, even more than among whites, is from that portion of the population least intelligent and fit, and least able to rear children properly. (p. 16)

In the 1940s the ABCL changed its name to Planned Parenthood and began to emphasize the problem of overpopulation, which, during the next two decades, would gain increasing currency (Hartmann, 1987).

The eugenicist theme of "less children from the unfit" also characterized the post-war discourses of the 1950s and 1960s, which established a connection among birth control, race, and welfare. Solinger (1992) described how public discourse during this time defined the meaning of unwed motherhood in race-specific terms, sanctioning the differential treatment of Black and White single mothers. For White women, unwed motherhood was understood in psychological as opposed to sexual terms and demanded intervention and treatment by social workers. By contrast, Black single pregnancy was attributed to the irresponsible hypersexuality of Black women. Black unmarried mothers were constructed by politicians, judges, civic leaders, journalists, and White citizens as women for whom producing babies was a business (S. Brown & Eisenberg, 1995; Solinger, 1992; Weisbord, 1975). Remarks such as those made by Mississippi State Representative David Glass were typical:

> During the calendar year 1957, there were born out of wedlock in Mississippi, more than seven thousand negro children . . . The negro woman because of child welfare assistance [is] making it a business, in some cases, of giving birth to illegitimate children . . . The purpose of my bill was to try to stop, slow down, such traffic at its source. (cited in S. Brown & Eisenberg, 1995, p. 199)

Thus, the 1950s and 1960s witnessed the development of a discourse of extreme hostility and punitiveness toward Black unmarried mothers. According to Solinger (1992), the latter were "blamed for the population explosion, for escalating welfare costs . . . and blamed for the tenacious grip of poverty in black America" (p. 25). For this they deserved not treatment but punishment. Neither imprisonment nor sterilization was deemed inappropriate retribution for the burden and chaos Black women were accused of thrusting on the larger society. Beginning in the 1950s and intensifying in the 1960s, numerous state and local legislatures enacted or attempted to enact punitive laws that would either deny public assistance to unwed mothers or mandate the imprisonment or sterilization of those who had more than a specified number of "illegitimate" children (Littlewood, 1977; Shapiro, 1985; Solinger, 1992; Weisbord, 1975). Although efforts to legislate the punitive sterilization of women were by and large unsuccessful, some states pursued this practice de facto.

By the mid-1970s the character and widespread nature of such abuses gained public notoriety as a result of the publicity surrounding several celebrated cases of forcible sterilization and the investigative reports they prompted. Of these, the most notable was that of the Relf sisters. At the ages of 12 and 14, these two sisters, daughters of a Black Alabama family receiving public assistance, were sterilized without their consent and under the pretense that they were being taken to a doctor for shots. Numerous other reports of sterilization abuse, such as those in Aiken County South Carolina, Los Angeles County, and North Carolina also surfaced (S. Brown & Eisenberg, 1995; Petchesky, 1984; Shapiro, 1985; Weisbord, 1975). Moreover, surveys of sterilization practices and physicians' attitudes during this time demonstrate just how pervasive and entrenched was support for and the practice of punitive sterilization. One survey found that compulsory sterilization was endemic in U.S. teaching hospitals reporting that "some women desiring an abortion were required to have a simultaneous sterilization as a condition of the abortion . . . In all, 53.6 percent of teaching hospitals made this requirement for some of their patients," with Black women particularly susceptible to such coercion (cited in Shapiro, 1985, p. 92). Studies of physicians' attitudes during this time showed that a significant majority believed public assistance patients were not intelligent or motivated enough to use contraceptives like the pill, and tended to favor such punitive measures as compulsory sterilization and the withholding of public assistance. This position was most characteristic of obstetrician–gynecologists, with 94% favoring such measures (Shapiro, 1985).

Although the introduction of oral contraceptives in the 1960s allowed for an alternative to punitive treatment, their implementation was far from value neutral. A confluence of interests served to perpetuate the relationship between welfare and contraception and the idea that Black women's fertility was a threat to the social, political, and economic stability of U.S. society. Advocates of the "population bomb"—political elites and Whites fearful of what they perceived to be a growing Black welfare class —the growing strength of the Civil Rights Movement, and riots in the inner cities convinced many of the necessity to curtail Black women's fertility (S. Brown & Eisenberg, 1995; Littlewood, 1977; Ross, 1992; Solinger, 1992).

With the establishment of Medicaid in the 1960s, publicly supported birth control became policy, making contraceptives an accessible reproductive alternative for poor women. Family planning programs enabled by federal funds spread, but were disproportionately directed at predominately Black urban areas, fueling charges of Black genocide. Even the war on poverty placed strong emphasis on family planning for Black Americans (Littlewood, 1977; Ross, 1992). Hence, family planning initiatives were a contradictory blessing for Black women, providing them greater opportunity to exercise reproductive control but in the context of a subtly coercive and racist population-control establishment. According to Solinger (1992),

> for black women the early history of the new contraceptive technology was controlled not by a value-free technological development, or by a discourse of women's rights, but by public discussion that blamed black women for the problems of their community and demands that these women accept measures to halt the "excess reproduction" ... The rhetoric promoting their [oral contraceptives] efficacy often had more in common with public justifications of sterilization of black women than it did with discussion of reproductive rights. (p. 211)

With the Food and Drug Administration's (FDA) approval of Norplant in 1990 we are again witnessing the imposition of punitive and coercive measures against poor women and women of color. These measures take two forms, legislative proposals targeted at women on public assistance and judicial actions that mandate the insertion of Norplant as a condition of sentencing or parole. Within days after Norplant received FDA approval, an editorial in the *Philadelphia Inquirer* suggested it be used as a mechanism to reduce Black poverty (Lewin, 1991; Scott, 1992). Similarly, Mathew Rees (1991) writer for *The New Republic*, argued that

> the current threat to children in our inner cities makes it an option that the morally serious can no longer simply dismiss ... The children born of drug abusing and violent women deserve our attention. And right now, Norplant may be the only practical option we've got. (p. 17)

Following this logic, Kansas State Representative Kerry Patrick introduced legislation that would mandate the insertion of Norplant in women convicted of felony drug crimes. He also proposed an incentive plan to pay women on welfare a one time payment of $500 to use Norplant, with an additional $50 a year contingent on a free medical checkup. Emulating Senator Patrick is Louisiana State Representative David Duke who would offer poor women $100.00 a year for using Norplant. According to Cockburn (1994), "there are efforts in at least 30 states to prohibit welfare increases for recipients who have additional children while on the dole as well as attempting to make Norplant a condition for many forms of social benefits" (p. 18). In a more perspicacious move, California Governor Pete Wilson had $5 million allocated to his Office of Family Planning for the specific purpose of making Norplant available to poor women. Currently, in all but two states, Norplant is being funded by Medicaid. Hence, political initiatives to link welfare with contraception continue into the present.

Making Norplant accessible to poor women or providing incentives for its use are not inherently pernicious. But, as Scott (1992) explained, "in these instances, the line between incentive and coercion is fuzzy. The incentives are only being offered for one contraceptive—Norplant—to one class of women—poor single mothers on welfare, who are more than likely women of color" (p. 45). Clearly, such initiatives bespeak stereotypes about poor and minority women's inability to control their reproductive lives and an approach to the problems of poverty and crime that is overly simplistic and eugenic in undertone. Because of this historical legacy and contemporary reality, it is not difficult to understand why birth control and abortion may be viewed by Blacks as racial genocide.

BLACK WOMEN AND THE STRUGGLE FOR REPRODUCTIVE RIGHTS

Ross (1990) estimated that fewer than 5% of Black women are involved in the White-led pro-choice movement. How can we understand this relative absence of Black women? A variety of factors appear to be at play here. As the above discussion illustrates, the continuing history of reproductive abuse is certainly a source of ambivalence toward White-led reproductive movements. To this point, Gamble and Houck (1994) commented that

> historical analysis makes clear why issues surrounding birth control touch . . . such high voltage sensitivity among black people. They provoke fears of genocide; they prompt concerns about who should make decisions and control the direction of the African American community; [and] they expose the perniciousness and tenacity of racial stereotypes. (p. 31)

But as problematic, if not more so, than this history of abuse is the political agenda and racism/elitism of the contemporary pro-choice movement. The latter is visible when the pro-choice movement argues that abortion is more cost effective than paying for the birth and upbringing of a child through welfare dollars, or when it makes appeals for support based on the threat of "overpopulation" (Ross, 1990). Equally egregious is the pro-choice movement's willingness to trade away the rights of poor and minority women to preserve those of the more privileged (Fried, 1990). Such a move was made by the Coalition for Choice in Massachusetts, representing among others Planned Parenthood and the National Organization for Women (NOW), when they decided to seek the backing of "soft supporters" by relinquishing a woman's right to abortion after the 24th week. Such legislation would impact significantly on Black women who are more likely than White women to seek late-term abortions (Lynxwiler & Wilson, 1994; Nsiah-Jefferson, 1989). The reasons for this are varied but are related to the decline in the number of providers, the general ambivalence and silence in the Black community on the issue of abortion, and the loss of Medicaid funding and the attendant difficulties this creates in raising money to pay for the service (Campbell, 1981; Henshaw & Van Vort, 1994; Torres & Forrest, 1988; Women of Color Partnership Program, 1992). Late abortions are also associated with greater financial costs and greater health and psychological risks (Lynxwiler & Wilson, 1994).

The conservative, narrowly focused, single-issue politics of the mainstream pro-choice movement also serves to perpetuate its predominantly White base and leadership. Responding to the allegation that Black women's lack of participation in the reproductive rights movement of the 1970s was due to their own lack of interest, Angela Davis (1981) asserted,

> The real meaning of the almost lily-white complexion of the abortion rights campaign was not to be found in the ostensibly myopic or underdeveloped consciousness among women of color. The truth lay buried in the ideological underpinnings of the birth control movement itself. (p. 203)

This statement is as relevant today as it was in the 1970s. In a defensive reaction to the numerous assaults on abortion rights, the current pro-choice movement has narrowed its agenda. Seeking greater popular support, the movement employs the language of "choice" and "personal freedom." Expunged are references to women's rights, social justice, and women's rightful claim to sexual autonomy. Commenting on the pro-choice movement's restricted political agenda, Fried (1990) wrote,

> A defensive stance implies we will settle for less. The decision to fight for choice as opposed to justice is a decision to appeal to those who already have choices. This keeps the visible movement white and middle class despite the fact that the abortion rights of poor women, of whom a disproportionate number are women of color, have been, and continue to be, the most vulnerable. (p. 6)

Indeed, there was no visible outcry or mobilization by the pro-choice movement in opposition to the passage of the Hyde Amendment in 1977, which eliminated federal Medicaid funding for abortion. It was not until the Webster decision in 1989, which prohibited abortions in public hospitals or private facilities that receive public funds, that the movement mobilized against legislation limiting access. This fact was not lost on women of color, who argue that the White-dominated pro-choice movement fails to act until the interests of White middle-class women become threatened (Redmond, 1990). Moreover, unlike the antiabortion movement, which has broadened its base by making links between abortion and many other issues such as school prayer, crime, and sexuality, the pro-choice movement has shied away from such alliances and in so doing has alienated several constituencies. In its singular and defensive emphasis on the right to "choice," the pro-choice movement has failed to connect abortion rights to struggles for basic health care, the AIDS epidemic and its devastating effects on communities of color, or the economic plight of poor women and women of color (Fried, 1990; Lee, 1990; Redmond, 1990).

Dismayed by the myopic vision of the dominant pro-choice movement and its marginalization of their concerns, Black women and other women of color have come together in mutual support and activism to construct a reproductive rights agenda of their own. In contrast to the dominant movement's emphasis on choice—that is, legal rights—women of color emphasize access and safeguards from abuse. For them, access is not only about access to safe and affordable abortions, but also access to basic health care services, prenatal care, birth control information and services, AIDS and drug rehabilitation services, and financial resources (Fried, 1990; Lee, 1990; Nsiah-Jefferson, 1989; Redmond, 1990; Roberts, 1990). The notion of choice advocated by the dominant White-led pro-choice movement is vacuous when the social and economic conditions within which women of color exercise reproductive choices are ignored. Dazon Dixon, director of Sisterlove, declared, "We can't have just choices; we have to have a way of accessing those choices" (cited in Redmond, 1990, p. 3).

For women of color involved in the multiracial pro-choice movement, protection of the reproductive rights of women with AIDS and maternal drug users is a central and growing concern, one they believe should have long ago been addressed by mainstream pro-choice organizations. The fear here is of punitive legal or medical action taken against such women in the name of "fetal rights." A recent trend is the sanctioning, through criminal proceedings, of women who give birth to infants that test positive for controlled substances. Legislation was proposed in Ohio, for example, that defined causing a child to be born drug addicted as second degree aggravated assault. A similar bill in South Carolina would charge pregnant women who test positive for illegal drugs with child abuse (Scott, 1992). Some judges are also allowing the prosecution of pregnant drug-addicted women for either child abuse or passing drugs to a minor (Berrien, 1990; Feringa, Iden, & Rosenfield, 1992). Such state intervention most severely threatens the lives and reproductive options of Black women, because they are significantly more likely than White women to be prosecuted for drug abuse while pregnant or of child abuse when newborns test positive for illegal substances (Scott, 1992). Moreover, Black women's greater dependency on public facilities and assistance make them more vulnerable to supervision and surveillance.

Currently, there is a dearth of drug treatment facilities, particularly those willing to accept pregnant women. Berrien (1990) cited examples of drug-addicted pregnant women who have sought but failed to find a drug treatment program that would admit them. Clearly, incarceration as a solution to maternal drug use is unlikely to result in healthier outcomes for either women or their newborns. Rather, as drug-addicted pregnant women seek to avoid legal penalties, they are less likely to seek help or prenatal care (Berrien, 1990; Roberts, 1990).

Similarly, AIDS infected women, the majority of whom are Black or Latina, face the potential of abuse. Routine testing and counseling of pregnant women seeking family planning services has been called for by the *Public Health Service Guidelines* (cited in Amaro, 1990). Such testing is confidential rather than anonymous. Anonymous testing would make test results available only to the individual being tested. Confidential testing, on the other hand, is likely to become part of an individual's medical record. All those who have access to these records, such as social workers or medical personnel, could gain knowledge of the test results. Given the hysteria surrounding AIDS and the trend toward privileging fetal rights over the rights of women, women at risk for HIV infection may fear punitive reactions, such as job loss, loss of custody of their children, coerced abortions, or legal sanctions for child abuse. Such fear is likely to deter women at risk from seeking prenatal and family planning services. On the other hand, pregnant women with AIDS who wish to terminate their pregnancy have been denied access to abortion services (Amaro, 1990; Henshaw, 1991). These threats to the reproductive rights of women with AIDS thus demand the attention of pro-choice organizations.

Women of color are also overwhelmingly the targets of coerced obstetrical interventions. Under the guise of child neglect statutes that equate a woman's refusal of a cesarean with fetal neglect, courts can mandate cesarean deliveries when requested by a physician as necessary to protect the health of the fetus and mother. One study found that 81% of women ordered by the courts to undergo such surgery were either Black, Hispanic, or Asian (cited in Daniels, 1990; Nsiah-Jefferson, 1989). Medical and judicial intervention in the name of fetal rights raise a number of legal and ethical issues. Nsiah-Jefferson (1989) addressed some of these when she wrote,

> A basic question is whether it is right to hold individual women responsible for poor outcomes at birth when many women are not able to live under healthful conditions. This topic thus implicates the general socioeconomic conditions poor women and women of color experience that result in lack of access to basic prenatal care, and advanced prenatal, perinatal, and neonatal technologies. Holding individual women responsible under present circumstances is morally unjust and diverts attention from the need to correct the serious inequities that permeate today's society. (p. 24)

BLACK WOMEN'S POLITICAL AGENDA AND ACTIVISM

A popular misconception is that Black women have little interest and hence, show little political activism around issues of reproductive rights.

This presumption, in part, reflects the fact that historical accounts of struggles for reproductive freedom tend to ignore the contributions of Blacks (Ross, 1992). Similarly, because abortion is not defined as a "minority issue," the mainstream media fail to seek out the views of Blacks on the abortion debate or to report on their activism in this regard (F. Brown, 1990).

However, a vibrant multiracial movement for reproductive freedom, sustained by numerous organizations like Sisterlove, the National Black Women's Health Project, the Multicultural Alliance for Reproductive Freedom, and the Women of Color Partnership Program, is underway and has sponsored a variety of forums, conferences, and conventions (Banks, 1986; Fried, 1990; Redmond, 1990). Yet their agenda and activities remain largely undocumented by the media establishment. Because of the inclusive political agenda of women of color, which is framed more in terms of basic health rights than abortion rights, much of the activism on behalf of reproductive freedom may not be defined as such. As discussed earlier, there are a variety of reasons for Black women's ambiguous stance toward abortion and toward the dominant White-led pro-choice movement. However, this should not be construed as a lack of concern for issues of reproductive freedom.

It is not necessarily the case that Black women place "race issues" ahead of reproductive rights issues. Rather, because race so structures the reproductive lives of Black women this distinction is unintelligible. Too often Black women are depicted as the passive victims of hegemonic elites who endeavor to control their fertility through population or eugenicist initiatives. It is such totalizing constructions of Black women that Ross (1992) and Rodrigue (1990) attempted to dispel in their discussions of Black women's long history of struggle for reproductive freedom.

These authors documented the support for family planning by the Black community during the 1920s. This support meshed with the efforts of Blacks to enhance the economic, political, and social status of Blacks. The Colored Women's Club Movement during this time, while denouncing the rampant sterilization of Black women, actively supported the establishment of family planning clinics in Black neighborhoods. In the 1950s it was Dorothy Brown, the first Black female general surgeon, who introduced in the Tennessee State Legislature the first bill to legalize abortion. In the context of the politics of population control in the mid-1960s, Black women made the distinction between birth control and population control and coopted racist family planning initiatives to serve their own interests. When Black men labeled family planning and abortion as genocide and closed down clinics in Cleveland and Pittsburgh, Black women organized to reopen them. With their right to reproductive freedom assailed on the right by the population control establishment and on the left by radical Black nationalists, Black women developed a novel perspective and holistic approach to the movement for reproductive rights. This legacy continues into the present and does much to inform contemporary race and gender politics.

SUMMARY AND CONCLUSION

In her discussion of African American women and abortion, Ross (1992) asserted, "The question is not *if* [Black women] support abortion, but *how*, and when, and why" (p. 141). As to the question why, Black women support abortion not because of its symbolic signification for gender politics but because of its practical necessity in their everyday lives. The research previously reviewed supports this judgment. The study I conducted in 1991 shows that attitudes toward sexual morality, gender roles, and family are weak predictors of Black women's abortion attitudes. Wilcox and Thomas (1992) finding that religiosity influences Black women's abortion attitudes but not their attitudes toward feminism is also consistent with this interpretation. Particularly significant is Lynxwiler and Gay's (1994) research demonstrating that Black women of childbearing age are as likely to be pro-choice as their White counterparts. We also know that married Black women are more likely to resolve pregnancy through abortion than are married White women, as are Black women who have had a previous live birth, regardless of marital status (Trent & Powell-Griner, 1991). The fact that Black married women, particularly those with children, are more likely than White women to be in the labor force and to be the primary source of family income may account for these racial differences in abortion use (Taeuber & Valdisera, 1986). The importance of economic realities to Black support for choice is further underscored by Hall and Ferree's (1986) finding that Blacks are more likely than Whites to view the inability to afford another child as a legitimate and compelling reason for a woman to seek an abortion. It appears then that racial differences in abortion attitudes are due to the greater opposition to legal abortions by Black men and older Black women.

It is not only concern about the economic consequences of unwanted pregnancy that spurs Black women's support for legalized abortion. As significant is the fact that any abridgment of reproductive freedom most severely impacts poor women and women of color. Historically, the criminalization of abortion has taken the worst toll on women of color, and can be expected to do so in the future (Carr & Wattleton, 1989; Nsiah-Jefferson, 1989; Ross, Ifill, & Jenkins, 1990). Prior to *Roe v. Wade* (1973), women of color constituted 64% of all deaths caused by illegal abortions. Since 1973, 80% of all women who have died from such abortions have been either Black or Puerto Rican (F. Brown, 1990; Christmas, 1981). Moreover, the context in which Black women live their lives continues to be characterized by coercive attempts to control their fertility, making reproductive freedom vital to their health and well-being. Collectively, these realities justify Ross's (1992) claim that "it was not persuasive analysis, arguments, or ideology that influenced African American women to support abortion. We did so because we needed to. Necessity was the midwife to our politics" (p. 144).

Although scholarship attempting to explicate racial differences in support for legal abortions is abundant, we have little knowledge or understanding of the forces dividing African Americans on this issue. Extant research does indicate that certain demographic characteristics such as education, occupation, place of residence, sex, and age exert some influence on the abortion attitudes of both Blacks and Whites. Likewise, attitudes toward sexuality, family, and gender roles are also relevant to the views of Blacks on legal abortion, though they are of less import than they are for Whites. As previously noted, Wilcox (1990, 1992) provided convincing evidence that the greater religiosity and religious fundamentalism of Blacks are important forces in structuring their opposition to legal abortion. Yet, a consistent finding is that the above factors, both individually and collectively, explain relatively little of the variance in the abortion attitudes of Blacks as compared with those of Whites. This indicates that there is a lot more at work in the structuring of Black's abortion attitudes about abortion than is captured by current research. Part of the problem here is that studies of the abortion attitudes of Blacks have been done primarily in the context of comparisons with Whites. Consequently, issues that may be unique to Black perspectives on abortion remain undetected. So what becomes the salient issue is how the abortion attitudes of Blacks, as well as the determinants of these attitudes, differ or are similar to those of Whites. A fuller understanding of the abortion debate in the Black community awaits the kind of in-depth probing of the worldviews of proponents and opponents of legal abortion such as those conducted by Luker (1984) and Gerson (1985).

In lieu of such research, a cursory sampling of the abortion debate in the Black community gleaned mostly from editorials in popular Black magazines provides some clues. Two themes are particularly recurring here. Consistent with Wilcox's (1990) contention, several commentators cite the strong religious background and religious fundamentalism of Blacks as at the core of their ambivalence toward abortion. The second theme is that of abortion as Black genocide (Bray, 1982; F. Brown, 1990; Campbell, 1981; Carr & Wattleton, 1989; Jackson, 1981; Lee, 1990; Malveaux, 1993; Smith, 1990). The following comment (cited in Lee, 1990) is representative:

> If we are for Black people we must be against abortion because it takes
> Black life. This is part of the population control motive—to keep the

Black and Latino populations at a minimum. We can't get equal hous-
ing. Black men can't get jobs. Yet look at the large amount of money
that is being spent solely to encourage Black women to have abortions.
(p. 51)

For some Black opponents, abortion is viewed as violating the very
principal that civil rights leaders strove so hard to achieve, that every life
is sacred and deserves equal protections and privileges under the law (Carr
& Wattleton, 1989; Jefferson, 1981). Black opponents reject the idea that
abortion can enhance the life chances of Blacks or solve the problems of
poverty, family disintegration, educational underachievement, or discrimination that they confront. Indeed, some view legal abortion as a threat to
Black family life because it promotes promiscuity, tells Black men that
pregnancy is a woman's concern and not theirs, and places individual self-
aggrandizement above the welfare of the black family and community
(Bray, 1982; Jefferson, 1981). However, even opponents argue for the necessity of sex education (F. Brown, 1990).

Black pro-choice advocates, like their opponents, also draw on the
history of reproductive abuse and genocidal attempts to control Black wom-
en's fertility to support their position. This history of abuse, they assert,
makes reproductive choice an absolute necessity. The dominant theme of
Black pro-choice advocates is the physical health and safety of Black
women, which any abrogation of their right to choose threatens. For them,
the charge of genocide is antithetical to the interests of Black women, and
antiabortion laws inherently discriminatory. This is so because Black
women, particularly teenagers, have higher proportions of unintended pregnancies than White women. And although their abortion rate is also
higher, Black women still deliver at over three times the rate of White
women (F. Brown, 1990). Because Black women seek abortions at a higher
rate than White women, and because they are significantly more likely to
die from illegal or self-induced abortions, antiabortion laws, contend pro-
choice advocates, are genocidal (Carr & Wattleton, 1989; F. Brown, 1990,
1991; Jackson, 1981; Lee, 1990; Strothers, 1989). While agreeing that legal
abortion is not the solution to the problems confronting the Black community, Blacks who support choice argue that laws that criminalize abortion will only exacerbate current conditions.

This limited review offers some insights as to the particularity of the
abortion debate in Black communities. The ideological context of the debate appears more grounded in the tradition and language of civil rights
than gender politics, though the opposing sides construe the meaning of
this legacy differently. The significance of Black women's ongoing history
of reproductive abuse is a dominant motif that informs the views of those
on both sides of the issue. As is the case for White opponents of legal
abortion, Black opponents also point to the threats to family that abortion
poses, though with a slightly different twist. Here the emphasis is not on

preserving traditional definitions of womanhood or gender roles, but on abortion as yet another force hostile to the stability of Black families. These commentaries further support the contention that, for Black women, abortion is primarily a practical consideration. They also indicate that the ideological context of the abortion debate in Black communities differs from that found in White communities, reflecting the specificity of their struggles against racism, particularly as manifested in the reproductive history of Black women.

By calling attention to the race and class context in which women exercise their reproductive options, women of color offer a wider vision of the conditions necessary for reproductive freedom. Regard for their agenda promises a more unified and potent abortion rights movement. When Medicaid will pay for sterilization but not for abortion, when Black women are significantly more likely than White women to "choose" sterilization as a method of contraception, when medical and legal actions in the name of fetal rights overwhelmingly coerce poor women and women of color to accept obstetrical interventions, racism and classism must become part of any agenda for reproductive freedom. As Fried (1990) remarked,

> Women of color are participating in the struggle for reproductive rights; women of color are prepared to take the leadership in the struggle for abortion rights so long as that struggle is not separated from other aspects of reproductive freedom. The struggle must be about women's survival in all of its breadth. (p. 13)

REFERENCES

Amaro, H. (1990). Women's reproductive rights in the age of AIDS. In M. G. Fried (Ed.), *From abortion to reproductive freedom: Transforming a movement* (pp. 245–254). Boston: South End Press.

Banks, J. (1986, December). Women of color forum stressed choice-education. *Off Our Backs*, p. 16.

Barnartt, S., & Harris, R. (1982). Recent changes in the predictors of abortion attitudes. *Sociology and Social Research*, 66, 320–334.

Berrien, J. (1990). Pregnancy and drug use: Incarceration is not the answer. In M. G. Fried (Ed.), *From abortion to reproductive freedom: Transforming a movement* (pp. 263–267). Boston: South End Press.

Blake, J., & Del Pinal, J. H. (1980). *Predicting polar attitudes toward abortion in the United States.* In J. Burtchaell (Ed.), Abortion parley (pp. 25–56). Kansas City, KS: Andrews & McNeel.

Bray, H. (1982, April). Abortion: One man's view. *Essence*, pp. 26–27.

Brown, F. D. (1990). More fuel for the abortion fire. *Black Enterprise*, 21, pp. 31–32.

Brown, F. D. (1991, April). We too must choose. *Essence*, pp. 26–27.

Brown, S. S., & Eisenberg, L. (Eds.). (1995). *The best of intentions*. Washington, DC: Institute of Medicine, National Academy Press.

Campbell, B. M. (1981, September). Abortion: The facts of life. *Essence*, pp. 86–130.

Carr, P., & Wattleton, F. (1989, October). Which way black America? Anti-abortion and pro choice. *Ebony*, pp. 134–138.

Cary, L. (1992, April). Why it's just not paranoia: An American history of "plans" for blacks. *Newsweek*, p. 23.

Centers for Disease Control and Prevention. (1994). Abortion surveillance: Preliminary data—United States, 1992. *Morbidity and Mortality Weekly Report, 43*, 930–939.

Christmas, J. J. (1981, October). Pro-choice is pro-life. *Encore American and Worldwide News*, pp. 14–16.

Cockburn, A. (1994). Social cleansing. *New Statesman and Society, 7*, 16–18.

Combs, M., & Welch, S. (1982). Blacks, whites, and attitudes toward abortion. *Public Opinion Quarterly, 46*, 510–520.

Conover, P., & Gray, V. (1983). *Feminism and the new right: Conflict over the American family*. New York: Praeger.

Cook, E., Jelen, T., & Wilcox, C. (1993). Generational differences in attitudes toward abortion. *American Politics Quarterly, 21*, 33–53.

Daniels, J. A. (1990). In M. G. Fried (Ed.), *Court-ordered caesareans: A growing concern for indigent women* (pp. 255–261). Boston: South End Press.

Davis, A. (1981). *Women, race and class*. New York: Random House.

Dugger, K. (1991). Race differences in the determinants of support for legalized abortion. *Social Science Quarterly, 72*, 570–587.

Feringa, B., Iden, S., & Rosenfield, A. (1992). Norplant: Potential for coercion. In S. E. Samuels & M. D. Smith (Eds.), *Norplant and poor women*. Menlo Park, CA: The Henry J. Kaiser Family Foundation.

Fried, M. G. (1990). Transforming the reproductive rights movements. In M. G. Fried (Ed.), *From abortion to reproductive freedom: Transforming a movement* (pp. 1–14). Boston: South End Press.

Gamble, V. N., & Houck, J. A. (1994). *A high voltage sensitivity: A history of African Americans and birth control*. Paper presented at the Committee on Unintended Pregnancy, Institute of Medicine, Washington, DC.

Gerson, K. (1985). *Hard choices: How women decide about work, career, and motherhood*. Berkeley, CA: University of California Press.

Gordon, L. (1977). *Woman's body, woman's right*. New York: Penguin.

Gordon, L., & Hunter, A. (1977). Sex, family and the new right: Anti-feminism as political force. *Radical America, 11*, 9–25.

Granberg, D. (1978). Pro-life or reflection of conservative ideology? An analysis of opposition to legalized abortion. *Sociology and Social Research, 62*, 414–429.

Granberg, D., & Granberg, B. (1980). Abortion attitudes, 1965–1980: Trends and determinants. *Family Planning Perspectives, 12,* 250–261.

Gump, P. (1980). The school as a social situation. *Annual Review of Psychology, 31,* 553–582.

Hall, E., & Ferree, M. M. (1986). Racial differences in abortion attitudes. *Public Opinion Quarterly, 50,* 193–207.

Harding, S. (1981). Family reform movements: Recent feminism and its opposition. *Feminist Studies, 7,* 57–75.

Hartmann, B. (1987). *Reproductive rights and wrongs: The global politics of population control and contraceptive choice.* New York: Harper & Row.

Henshaw, S. K. (1991). The accessibility of abortion services in the United States. *Family Planning Perspectives, 23,* 246–263.

Henshaw, S. K., & Van Vort, J. (1994). Abortion services in the United States. *Family Planning Perspectives, 26,* 100–112.

Hyde Amendment. Public Law 95-205, 95th Congress, Joint Resolution, H. R. Res. 662, December 9, 1997.

Jackson, J. (1981, December). Pro-choice is pro-life. *Encore American & Worldwide News,* pp. 14–16.

Jefferson, M. (1981, October). For-life—against abortion. *Encore American & Worldwide News,* pp. 18–19.

Lee, F. R. (1990, May). Empty womb. *Essence,* pp. 51–52.

Lewin, T. (1991, February 9). A plan to pay welfare mothers for birth control. *New York Times,* p. A10.

Littlewood, T. B. (1977). *The politics of population control.* Notre Dame, IN: University of Notre Dame Press.

Luker, K. (1984). *Abortion and the politics of motherhood.* Berkeley, CA: University of California Press.

Lynxwiler, J., & Gay, D. (1994). Reconsidering race differences in abortion attitudes. *Social Science Quarterly, 75,* 67–84.

Lynxwiler, J., & Wilson, M. (1994). A case study of race differences among late abortion patients. *Women and Health, 21,* 43–56.

Malveaux, J. (1993, February). Black America's abortion ambivalence. *Emerge,* pp. 33–34.

Nsiah-Jefferson, L. (1989). Reproductive laws, women of color, and low income women. *Women's Rights Law Reporter, 11,* 15–38.

Petchesky, R. P. (1984). *Abortion and a woman's choice: The state, sexuality, and reproductive freedom.* New York: Longman.

Plutzer, E. (1988). Work life, family life, and women's support of feminism. *American Sociological Review, 53,* 640–649.

Redmond, P. (1990). Women of color set agenda. *New Directions for Women, 19,* 1–8.

Rees, M. (1991, December 9). Shot in the arm. *The New Republic,* pp. 16–17.

Roberts, D. E. (1990). The future of reproductive choice for poor women and women of color. *Women's Rights Law Reporter, 12*, 56–67.

Rodman, H., Sarvis, B., & Walker, J. (1987). *The abortion question*. New York: Columbia University Press.

Rodrigue, J. M. (1990). The black community and the birth control movement. In E. C. DuBois & V. L. Ruiz (Eds.), *Unequal sisters: A multicultural reader in U.S. women's history* (pp. 333–342). London: Routledge.

Roe v. Wade, 410, U.S., 113 (1973).

Ross, L. J. (1990). Raising our voices. In M. G. Fried (Ed.), *From abortion to reproductive freedom: Transforming a movement* (pp. 139–143). Boston: South End Press.

Ross, L. J. (1992). African-American women and abortion: A neglected history. *Journal of Health Care for the Poor and Underserved, 3*, 274–284.

Ross, L. J. (1993). African-American women and abortion: 1800–1970. In S. M. Jones & A. P. Busia (Eds.), *Theorizing black feminism* (pp. 141–159). London: Routledge.

Ross, L. J., Ifill, S., & Jenkins, S. (1990). Emergency memorandum to women of color. In M. G. Fried (Ed.), *From abortion to reproductive freedom: Transforming a movement* (pp. 147–150). Boston: South End Press.

Sarvis, B., & Rodman, H. (1974). *The abortion controversy* (2nd ed.). New York: Columbia University Press.

Schulder, D., & Kennedy, F. (1971). *Abortion rap*. New York: McGraw-Hill.

Scott, J. R. (1992). Norplant and women of color. In S. E. Samuels & M. D. Smith (Eds.), *Norplant and poor women* (pp. 39–52). Menlo Park, CA: The Henry J. Kaiser Family Foundation.

Sears, D. O. (1988). Symbolic racism. In P. A. Katz & D. A. Taylor (Eds.), *Eliminating racism: Profiles in controversy* (pp. 53–84). New York: Plenum.

Sears, D. O. (1975). Political socialization. In F. I. Greenstein & N. W. Polsy (Eds.), *Handbook of Political Science* (Vol. 2, pp. 96–136). Reading, MA: Addison-Wesley.

Shapiro, T. (1985). *Population control politics: Women, sterilization and reproductive choice*. Philadelphia, PA: Temple University Press.

Smith, B. (1990). Choosing ourselves: Black women and abortion. In M. G. Fried (Ed.), *From abortion to reproductive freedom: Transforming a movement* (pp. 83–86). Boston: South End Press.

Solinger, R. (1992). *Wake up little Sussie: Single pregnancy and race before Roe v. Wade*. New York: Routledge.

Strothers, E. (1989, July). Our big choice. *Essence*, p. 116.

Taeuber, C., & Valdisera, V. (1986). *Women in the American Economy*. Washington: United States Government Printing Office.

Torres, A., & Forrest, J. D. (1988). Why do women have abortions. *Family Planning Perspectives, 20*, 169–176.

Trent, K., & Powell-Griner, E. (1991). Differences in Race, Marital Status, and

Education Among Women Obtaining Abortions. *Social Forces, 69,* 1121–1141.

Turner, P. A. (1993). *I heard it through the grapevine.* Berkeley, CA: University of California Press.

Walters, J. (1985). Parenthood is a question of free choice and there should be no societal pressure. In H. Feldman & M. Feldman (Eds.), *Current controversies in marriage and family* (pp. 183–192). Beverly Hills, CA: Sage.

Webster v. Reproductive Health Services, 492 U.S., 490 (1988).

Weisbord, R. G. (1975). *Genocide? Birth control and the black American.* Westport, CT: Greenwood Press.

Wilcox, C. (1990). Race differences in abortion attitudes: Some additional evidence. *Public Opinion Quarterly, 54,* 248–255.

Wilcox, C. (1992). Race, religion, region and abortion attitudes. *Sociological Analysis, 53,* 97–105.

Wilcox, C., & Thomas, S. (1992). Religion and feminist attitudes among African-American women: A view from the nation's capital. *Women & Politics, 12,* 19–40.

Willie, C. (1970). Institutional vitality and institutional alliances. *Sociology and Social Research, 54,* 249–259.

Women of Color Partnership Program. (1992). Women of color reproductive health poll. *Womens International Network News, 18,* 40.

6

LATINAS AND ABORTION

PAMELA I. ERICKSON AND CELIA P. KAPLAN

Although popular wisdom suggests that Latina women, being predominantly Catholic and highly invested in maternal roles, would tend not to use abortion (Amaro, 1988), recent statistics suggest that Latinas have a higher abortion rate than Whites (Henshaw & Silverman, 1988; Koonin, Smith, & Ramick, 1995).[1] This chapter investigates the use of abortion by Latina women in the United States. Our goal is to provide a broader understanding of the role of abortion in the fertility behavior of Latina women. To provide a context for interpretation of the statistical information on use of abortion by Latina women in the United States, we begin by describing the U.S. Latino population.

WHO ARE THE LATINOS LIVING IN THE UNITED STATES?

Latinos are the second largest and fastest growing ethnic group in the United States (Molina & Aguirre-Molina, 1994). Officially, they account

The authors thank Louise Badiane, Jong-In Lee, and Heidi Zavatone-Veth for their assistance in identifying and accumulating the bibliographic resources on abortion in Latin America and the United States. Special thanks go to Ms. Zavatone-Veth who summarized the literature available through 1992.
[1]*Latino/a* is the currently preferred term for persons previously described as Hispanic. The U.S. Bureau of the Census defines Hispanic (i.e., Latino) as those persons of Mexican, Puerto

for about 21.4 million Americans, almost 9% of the population. Despite the growing presence of Latinos in the United States, it was not until the 1980s that national, state, and local reporting systems began to designate Latino as a separate ethnicity, and data on their health and demographic characteristics became available.

The term *Latino* encompasses a wide variety of subgroups. The largest subgroups include persons of Mexican origin (63% of the Latino population), Puerto Ricans (11%), and Cubans (5%). The remaining 21% are primarily from Central and South America (Molina & Aguirre-Molina, 1994).

Most Latinos in the United States, about 61%, live in the southwest. In New Mexico, California, and Texas, Latinos make up more than 25% of each state's population. Here, persons of Mexican origin or descent are predominant. About 25% of the Latino population live in New York, New Jersey, Illinois, and Florida. In New York and New Jersey, Latinos tend to be of Puerto Rican origin; in Florida, Cubans predominate; and in Illinois, Latinos tend to be of Mexican origin or descent. The rest of the states have only small Latino populations.

Latinos, as a group, are a younger population than any other racial or ethnic group except Native Americans. The median age of Mexican Americans is 24.3 and of Puerto Ricans 26.7, compared with 33.7 for non-Latino Whites. In contrast, Cubans are an older group with a median age of 39.3 (Molina & Aguirre-Molina, 1994).

Latinas have higher fertility than non-Latinas. In 1990, the Latina birth rate was 93.2 per 1,000 women age 15 to 44, compared with 64.4 for non-Latinas (Molina & Aguirre-Molina, 1994).[2] Teenage childbearing is also higher among Latinas than among Whites, but lower than that among African Americans. Among the Latino subgroups, Puerto Ricans (21%) and Mexicans (17%) have the highest proportion of births to teen mothers, whereas Cubans have a lower proportion of teen births (7%) than do Whites (9%; Molina & Aguirre-Molina, 1994).

Latinos are more likely to live in poverty than Whites. Twenty-eight percent of Latinos live in poverty compared with 11% of Whites and 32% of African Americans (Molina & Aguirre-Molina, 1994). Of the Latino subgroups, the highest poverty rates are among Puerto Ricans (41%) and Mexicans (28%), and the lowest among Cubans (17%). Education completed mirrors poverty status with the lowest levels of educational attainment among Mexicans (especially the foreign born) and Puerto Ricans.

Rican, Cuban, Central or South American, or other Spanish culture or origin regardless of race (Molina & Aguirre-Molina, 1994). In this chapter we use the feminine form, *Latina*, when referring to women only and *Latino* when referring to both men and women.
[2]Comparisons by race or ethnic group are made in different ways in the different works cited. Unless a specific race or ethnic group is specified (e.g., non-Latina White, African American, etc.) the term *non-Latina* covers all other groups in the study.

In summary, Latinos in the United States are a varied group, with distinct differences in geographic distribution, age structure, fertility behavior, and socioeconomic status by subgroup. Because the Latino population is a young population, patterns of fertility control in this group will affect American society substantially in the future. Having a clear understanding of abortion use among Latinas is important for the delivery of reproductive health and family planning services to the fastest growing ethnic group in the United States today.

In the following discussion, we provide an overview of abortion use patterns among Latinas from published data and from original analyses of abortion use by Latino subgroups based on estimates from the Hispanic Health and Nutrition Examination Survey (H-HANES).[3] We then discuss cultural perspectives on abortion, including the ways in which gender, religion, country of origin, and class influence Latinas' use of abortion. We conclude the chapter by outlining priorities for future research on Latina abortion and by describing the reproductive health implications of U.S. Latina abortion patterns.

ABORTION AMONG LATINAS IN THE UNITED STATES

Reliable statistical information on legal abortion in the United States has been available since 1969 when the Centers for Disease Control and Prevention (CDC) began surveillance of the number and characteristics of women obtaining legal abortions from 52 reporting areas: the 50 states, the District of Columbia, and New York City. The other major source of information on abortion in the United States is the Alan Guttmacher Institute's (AGI)[4] periodic survey of all identified abortion providers in the United States (for more information see Henshaw, chap. 3, in this volume). Abortion data are reported by race, but until recently, information on the use of abortion by Latinas was unavailable. In the late 1980s, AGI began to include information on Latina ethnicity on its surveys, and in 1990,

---

[3] The H-HANES was undertaken by the National Center for Health Statistics between 1982 and 1984 to obtain a representative sample of 12,000 Latinos from three geographic regions in the United States: (a) Mexican Americans in the Southwest (Arizona, California, Colorado, New Mexico, and Texas), (b) Puerto Ricans in the New York metropolitan area, and (c) Cuban Americans in Dade County, Florida. The survey is estimated to be representative of about 76% of the 1980 civilian, noninstitutionalized Latino population between the ages of 6 months and 74 years.

[4] The Alan Guttmacher Institute (AGI), an independent, nonprofit, corporation for research, policy analysis, and public education, has conducted a periodic survey of abortion providers in the United States since 1973 to monitor the availability of abortion services and to collect information about abortion providers and the services they offer. The survey produces the most complete count of the number of abortions performed in the United States, by state, metropolitan area, and county (AGI, 1992). The Centers for Disease Control and Prevention (CDC) reports consistently identify fewer abortions than the AGI surveys. For example, the 1988 CDC count was 86% of the AGI count. This is thought to be due largely to incomplete reporting and to nonrequired reporting of abortions in some states.

CDC data on Latina women became available for 20 of the 52 reporting areas.

According to AGI's 1987 survey of abortion providers, an estimated 13% of abortion patients in the United States were Latina (Henshaw & Silverman, 1988). The abortion index for Latina women (1.44) fell between that of Whites (0.83) and non-Whites (1.80), and controlling for age did not change these results (Henshaw & Silverman, 1988).[5]

The most recent published data from CDC are for 1991.[6] In that year, the abortion rate was 24 per 1,000 women 15 to 44 years of age, and the abortion ratio was 339 per 1,000 live births (Koonin et al., 1995). Twenty states, the District of Columbia, and New York City reported abortion data by Hispanic ethnicity.[7] These areas account for only 44% of Latina women of reproductive age (Koonin et al., 1995). Nevertheless, in these reporting areas, 13% of all abortions were to Latina women, identical to the AGI results (Henshaw & Silverman, 1988). The abortion ratio for Latinas was 300 per 1,000 live births, slightly lower than the ratio for non-Latinas in the same reporting areas (332 per 1,000 live births). The abortion rate, however, was somewhat higher for Latina (28 per 1,000) women than that for non-Latina women (22 per 1,000; Koonin et al., 1995). The percentage of abortions by 5-year age groups was almost identical for Latina and non-Latina women. A slightly greater proportion of abortions among Latinas was to married women (26.3%) than among non-Latinas (21.3%). The majority of abortions in both groups was to unmarried women (Koonin et al., 1995).

The AGI study included information on contraceptive use for 1,900 abortion patients. The higher use of abortion among Latinas appears to be due to their lesser use of contraception overall and to greater reliance on less effective methods. Fifty-eight percent of Latina women who had had an abortion were not using a method of birth control, compared with 42% of White women. More than 33% of the never-married Latina adolescents under age 18 who had had an abortion had never used contraception,

---

[5] The two abortion statistics most commonly reported are the *abortion rate* (the number of abortions per 1,000 women of childbearing age) and the *abortion ratio* (the number of abortions per 1,000 births). The *abortion index* is the ratio of the proportion of women who had abortions to their proportion in the population, and approximates the abortion rate.

[6] The CDC information comes from central health agencies in 45 states, the District of Columbia, and New York City. In the other five areas the data come from hospitals and other medical facilities.

[7] States reporting Latina ethnicity include Arizona, Arkansas, Georgia, Idaho, Kansas, Mississippi, Nevada, New Jersey, New Mexico, New York, North Dakota, Oregon, Pennsylvania, Rhode Island, South Carolina, Tennessee, Texas, Utah, Vermont, and Wisconsin. Three states with large Latino populations—California, Colorado, and Illinois—do not report abortion statistics by Latina ethnicity. Lack of reporting from California is notable, both because California has the highest abortion ratio and rate of all the states reporting (Koonin et al., 1995) and because over one quarter (25.8%, more than 7.5 million people) of the state's population is Latino (1990 Census). Thus, the CDC abortion statistics for Latina women may not be representative of the overall Latino population in the United States, although they are, in fact, quite similar to those of the 1987 AGI study.

compared with more than 25% of White adolescents. Among those using contraception when they became pregnant, Latina women (12.3%) were more likely than White women (6.7%) to be using the rhythm method, and more likely (12.4%) than White women (11.9%) to be using withdrawal (Henshaw & Silverman, 1988).

Analysis of the AGI survey also suggested that Latina women generally use abortion to end childbearing (Torres & Forrest, 1988). This interpretation is supported by several studies on the use of abortion among young Latina women that used data from the National Longitudinal Survey, Youth Cohort (NLSY). These studies all reported that young Latinas were less likely to abort than their non-Latina White counterparts (Cooksey, 1990; King, Myers, & Byrne, 1992; Stevans, Register, & Sessions, 1992). For example, Cooksey (1990) found that in a sample of 1,946 women under 24 years of age at first conception in the 1979 to 1986 rounds of the NLSY, the Latina women had a lower rate of abortion (24% of pregnancies were terminated) than non-Latina Whites (37%) but a higher rate than African Americans (13%). This study also found that higher parental education was a strong predictor of abortion among young Latina women (Cooksey, 1990).

Although these studies support the idea that Latina women may use abortion to end childbearing, the analysis presented by Cooksey (1990) suggests that socioeconomic status (as measured by parental education) also has a significant effect on young, unmarried Latina women's pregnancy resolution decisions (i.e., the higher the socioeconomic status, the more likely abortion will be chosen). As a further caution to interpretation of these data, Jones and Forrest (1992) found that abortion reporting in the NLSY surveys was "highly deficient" and that Whites were more likely to report abortions than non-Whites.

In summary, the results from the CDC and AGI surveys are quite similar and suggest that use of abortion by Latina women in the United States is intermediate between the lower rate of Whites and the higher rate of non-Whites. There appear to be no differences regarding age, although there is some indication that Latina women who abort are slightly more likely to be married than non-Latina Whites, and they may be more likely to use abortion to end childbearing. Finally, Latina adolescents are less likely than White teens to have had an abortion. This is consistent with data suggesting that Latinas use abortion more frequently to end than to delay childbearing. At least one study found that Latina adolescents of higher socioeconomic status were more likely to abort than those of lower socioeconomic status. Because, in general, Latinas are overrepresented in lower socioeconomic groups, overall abortion trends among Latinas may mask significant variation in adolescent abortion use by socioeconomic class.

Use of Abortion by Latina Subgroups

Very little is known about differences in use of abortion among subgroups of Latinas in the United States (Amaro, 1988; Aneshensel, Becerra, & Fielder, 1990; Fennelly, 1993; Joyce, 1988). Fertility differences by subgroup are marked, however. For example, women of Mexican origin in the United States have the highest mean numbers of children born in both first (2.74) and second or later generations (2.34). Puerto Rican women have a high first-generation mean (2.53), but a mean (1.59) lower than that of non-Latina Whites (1.83) for second or later generation. Cuban women have rates for both first generation (1.66) and second or later generation (0.67) lower than those of non-Latina Whites (Bean & Tienda, 1987).[8] It is likely that aggregate statistics on use of abortion by Latina women in the United States, like aggregate statistics on fertility variables, mask subgroup differences and may reflect patterns of use of abortion in the largest Latino group (i.e., those of Mexican origin).

There are, however, very few studies that address the use of abortion by Latina women that separate statistical information by subgroup. Those studies that do exist tend to use small-scale, geographically distinct samples, and to address particular age groups or clinic populations. Many limit study to adolescents. Thus, important subgroup differences may be masked by use of aggregate data on Latinas, and studies of selected populations or age groups, while providing important insights into abortion in these groups, are not generalizable to other Latina subgroups or age groups. Keeping these caveats in mind, we summarize the literature available on use of abortion by Latina subgroups.

Mexican American Women's Use of Abortion

Existing studies tend to show that Mexican women do not differ greatly from White women in their use of abortion. In one study of women along the United States–Mexican border, 24% of Mexican compared with 28% of non-Latina White women reported having had an abortion (Rochat, Warren, Smith, Holck, & Friedman, 1981). A study in a family planning clinic in Texas with a predominantly Mexican American (81%) clientele found that among 471 women with positive pregnancy tests in 1975 to 1976, 46% aborted (Urdaneta, 1980). After the Hyde Amendment restricting public funding of abortion, the proportion of pregnancies aborted dropped to 24% in 1978. This is ironic, as Urdaneta (1980) reported that economic hardship was a primary reason for abortion among the clinic clients she studied.

---

[8]In most of these fertility studies, the Cuban population represented is that of the Cuban refugees and their descendants who immigrated after the 1959 Cuban Revolution rather than the more recently arrived immigrants.

Among adolescents, abortion appears to be used less often by Mexican American than by non-Latina White teens (Aneshensel et al., 1990; Rochat et al., 1981). In a study of 450 Latina teen mothers under age 18, delivering at a public hospital in East Los Angeles, only 2% had had an abortion before having their first child (Erickson, Ovalle, Diaz, Gillette, & Martorana, 1995). Follow-up with 145 teen mothers still in family planning care 12 months postpartum, however, suggested that abortion was more acceptable for a rapid repeat pregnancy. Among 23 teens faced with an unintended pregnancy within 1 year of a birth, 6 teens (26%) had a therapeutic abortion (Erickson et al., 1995). Another study of young, primarily Mexican-origin Latina women using state-funded Family Planning clinics in Los Angeles also found very low rates of prior abortion (Kaplan & Erickson, 1996). Of 1,411 women age 18 to 24 interviewed, 93% had been pregnant one or more times, but only 7% reported having had a therapeutic abortion. U.S.-born Latinas in this study were more likely to have had an abortion (13%) than were those born in Central America (6%) or Mexico (4%; Kaplan & Erickson, 1996).

In summary, attitudes about and use of abortion among Mexican-origin women appear to be similar to that of non-Latina Whites. Unlike Whites, however, Mexican-origin adolescents appear to use abortion less to resolve unintended pregnancy. This suggests that among Mexican-origin women, abortion may be used primarily to control fertility or space children after having at least one child. Some of these studies suggest that acculturation, education, and socioeconomic status may mediate abortion decisions among Mexican Americans.

Puerto Rican Women's Use of Abortion

Several older studies in New York indicate that Puerto Rican women are less likely to terminate a pregnancy and more likely to hold more negative attitudes regarding induced abortion than non-Latina Whites in the United States (Borras, 1984; Gold, Erhardt, Jacobziner, & Nelson, 1965; Parker & Nelson, 1971, 1973; Steinhoff, 1973). Use of abortion by White women from 1943 to 1962 in New York City was 26 times that of Puerto Rican women (Gold et al., 1965). Following legalization of abortion in New York in 1970, Parker and Nelson (1971) found that the ratio of abortions to live births over a 9-month period was much lower for Puerto Rican women than for Whites and non-Whites, but nowhere near the magnitude of the years prior to legalization: 422 per 1,000 for White, 594 for non-White, and 258 for Puerto Rican women. Parker and Nelson (1973) later analyzed data on abortions from 1970 to 1973 in New York City and found similar results. The abortion ratio for Puerto Ricans was 250 per 1,000 live births compared with 373 for Whites and 563 for non-Whites (Parker & Nelson, 1973).

A more recent study of adolescent use of abortion in New York City suggested that White teens in the sample were the most likely to abort, followed by African Americans, Puerto Ricans, and other non-Puerto Rican Latinas (Joyce, 1988). Among the non-Puerto Rican Latina teenagers, Cuban teens were the most likely and Mexican teens the least likely to abort (Joyce, 1988). Another study found that Puerto Rican adolescents who chose to have an abortion were more religious and had less family support (Ortiz & Nuttall, 1987). The authors suggested that the seeming paradox regarding religiosity was explained by the fact that an "unpublicized" abortion allowed continuation of church attendance. In sum, there is only limited and somewhat dated information on Puerto Rican women that suggests they use abortion less often and may also be less approving of abortion than Whites.

Cuban Women's Use of Abortion

There is almost no information about Cuban American women's use of abortion. One study in Miami suggested that, whereas Cuban women had the least favorable attitudes about abortion, they had used abortion more than other Latina, African American, and non-Latina White women in the study (Linn, Carmichael, Klitenick, Webb, & Gurel, 1978). As indicated above, among adolescents in New York City, Cubans were more likely than Mexicans, but less likely than Puerto Ricans, to abort (Joyce, 1988).

The studies that are available suggest that Cubans are more similar to non-Latina Whites in their fertility patterns, but their use of abortion may be higher than that of both other Latinas and non-Latina Whites. Puerto Ricans and Mexicans have higher fertility than both Cubans and non-Latina Whites, and they tend to use abortion less. Among adolescents, Mexicans use abortion less than other Latinas. Use of abortion among Mexican women, thus, may tend to occur at older ages as a means of ending childbearing. The studies addressing Latina adolescent fertility behavior suggest the importance of generation in the United States, level of acculturation or assimilation into American society, and socioeconomic status as mediators of abortion use.

ESTIMATING ABORTION FROM THE H-HANES

Because so little information was available on use of abortion by Latina subgroup, we analyzed data from the 1982 to 1984 H-HANES to estimate use of abortion by Latinas of different heritage. The Adult Supplement to the H-HANES included reproductive information for 4,365 Latina women age 18 to 74, 60% of whom were Mexican American, 26%

Puerto Rican, and 14% Cuban. The H-HANES contains information on demographic and reproductive variables.[9] Respondents were only asked to report live births, spontaneous abortions, and still births, and we computed therapeutic abortion from these data, excluding currently pregnant women.[10] This calculation estimates lifetime abortions at the time of the interview. The data presented here are weighted.[11]

Table 1 provides demographic characteristics of the sample of 4,365 women. Cubans were slightly older than the other groups, having fewer women in the under 30 age groups—a reflection of the older age structure of Cubans in the United States. Puerto Rican women (39%) were less likely to be married than Mexican (59%) and Cuban (62%) women. The majority of both Mexicans (64%) and Puerto Ricans (60%) had less than 12 years of schooling, compared with about half (51%) of Cubans. Cubans had the largest proportion who had attended college.

Cubans also had the highest proportion of foreign-born (91%) and primarily Spanish-speaking (41%) women, reflecting their older age structure and migration patterns from Cuba after the revolution. About two thirds of Puerto Ricans (62%) were born on the island, but less than one fifth were primarily Spanish speaking (19%). Mexicans had the lowest proportion of foreign-born women (31%) and the highest proportion of primarily English-speaking (53%) women. All of the groups had a majority with English-speaking or bilingual ability, however.

About 75% of each group had been pregnant and given birth at least once. About 33% of each group had had a spontaneous abortion. Stillbirth was slightly more prominent among Mexican (4.2%) and Puerto Rican (4.1%) women than among Cubans (1.1%).

Among the ever-pregnant women in the sample, the Mexican women were the least likely of the three groups to have had a therapeutic abortion. Only 12% of the Mexican women compared with 30% of Puerto Rican and 32% of the Cuban women had had an abortion. The Cuban women were the most likely to have had two or more therapeutic abortions (see Table 2). The ratio of abortions to pregnancies suggests that only 3% of pregnancies among Mexican American women were terminated compared

---

[9]Demographic variables of interest included age at interview, marital status, number of years of education completed, ethnic identity, language preference, and poverty status (above or below the official U.S. poverty level). Reproductive history variables included number of pregnancies, live births, still births, and spontaneous abortions and whether the respondent was currently pregnant.

[10]The number of therapeutic abortions was calculated as follows: number of pregnancies resolved by the time of the interview minus the number of live births plus the number of still births plus the number of spontaneous abortions. The formula may underestimate abortion because of multiple gestation (e.g., twins), which was not distinguished in the data set.

[11]In the sampling design for the H-HANES, each respondent does not represent the same number of individuals in the population due to oversampling and undersampling of certain age groups. All results presented are weighted with the weights provided in the H-HANES Public Use Data Tape.

TABLE 1
Demographic Characteristics of the Sample:
H-HANES Weighted Percentages

Variable	Mexican (n = 2,619)	Puerto Rican (n = 1,149)	Cuban (n = 597)
Age at time of interview			
<19	20.4	21.5	11.5
20–29	29.0	26.2	16.9
30–39	21.9	22.6	21.8
40–49	11.9	15.5	18.8
50–59 and over	16.8	14.1	31.1
Marital status			
Single	24.1	35.5	17.3
Married	58.8	38.8	61.7
Widowed/separated/divorced	17.0	25.8	21.1
Years of education			
<6 years	27.3	15.6	22.3
7–11 years	36.9	44.3	28.6
12 years	22.3	25.4	25.4
>13	13.5	14.7	23.7
Place of birth			
Foreign born	31.1	62.0	91.4
U.S. born	68.9	38.0	8.6
Language ability			
Primarily Spanish	21.6	18.8	40.6
About equal	25.1	39.0	43.7
Primarily English	53.3	42.2	15.8
Ever pregnant	74.3	73.1	75.1
Ever have abortion	12.0	30.1	32.1

Note. H-HANES = Hispanic Health and Nutrition Examination Survey.

with 11% of those to Puerto Rican women and 23% of those to Cuban women.

Table 2 shows the proportion of women ever having had an abortion at the time of the survey by 10-year age groups. In all age groups, Mexican women had the lowest proportion having terminated a pregnancy, half or less of the proportion among Puerto Ricans and Cubans for all groups but those under age 20. Only among Cubans was there a high use of abortion among women 50 years and older at the time of the survey. This is consistent with migration patterns from Cuba after the revolution and the trend to use abortion to control fertility in Cuba documented by Henshaw (1990).

Among all three Latina groups there appears to be a trend toward greater use of abortion among women in the younger age groups. The increase appears to be strongest among women under age 30 at the time of the interview. These women would have been in their 20s or younger at the time abortion was legalized in the United States in 1973, and this

TABLE 2
Estimated Number of Abortions by Demographic Characteristic Among Ever-Pregnant Women (Weighted Percentages): 1982 to 1984

Variable	Mexican (*n* = 2,619)	Puerto Rican (*n* = 1,149)	Cuban (*n* = 597)
Percentage of each subgroup having had an abortion			
Age	(*n* = 1,887)	(*n* = 821)	(*n* = 439)
<19	32.8	48.1	49.2
20–29	21.4	48.1	47.3
30–39	10.6	26.2	29.6
40–49	5.0	19.8	22.8
50 and over	1.6	15.5	34.3
Marital status	(*n* = 1,871)	(*n* = 814)	(*n* = 437)
Single	35.1	50.0	48.7
Married	10.6	25.5	29.6
Widowed/separated	9.0	23.2	36.6
Years of education	(*n* = 1,859)	(*n* = 809)	(*n* = 436)
0–6	8.2	20.3	30.1
7–11	12.0	30.8	38.9
12	13.6	29.0	30.1
>12	17.1	36.8	28.7
Birth place	(*n* = 1,871)	(*n* = 805)	(*n* = 436)
U.S. born	12.3	45.1	43.3
Foreign/Island born	11.1	23.6	31.1
Language preference	(*n* = 1,756)	(*n* = 714)	(*n* = 413)
Mostly Spanish	10.3	21.6	34.5
About equal	7.2	25.8	29.5
Mostly English	15.2	41.7	33.1
Number of abortions			
None	88.0	69.9	67.9
One	10.1	18.3	15.8
Two or more	1.9	11.8	16.3

may have been a factor in their increased use of abortion over women in older cohorts.

It should be noted that almost 50% of the ever-pregnant Puerto Rican and Cuban teens and almost 33% of ever-pregnant Mexican teens had had an abortion. About 15% of both Mexican (13.7%) and Puerto Rican (14.7%) adolescents had been pregnant compared with less than 5% of Cuban teens (4.4%). This indicates a significant need for family planning services and encouragement of contraceptive use among Latina adolescents, especially among those of Mexican and Puerto Rican origin. The proportion having had an abortion among Cuban and Puerto Rican women in their 20s was almost identical to that of teenagers (about 50%), further indicating the need to target family planning efforts to young Latina women. Among the Mexican women, the proportion in their 20s having had an abortion was less than half that of the other two groups. Only about 20% of ever-pregnant Mexican women in their 20s had had an abortion, and the proportion having had an abortion dropped off rapidly among Mexican women in the older age groups, unlike Cubans and Puerto Ricans.

Single women accounted for the largest proportion of ever-pregnant women who had had an abortion in all three groups. About 50% of single Puerto Rican and Cuban women compared with about 33% of single Mexican women had had an abortion. Among married women, Mexicans had the lowest proportion (10%) who had had an abortion. Among married Puerto Rican and Cuban women about 25% had had an abortion.

Among Mexicans and Puerto Ricans, women with a higher completed education level, a proxy for socioeconomic status, were more likely to have had an abortion than those with less education. Mexican women with less than a 12th-grade education were about one third less likely than Cubans and Puerto Ricans of the same education level to have had an abortion. Although the gap between Mexican women and the other two groups narrows with increasing education level attained, at all levels Mexican women were less likely to have availed themselves of therapeutic abortion than were Cuban or Puerto Rican women.

Among Cubans and Puerto Ricans, mainland U.S.-born women were more likely than island-born women to have had an abortion. Among Mexican women, there was no apparent difference between U.S.-born and foreign-born women in their use of abortion. Among Cuban women, there was no apparent difference in the use of abortion among Spanish speakers, bilinguals, and English speakers. Among Puerto Rican women, there was a greater tendency for English speakers to have had an abortion. Among Mexican women, bilingual women seem to have been the least likely to have had an abortion, although the differences among the language groups were not at all large.

In sum, these data suggest that there are differences in the use of abortion among these three Latina groups, illustrating the need to disaggregate Latina subgroups in the analysis of reproductive data. The Mexican women in this sample were the least likely to have used abortion, Cubans the most likely, and Puerto Ricans intermediate. The mean number of live births among the three groups followed an opposite pattern, with Mexicans having the highest mean, Cubans the lowest, and Puerto Ricans intermediate. The total number of pregnancies among Mexican and Puerto Rican women was similar, but was lower among Cubans. In all, then, Mexican women have higher fertility and use abortion less; Puerto Rican women have intermediate fertility, use abortion more than Mexican women, and rely on abortion to keep their fertility low; and Cubans have the lowest fertility of all three groups and use abortion the most, keeping their fertility lowest of all groups.

LATINOS' ATTITUDES TOWARD ABORTION

There have been only a few studies of abortion attitudes among Latinos in the United States. In a 1985 Harris poll, 47% of Latinos approved of the *Roe v. Wade* (1973) decision, only slightly lower than the proportion of non-Latino Whites who did so (51%), and higher than the 42% of African Americans who favored the decision (Rossi & Sitaraman, 1988). Approval rates among Latinos were identical to those among Catholics (47%), which were slightly lower than those of Protestants (49%) but higher than those for White, born-again Christians (31%). They were also more similar to those with high school education or less (49% and 32%, respectively) compared with those with a college education (62% of those with some college and 67% of college graduates).

A telephone survey of 341 Whites, African Americans, and Latinos in New York City indicated that Latinos (51%) were less likely than Whites (79%) or African Americans (77%) to say that it would be all right for information about abortion to be included in sex education programs (Namerow & Philliber, 1983). Another study including abortion attitudes suggested that Mexican Americans were more conservative than non-Latino Whites or African Americans regarding approval of abortion for reasons of poverty (34% of Mexican Americans *vs.* 51% of Whites and 40% of African Americans); being unmarried (26% of Mexican Americans *vs.* 48% of Whites and 33% of African Americans); and wanting no more children (25% of Mexican Americans *vs.* 45% of Whites and 37% of African Americans). Mexican Americans were similar to non-Latino Whites and more liberal than African Americans, however, in approving abortion for reasons of maternal health (86% of Mexican Americans *vs.* 90% of Whites and 80% of African Americans); fetal defect (77% of Mexican Americans *vs.* 83% of Whites and 65% of African Americans); and in cases of rape or incest (77% of Mexican Americans *vs.* 82% of Whites and 65% of African Americans; Darabi, Namerow, & Philliber, 1983).

Another study of 137 Mexican American women in a community health center in East Los Angeles found that the women favored abortion for fetal abnormalities (72%), for maternal life or health reasons (71%), and in cases of rape (64%; Amaro, 1988). They were much less likely to favor abortion for social and economic reasons. About one third approved of abortion when the family is economically unable to support the child (37%), when the pregnancy is unwanted (34%), and when the mother is not married or in union (29%). These women indicated that the people most likely to influence their decision regarding having an abortion were their husbands or boyfriends (69%), their own mothers (41%), physicians (34%), and friends (32%). About 25% of the ever-pregnant respondents in the sample had thought about having an abortion at some time in their lives, although only 14% of the women had ever had an abortion (Amaro, 1988).

Aviaro (1981) characterized attitudes toward abortion in a study of 120 Mexican women in Los Angeles as falling into three general categories: those who were unwavering in their opposition to abortion even if the woman's life were threatened; those who were completely pro-choice; and the largest group, those who approved for maternal health, fetal defect, or rape and incest.

The results for Mexican Americans in each of these studies parallel those of opinion polls in Mexico, where there is also high approval of abortion in cases of threat to maternal health, for fetal defects, and in cases of rape or incest, but much lower approval for socioeconomic reasons (Nuñez-Fernández, Shrader-Cox, & Benson, 1994). The extent to which attitudes of Mexican Americans reflect those of Puerto Ricans and Cubans is not known.

CULTURAL PERSPECTIVES ON ABORTION

The stereotype of Latina women is that they are "dominated by Catholic doctrine, passive in fertility decisions, and desirous of large families" (Amaro, 1988, p. 6). Women are socialized for the wife and mother role from an early age and taught to value others before themselves. Williams (1990), in her study of the Mexican American family, described this traditional, religion-based cultural pattern as follows:

> It was taken for granted that all men and women would marry and have children, and many did so in their teens. This was reinforced by the Catholic Church, where marriage and childbearing are considered to be part of God's plan for human beings. Marriage was vital, for homemaking and the bearing of children were considered the ultimate fulfillment of a woman's life in this world. (p. 27)

In the United States, Latina women tend to enter into marriage and childbearing at earlier ages, and to want and to have more children than White women (Bean & Tienda, 1987; Marin, Gerardo, & Padilla, 1981; Molina & Aguirre-Molina, 1994). Indeed, by age 20, 34% of Latinas are already married (Fennelly, 1993). Family is thought to be extremely important to Latinos, and men and women adhere to traditional gender roles to a greater extent than do Anglo Americans. These family patterns are reinforced by *machismo*, respect, and the subordination of younger to older persons (Pavich, 1986). Although these stereotyped versions of gender behavior are still influential in Latino culture throughout Latin America and the United States, changes in socioeconomic realities necessitating female labor participation, lower fertility norms, the emergence of an educated

Latino middle class, the feminist movement, and exposure and to the more egalitarian gender norms characteristic of the United States result in great variation in actual gender behavior among Latinos. Thus, although family and children are important to Latinas, as they are to women in every culture, Latinas are less defined by their fertility today than they were in the past.

Latina women are also thought to hold religious values that buttress the primacy of the wife/mother role and that "promote attitudes favorable to continuous childbearing, opposition to contraception, and opposition to abortion" (Amaro, 1988, p. 6). Several studies do suggest that birth control is rarely used before the first birth, but becomes more acceptable for child spacing and to end childbearing (Erickson, 1994; Erickson & Scrimshaw, 1985; Kay, 1978; Shedlin & Hollerbach, 1981). Most Latinos, indeed most Catholics, are not opposed to contraception and readily disregard the Church's teaching on contraception. In fact, fertility patterns of Catholics and Protestants have converged (Goldscheider & Mosher, 1991; Mosher, Williams, & Johnson, 1992), and attitudes of American Catholics toward abortion are similar to those of the general population (Rossi & Sitaraman, 1988).

As we have already seen, the limited information available on Latinos' attitudes toward abortion suggests that the majority of Latinos are not opposed to abortion under all circumstances, the official position of the Catholic Church, but generally approve of abortion in cases of threat to maternal or fetal health and in cases of rape. There tends to be less approval of abortion for socioeconomic reasons, yet these are the reasons Latina women undergoing abortion cite most often for actually having an abortion. Thus, overall, Latino attitudes toward abortion tend to be more similar to those of the general American population than to those of the Catholic Church. Moreover, despite the hegemony of Catholicism among Latinos in the United States and in Latin America, Latina women throughout the Americas do use abortion to limit their fertility. And, in all but a few countries where abortion is legal, they do so at great risk to their health and well-being, especially if they are poor (Frejka & Atkin, 1990; Henshaw, 1990; Paxman, Rizo, Brown, & Benson, 1993).[12] Broader changes in lifestyle accompanying the modernization process in Latin America and the immigration process in the United States (i.e., urbanization, female labor

---

[12]With the exception of Cuba and Puerto Rico, which have abortion on demand like the United States, abortion is highly restricted by law in every other country in Latin America, which limits its practice to saving the life or health of a woman (Henshaw, 1990; Paxman et al., 1993). Yet, since the 1960s, abortion has played an important role in fertility reduction throughout Latin America, accounting for as much as 25% of the reduction in fertility in the region over the past three decades (Frejka & Atkin, 1990). Although it is difficult to obtain accurate data, it is estimated that there are between 4 and 5 million abortions in Latin America annually; that between 25% and 33% of all pregnancies in Latin America are

force participation in a cash economy, lower fertility, emphasis on education and employment, exposure to Anglo American culture) are changing the traditional cultural and religious values that perpetuated large families, traditional gender roles, and opposition to contraception and abortion.

Earlier in this century, there was contentious debate over the morality of contraception. Today, all but a minority of very religious persons approve of contraception. The current debate over abortion is an extension of the debate about contraception, the right of women to control their fertility, and the role of women in society. Most people in the United States already approve of abortion in cases of rape, incest, and threat to the woman's health. With increasing education levels among the general population and with increasing secularization of society, attitudes toward abortion are becoming more liberal in the United States and in Latin America. In a world of imperfect contraceptive methods and imperfect method use, women (and men) will be faced with unintended pregnancy. Abortion is used because it is the only acceptable means of limiting fertility after conception.[13]

Cultural values and attitudes change, albeit slowly, to catch up to changed behavior patterns. We are currently in the painful transition period between traditional religious values generated in a prior historical era when high fertility was more adaptive. The realities of the modern world make low fertility adaptive. In a sense, the abortion patterns in Cuba, Puerto Rico, and Mexico exemplify stages in the liberalization of abortion attitudes and behavior accompanying modernization and associated fertility declines in Latin America. Only in Cuba does abortion have the full support of the government and medical institutions, and the Catholic Church is weak. As in many former communist countries, safe, legal abortion has played a major role in fertility decline for several decades, and abortion use is high, with an estimated 43% of pregnancies ending in termination (Hollerbach, 1988; Hollerbach & Diaz-Briquets, 1983).

In Puerto Rico, although abortion is legal, it has received less support from government and medical institutions and has been openly opposed by the Catholic Church. Although public attitudes are ambivalent, use of abortion is similar to that in the United States. The abortion ratio on the island of Puerto Rico, where 25% of pregnancies end in abortion, is intermediate between that of Cuba and Mexico and is most similar to the ratio for the United States, 30% (Acosta, 1990; Acosta-Belén, 1986; Henshaw, 1990; Ramirez de Arellano & Seipp, 1983).

---

aborted; and that between 20% and 46% of Latin American women have had an abortion at some time in their lives (Frejka & Atkin, 1990; Henshaw, 1990; Paxman et al., 1993). Many abortions are thought to be self-induced or performed by nonmedical practitioners, and access to high-quality abortion services is particularly limited among the poor and in rural areas (Henshaw, 1990; Paxman et al., 1993). Thus, complications of abortion are a principal cause of death among Latin American women aged 15 to 39, and the cost of treatment of the sequelae of illegal abortion is substantial (Paxman et al., 1993).

[13]Throughout human history, infanticide, now illegal throughout the world, is thought to have been a major method of fertility control (Scrimshaw, 1984).

In Mexico, abortion is illegal, the Catholic Church is strong, and maternal morbidity and mortality due to abortion are high (Aguayo-Hernandez, 1991; Infante-Castañeda & Cobos-Pons, 1989; Paxman et al., 1993; Pick de Weiss & David, 1990). Public support of abortion is low, although becoming more liberal especially for reasons of health and victimization (Hass, 1976; Nuñez-Fernandez et al., 1994). Abortion is used the least in Mexico, where an estimated 10% to 13% of pregnancies are terminated (Aguayo-Hernandez, 1991; Infante-Castañeda & Cobos-Pons, 1989; Paxman et al., 1993). In comparison to Cuba and Puerto Rico, Mexico is a less developed country with lower levels of education, higher levels of poverty, and larger rural, agricultural populations.

Abortion use by Latina subgroups in the United States, the majority of whom have origins in these three areas, tends to reflect the patterns of use and attitudes about abortion in the area of origin. Thus, American Latinos appear to be deeply affected by abortion attitudes and practices in the country of ancestry or origin, and the observed differences in Latina subgroups are consistent with a persistence of culturally learned fertility behavior.

In summary, it is apparent that Latinos in the United States are not a homogenous group. Different subgroups, although sharing a common base of language, religion, and Spanish colonization, can have strikingly different cultures shaped by the particular historical processes to which they were subject. Fertility behavior is only one example of the extent to which American Latinas differ among themselves. Although there appear to be strong effects of traditional Latino cultural values on their use of abortion, these effects appear to be mediated by country or area of ancestry or origin, acculturation or biculturalization in the United States, and socioeconomic status. Abortion use among Latinas must be understood in the context of subgroup difference and culture change.

CONCLUSION

If we have learned anything from this review of the use of abortion by Latinas in the United States, it is that there are enormous gaps in our knowledge of this aspect of Latina reproductive health behavior. We should begin to look more carefully at abortion patterns among Latinas, especially among the different subgroups, because Latinas' overall high reliance on abortion indicates need for family planning education, services, and contraceptive use. We especially need to understand differences in patterns of abortion use by age, acculturation, and socioeconomic status within subgroups. What little we know about abortion among Latinas in the United States and throughout Latin America suggests that Latina women will use abortion when faced with an unintended or unwanted pregnancy. Mexican-origin women may be less likely to choose abortion than Puerto Rican and Cuban women, perhaps because of more conservative cultural and religious attitudes toward abortion in Mexico and, possibly, their greater experience with or knowledge of adverse outcomes of illegal abortion. Latinas in the United States, especially those of Mexican and Puerto Rican origin, may be more conflicted about having an abortion for religious reasons and may need more extensive, culturally appropriate abortion counseling services.

An extensive literature search found only a handful of studies that addressed the more qualitative, meaning-centered aspects of abortion among Latinas. There is a great need for studies of abortion decision making and the psychological impact of abortion among Latinas. This is especially true because their use of abortion is relatively high; the data available suggest that approval of abortion for reasons other than health and victimization is low, yet most Latinas abort for socioeconomic reasons; and the dominant religion among Latinas, Catholicism, condemns abortion. Under such circumstances, Latina women undergoing abortion may feel particularly vulnerable and alone. This is an especially salient point for young Latinas and may be related to higher rates of adolescent childbearing among Latinas, an issue of increasing political and social importance in the United States today.

Another issue that has received little attention in the literature is the impact of HIV/AIDS on abortion decisions among Latinas. Latina women are overrepresented among U.S. women infected with HIV/AIDS, and the chance of delivering an infected infant is substantial, between 13% and 45% (Hatcher et al., 1994). For this reason, abortion is presented as an option for HIV-infected women who become pregnant. Such a decision may be particularly difficult for HIV-infected Latinas. Although most studies suggest that childbearing decisions among HIV-infected women do not differ from those of uninfected women, these studies have not distinguished among women of different racial and ethnic groups (Hatcher et al., 1994). Much more research into the psychological impact of reproductive decision making among HIV-infected women of different racial and ethnic groups is needed to provide appropriate care and counseling.

Although opinion polls suggest that the majority of Latinos approve of abortion for fetal abnormalities, in general there is more certainty in predicting the type and severity of genetic abnormalities from amniocentesis than there is predicting which infants will become infected with HIV. Special care must be taken in counseling HIV-infected Latinas regarding their options, especially with the new AZT regimen for HIV-positive pregnant women that reduces the risk of infection for the fetus. The abortion decision is a difficult one under any circumstances, but it is especially difficult when there is a risk for the fetus. Realizing the pain and suffering a child with HIV/AIDS will almost certainly undergo, health providers often exert subtle pressures favoring abortion under such circumstances (Kurth,

1993). Considering the myriad difficult social, cultural, and ethical issues surrounding HIV/AIDS, genetic testing, and abortion, further study of cultural differences in attitudes and behaviors is merited.

Finally, socioeconomic class, generation, and acculturation differences in abortion attitudes and use among Latinas are vastly underresearched. Because a high proportion of Latinas live below poverty, issues of access to abortion services (especially Medicaid funding) are paramount. The impact of racism and anti-immigrant sentiment (e.g., California's Proposition 187 denying public services to illegal immigrants) on fertility behavior is also an under-researched subject. Although, in general, Latinos seem not to have the same sense of fertility control as genocide, felt so keenly by African Americans and Native Americans, this may not be true for all Latino subgroups and may change if hostility toward Latinos increases. Certainly, racism limits opportunities and, in combination with poverty, may have a significant impact on Latinas' reproductive choices.

Latinas, like other women in the United States, hold a range of attitudes and opinions about abortion from pro-life to pro-choice. The majority, like the majority of the general population, are ambivalent about abortion, recognizing the need for it under certain circumstances, yet still regarding it as a serious moral issue. This ambivalence and the struggle over the morality of abortion will continue to be reflected in the abortion decisions made by women throughout the world.

Currently, Latinas tend to overutilize abortion in comparison to non-Latina Whites. In addition, Latinas, especially Mexican origin Latinas, may be more affected psychologically, emotionally, and socially by abortion than their non-Latina sisters due to greater cultural ambivalence about abortion. The first of these factors indicates that our health care system has failed to meet the reproductive needs of Latina women. The second argues strongly for attention to culturally appropriate counseling, education, and care by abortion providers.

REFERENCES

Acosta, E. P. (1990). El Aborto Inducido en Puerto Rico 1985. [Induced abortion in Puerto Rico, 1985]. *Puerto Rican Health Sciences Journal, 9*, 37–41.

Acosta-Belén, E. (1986). Puerto Rican women in culture, history, and society. In E. Acosta-Belén (Ed.), *The Puerto Rican woman. Perspectives on culture, history, and society* (2nd ed., pp. 1–29). New York: Praeger.

Aguayo-Hernandez, J. R. (1991). Aborto: Un Problema de Salud Pública o de Planificación Familiar? [Abortion: A problem of public health or family planning?] *Emisor Demográfico, 5*, 19–24.

Alan Guttmacher Institute. (1992). Facts in brief. In *Abortion factbook, 1992 edi-*

tion: Readings, trends, and state and local data to 1988 (pp. 37–38). New York: Author.

Amaro, H. (1988). Women in the Mexican American community: Religion, culture, and reproductive attitudes and experiences. *Journal of Community Psychology, 16*, 6–20.

Aneshensel, C. S., Becerra, R. M., & Fielder, E. P. (1990). Onset of fertility-related events during adolescence: A prospective comparison of Mexican American and non-Hispanic White females. *American Journal of Public Health, 80*, 959–963.

Aviaro, H. (1981). Latina attitudes towards abortion. *Nuestro, 5*(6), 43–44.

Bean, F. D., & Tienda, M. (1987). *The Hispanic population of the United States*. New York: Russell Sage Foundation.

Borras, V. A. (1984). *Birth knowledge, attitudes and practice: A comparison of working and middle class Puerto Rican and White American women*. Unpublished doctoral dissertation, University of Massachusetts.

Cooksey, E. C. (1990). Factors in the resolution of adolescent premarital pregnancies. *Demography, 27*, 207–218.

Darabi, K. F., Namerow, P. B., & Philliber, S. G. (1983, April). *The fertility-related attitudes of Mexican-Americans*. Paper presented at the Annual Meeting of the Population Association of America, Pittsburgh, PA.

Erickson, P. I. (1994). Lessons from a repeat pregnancy prevention program for Hispanic teen mothers in east Los Angeles. *Family Planning Perspectives, 26(4)*, 174–178.

Erickson, P. I., & Scrimshaw, S. C. M. (1985). Contraceptive knowledge and intentions among Latina teenagers experiencing their first birth (Working Papers in the Social Sciences, Vol. 1, No. 1). Los Angeles: University of California, Institute for Social Science Research.

Erickson, P. I., Ovalle, B., Diaz, A., Gillette, L. S., & Martorana, S. (1995). *Annual report 1994 to The William and Flora Hewlett Foundation*. Teen Pregnancy Prevention Project, Family Planning Program, Los Angeles County, University of Southern California, Medical Center, Women's and Children's Hospital.

Fennelly, K. (1993). Sexual activity and childbearing among Hispanic adolescents in the United States. In R. M. Lerner (Ed.), *Early adolescence: Perspectives on research, policy, and intervention* (pp. 335–352). Hillsdale, NJ: Erlbaum.

Frejka, T., & Atkin, L. C. (1990). El Papel del Aborto en la Transición de la Fecundidad de América Latina [The role of abortion in Latin America's fertility transition]. *Salud Pública de México, 32*, 276–286.

Gold, E. M., Erhardt, C. L., Jacobziner, H., & Nelson, F. G. (1965). Therapeutic abortions in New York City: A twenty year review. *American Journal of Public Health, 55*, 964–972.

Goldscheider, C., & Mosher, W. D. (1991). Patterns of contraceptive use in the United States: The importance of religious factors. *Studies in Family Planning, 22*, 102–115.

Hass, P. H. (1976). Contraceptive choices for Latin American women. *Populi, Journal of the United Nations Fund for Population Activities, 3(4)*, 14–24.

Hatcher, R. A., Trussell, J., Stewart, F., Stewart, G. K., Kowal, D., Guest, F., Cates, W., Jr., & Policar, M. S. (1994). *Contraceptive Technology 1994–1996 (16th rev. ed.)*. New York: Irvington.

Henshaw, S. K. (1990). Induced abortion: A world review, 1990. *Family Planning Perspectives, 22(2)*, 76–89.

Henshaw, S. K., & Silverman, J. (1988). The characteristics and prior contraceptive use of U.S. abortion patients. *Family Planning Perspectives, 20(4)*, 158–168.

Hollerbach, P. E. (1988). Cuba. In Paul Sachdev (Ed.), *International handbook on abortion* (pp. 112–123). New York: Greenwood Press.

Hollerbach, P. E., & Diaz-Briquets, S. (1983). *Fertility determinants in Cuba* (Rep. No. 26). Washington, DC: Committee on Population and Demography, National Academy Press.

Infante-Castañeda, C., & Cobos-Pons, Y. (1989). El aborto inducido en cifras: Análisis de la difusión de las estadísticas en la prensa [Induced abortion in statistics: Analysis of the dissemination of statistics in the press]. *Salud Publica de Mexico, 31*, 385–393.

Jones, E. F., & Forrest, J. D. (1992). Underreporting of abortion in surveys of U.S. women: 1976 to 1988. *Demography, 29*, 113–126.

Joyce, T. (1988). The social and economic correlates of pregnancy resolution among adolescents in New York City, by race and ethnicity: A multivariate analysis. *American Journal of Public Health, 78*, 626–631.

Kaplan, C. P., & Erickson, P. I. (1996). *The effects of acculturation, gender roles, and familism on abortion among young, Latina women.* Manuscript in preparation.

Kay, M. A. (1978). The Mexican–American. In A. L. Clark (Ed.), *Culture/childbearing/health professionals* (pp. 88–108). Philadelphia: F. A. Davis Co.

King, R. H., Myers, S. C., & Byrne, D. M. (1992). The demand for abortion by unmarried teenagers. *American Journal of Economics and Sociology, 51*, 223–236.

Koonin, L. M., Smith, J. C., & Ramick, M. (1995). Abortion surveillance—United States, 1991. *Morbidity and Mortality Weekly Report, 44*, 23–53.

Kurth, A. (1993). Reproductive issues, pregnancy, and childbearing in HIV infected women. In F. L. Cohen and J. D. Durham (Eds.), *Women, children, and HIV/AIDS* (pp. 104–133). New York: Springer.

Linn, M. W., Carmichael, J. S., Klitenick, P., Webb, N., & Gurel, L. (1978). Fertility related attitudes of minority mothers with large and small families. *Journal of Applied Psychology, 8*, 1–14.

Marin, B. V., Gerardo, M., & Padilla, A. M. (1981). Attitudes and practices of low-income Hispanic contraceptors (Occasional Paper No. 13). Los Angeles: Spanish Speaking Mental Health Research Center, University of California.

Molina, C. W., & Aguirre-Molina, M. (1994). *Latino Health in the U.S.: A growing challenge*. Washington, DC: American Public Health Association.

Mosher, W. D., Williams, L. B., & Johnson, D. P. (1992). Religion and fertility in the United States: New patterns. *Demography, 29*, 199–214.

Namerow, P. B., & Philliber, S. G. (1983). Attitudes towards sex education among black, Hispanic and white inner-city residents. *International Quarterly of Community Health Education, 3*, 291–299.

Nuñez-Fernández, L., Shrader-Cox, E., & Benson, J. (1994). Encuesta de opinión sobre el aborto en la ciudad de México. [Abortion polls in Mexico City]. *Salud Pública de México, 36*, 36–45.

Ortiz, C. G., & Nuttall, E. V. (1987). Adolescent pregnancy: Effects of family support, education, and religion on the decision to carry or terminate among Puerto Rican teenagers. *Adolescence, 22*, 897–917.

Parker, J., & Nelson, F. (1971). Abortion in New York City: The first nine months. *Family Planning Perspectives, 3(3)*, 5–12.

Parker, J., & Nelson, F. (1973). Two years experience in New York City with the liberalized abortion law: Progress and problems. *American Journal of Public Health, 63*, 524–535.

Pavich, E. G. (1986). A Chicana perspective on Mexican culture and sexuality. *Journal of Social Work and Human Sexuality, 4*, 47–65.

Paxman, J. M., Rizo, A., Brown, L., & Benson, J. (1993). The clandestine epidemic: The practice of unsafe abortion in Latin America. *Studies in Family Planning, 24*, 205–226.

Pick de Weiss, S., & David, H. P. (1990). Illegal abortion in Mexico: Client perceptions. *American Journal of Public Health, 80*, 715–716.

Ramirez de Arellano, A. B., & Seipp, C. (1983). *Colonialism, Catholicism and contraception: A history of birth control in Puerto Rico*. Chapel Hill: University of North Carolina Press.

Rochat, R. W., Warren, C. W., Smith, J. C., Holck, S. E., & Friedman, J. S. (1981). Family planning practices among Anglo and Hispanic women in U.S. counties bordering Mexico. *Family Planning Perspectives, 13*, 176–180.

Roe v. Wade, 410 U.S. 113 (U.S. Supreme Court, 1973).

Rossi, A. S., & Sitaraman, B. (1988). Abortion in context: Historical trends and future changes. *Family Planning Perspectives, 20*, 273–282.

Scrimshaw, S. C. M. (1984). Infanticide in human populations: Societal and individual concerns. In G. Hansfater & S. Hardy (Eds.), *Infanticide: Comparative and evolutionary* (pp. 439–462). New York: Aldine.

Shedlin, M. G., & Hollerbach, P. E. (1981). Modern and traditional fertility regulation in a Mexican community: The process of decision making. *Studies in Family Planning, 12*, 278–296.

Steinhoff, P. G. (1973). Background characteristics of abortion patients. In H. G. Osorfsky & J. D. Osorfsky (Eds.), *The abortion experience: Psychological and medical impact* (pp. 206–231). Hagerstown, MD: Harper & Row.

Stevans, L. K., Register, C. A., & Sessions, D. N. (1992). The abortion decision: A qualitative choice approach. *Social Indicators Research, 27,* 327–344.

Torres, A., & Forrest, J. D. (1988). Why do women have abortions? *Family Planning Perspectives, 20,* 169–176.

Urdaneta, M. L. (1980). Chicana use of abortion. In M. Melville (Ed.), *Twice a minority* (pp. 33–51). St. Louis, MO: C.V. Mosby Co.

Williams, N. (1990). *The Mexican American family: Tradition and change.* Dix Hills, NY: General Hall.

7

ABORTION AND ASIAN PACIFIC ISLANDER AMERICANS

SORA PARK TANJASIRI AND SONO AIBE

Asian Pacific Islander American (APIA) women face unique challenges in maintaining reproductive health in the United States. They must incorporate and reconcile American values, norms, and beliefs with their own cultural roots (Asians and Pacific Islanders for Reproductive Health [APIRH], 1995) while simultaneously navigating the complex system of health care delivery in the United States. Numerous barriers to attaining personal health exist, including factors associated with difficulties in immigration and settlement, transposition of reproductive health attitudes and practices learned in Asia and the Pacific Islands to the United States, acculturation from Asian cultural values of sexual and reproductive health to Western ideals and beliefs, and negotiation of health care services in this country. Given the paucity of information on abortion among APIA women, this chapter examines women's experiences in each of these facets. Although a definitive understanding of the role of, and need for, abortion among APIA women cannot be gained at this time, an initial portrait of abortion attitudes and practices is constructed to motivate and guide much needed future research.

NATIVITY AND IMMIGRATION HISTORY

APIAs represent the smallest but most rapidly growing racial category in the United States. Between 1980 and 1990, the number of APIAs grew 108% to 7.3 million persons (Chen & Hawks, 1995). Of this group, 6,908,638 (95%) were Asians and 365,024 (5%) were Pacific Islanders (U.S. Bureau of the Census, 1993a, 1993b). APIAs consist of a diversity of more than 25 recognized ethnic populations. Whereas the five largest Asian ethnic groups in 1990 were Chinese, Filipino, Japanese, Asian Indian, and Korean, also included are Vietnamese, Cambodian, Hmong, Laotian, Thai, Bangladeshi, Burmese, Indonesian, Malaysian, Okinawan, Pakistani, and Sri Lankan. Pacific Islanders include native Hawaiian, Guamanian (or Chamorros), Samoan, Tongan, Tahitian, Northern Mariana Islander, Palauan, and Fijian. Each of these API ethnic groups possesses a distinct language, culture, and social structure within its community.

Overall, APIA women and their families are relatively recent immigrants to the United States, the majority of whom arrived in this country within the past 15 years. According to the 1990 census, 74% of all APIAs are foreign born, with the majority having entered the United States between 1980 and 1990 (Lin-Fu, 1993). By ethnic group, however, the proportion of foreign-born individuals varies widely. Only 32.4% of Japanese were born abroad, due to their earlier immigration and longer history in this country. Conversely, 64.4% of Filipinos, 69.3% of Chinese, 72.7% of Koreans, and 75.4% of Asian Indians were foreign born in 1990, reflecting large numbers of recent immigrants, especially during the past 10 years (U.S. Bureau of the Census, 1993b). Refugee populations from Southeast Asia comprise the most recent waves of immigrants, as shown by their high proportions of foreign-born persons (e.g., 79.1% of Laotians and 79.9% of Vietnamese are foreign born).

Immigration history and settlement patterns represent crucial considerations when understanding many present demographic characteristics and corresponding health practices of APIA ethnic groups. By and large, APIA immigration to this country was characterized by centuries of discrimination, including exclusionary acts banning entry from many countries in Asia. In the following discussion, the unique immigration histories of Chinese, Filipinos, Vietnamese, Asian Indians, and Pacific Islanders are presented as examples of the diversity inherent in APIA populations.

Chinese Americans

Chinese male laborers came to this country beginning in the mid-1800s, during the years of the gold rush and construction of the transcontinental railroad. Discrimination against Chinese immigrants quickly increased, as they were blamed for periods of severe economic hardship in the United States. As a result, numerous bans and limitations were placed on Chinese immigration, including the 1882 Chinese Exclusion Act, the 1924 Immigration Act, and antimiscegenation laws (Uba, 1994). Other policies further prevented immigration from China, including such U.S. policies as the failure to recognize the newly founded People's Republic of China in 1949. Although the Immigration Act of 1965 marked the beginning of immigration from Taiwan and Hong Kong (Wang, 1991), it was not until diplomatic relations were established with the People's Republic of China in 1979 that mainland Chinese were able to immigrate and reunite with family members.

Filipino Americans

The relationship between the United States and the Philippines has been a turbulent one. The Philippines was illegally ceded to the United States at the Treaty of Paris after Spain's defeat in the Spanish-American War of 1898 for $20 million, together with Cuba and Puerto Rico. It became a U.S. colony after the Filipino-American War in 1903, a war that lasted for more than 10 years and killed more than 600,000 natives (Health Action Information Network, 1991). A period of U.S. occupation ensued, during which there were two waves of immigration to the United States (Melendy, 1981). The first wave began in 1903 and brought young male students, or *pensionados*, in search of college education. Between 1903 and 1930, a second wave of immigrants was recruited from the Philippines to labor as agricultural workers on Hawaiian plantations. In 1934, the Tydings-McDuffie Act drastically limited Filipino immigration to the United States to only 50 persons per year (U.S. Immigration and Naturalization Service, 1981). Immigration resumed again in the 1950s. Finally, a third wave of immigrants arrived after the 1965 Immigration Act. This last wave of immigrants differed from past waves in that both men and women entered the United States, many well educated and with families.

Vietnamese Americans

Since the fall of Saigon in 1975, large numbers of refugees from Vietnam, as well as from Cambodia and Laos, have entered the United States through provisions in the Refugee Act of 1980. The first wave of refugees after 1975 consisted of mostly well-educated upper- and middle-class Vietnamese fleeing due to political ties with the fallen regime. After 1979, a second wave of refugees began arriving in the United States, spurred by the Vietnamese invasion of Cambodia and military offenses against people in Laos (Muecke, 1983). This second wave of refugees differed from the previous, as the immigrants were generally less educated, less literate, and in poorer health. Escape from countries of origin for people during this wave was generally difficult and often fatal, and their entry into the United States often occurred only after several years of subsistence in refugee camps throughout Asia. In 1982, the Orderly Departure Program was established by the United States to admit Vietnamese directly from Vietnam and resulted in increased immigration by people from rural areas of the country (Chuong, 1994).

Asian Indians

Although South Asian American groups include immigrants from Bangladesh, Bhutan, Maldives, Myanmar, Nepal, Pakistan, and Sri Lanka, the largest population is Asian Indians from India. Around the time when anti-Chinese sentiment was raging in the late 1800s, a successful campaign was waged to exclude Indian immigrants. Congress passed the Immigration Regional Restriction Act of 1917, which prohibited immigration of Asians from "barred zones": India, Southeast Asia, Indonesia, New Guinea, and parts of Arabia, Afghanistan, and Siberia (Melendy, 1981). Furthermore, a movement was mounted to deny citizenship to Indians in the United States, take away the citizenship from Indians to whom it had already been granted, and apply the Regional Exclusion Act retroactively to deport all Indians in the United States. Renewed Indian immigration did not occur until after World War II, due to the relaxing of restrictions for Indians (and Filipinos). Starting in the 1950s, Asian immigrants consisted of mainly professionals and their families (Melendy, 1981). For instance, a number of Indian doctors immigrated to the United States in the late 1960s to fill the shortage of doctors created by the Vietnam War (Jensen, 1988). The immigration momentum increased during this time and has led to the continuing increase of particularly highly educated Indians. Although most immigrants come from large cities, there also exist immigrant laborers who come from rural areas in search of better economic opportunities in the United States.

Pacific Islanders

Although Pacific Islanders inhabit thousands of islands in the Pacific Oceans, they are generally categorized into three major groups: Melanesians, Micronesians, and Polynesians. Polynesians, including native Hawaiians, Tongans, and Samoans, comprise the largest of the Pacific Islander populations in the United States. Micronesia includes the Marshall Islands and Guam, the latter of which are populated by indigenous Chamorros people. Melanesia includes Fiji, the Solomon Islands, and Papua New Guinea, from which few migrate to the United States. Immigrants from the Pacific Islands generally have entered the United States seeking better economic conditions and educational opportunities. In Hawaii, arrival by the British occurred in

1778, annexation by the United States in 1898, and statehood in 1959. Today, although 115,000 people living in Hawaii claim varying degrees of Hawaiian blood lineage, experts estimate the number of pure Hawaiians at less than 1,000 (Bisignani, 1994). In 1900 and 1950, respectively, Samoa and Guam were declared American territories. Immigration from Pacific U.S. territories occurs relatively easily, primarily through entry via Hawaii (National Asian Women's Health Organization, 1995).

Summary

For all APIs, the Immigration Act of 1965 opened the doors to immigration from countries in Asia and the Pacific Islands. Through this act, U.S. immigration policy specifically favored younger professionals, allowing entry to largely working-age adults who possessed special skills deemed valuable in this country. However, family reunification has also been a major reason for the increase in immigration from Asian and the Pacific Island countries (U.S. Immigration and Naturalization Service, 1991).

SOCIODEMOGRAPHIC CHARACTERISTICS OF APIA WOMEN

Nativity and Age

Due in part to the recency of immigration and the selectivity of U.S. immigration policies, APIA women and their families are generally a young population. The median age for APIAs was 30 years in 1990 as compared with 33 years for the total population (U.S. Bureau of the Census, 1993a, 1993b). Consequently, APIA women of reproductive age comprise a large proportion of the U.S. female population. As shown in Table 1, compared with the proportions of White and Black women between the ages of 15 and 44 years (37.7% and 49.0%, respectively), 53.3% of all API women fall within these reproductive ages. These already high figures may even underrepresent the true number of women bearing children due to cultural differences in the interpretation of "reproductive age." Whereas the usual age for reproduction among Chinese, Korean, and Japanese women is close to the U.S. average, the age is much lower in Southeast Asian groups, particularly Cambodians and Laotians. Because these ethnic groups have large percentages of reproductive-aged women, the development of accessible family planning and perinatal care services for APIAs would be an effective use of scarce health care resources.

There exist many important differences among APIA women by nativity and acculturation level. In 1992, only 17% of API mothers giving birth were born in the United States (Martin, 1995). However, API families in the United States will increasingly comprise U.S.-born children

TABLE 1

Size and Percentage of Asian and Pacific Islander American
(APIA) Women of all Ages and of Reproductive Age
in the United States: 1990

Category	Total female population	Women 15–44 years	Women 15–44 years in each ethnic group (%)
United States	127,470,455	58,583,772	46.0
All APIAs	3,715,624	1,981,135	53.3
Chinese	824,348	55,984	55.3
Japanese	458,078	212,338	46.4
Filipino	445,139	406,039	53.7
Korean	756,334	239,694	53.8
Asian Indian	377,604	211,607	56.0
Vietnamese	289,303	165,928	57.4
Cambodian	75,724	35,673	47.1
Laotian	71,984	35,150	50.2
Hmong	44,192	15,220	34.4
Thai	53,696	34,965	65.1
Other Asian	138,247	74,210	53.7
Hawaiian	105,212	52,968	50.3
Samoan	30,978	15,341	49.5
Guamanian	24,140	13,817	57.2
Other Pacific Islander	21,645	11,201	54.3

Note. Table data from the U.S. Department of Commerce, Bureau of the Census, General Population Characteristics, 1990.

and young adults, and their foreign-born parents. By the year 2020, adolescents and young adults will make up approximately 34% to 38% of the total API population. Of this group, 82% to 85% will be U.S. born (Ong & Hee, 1993). In comparison, approximately 67% of working age APIA adults (25 to 64 years) were foreign born in 1990, and this will increase to a predicted 71% by the year 2020.

Education and Income

Educational attainment by APIA women is roughly equal to the overall U.S. average. For instance, in 1990 73.9% and 75.0%, respectively, of Asian American and Pacific Islander women 25 years and older were at least high school graduates, and the U.S. average was 74.8%. However, considerable variation lies hidden within these figures. By ethnic group, the Japanese had the largest proportion of women with high school degrees (85.6%), whereas Asian Indians had the greatest proportions of women completing at least a bachelor's degree (48.7%). Conversely, Southeast Asians had some of the lowest levels of educational attainment by females, with only 19% and 3% of Hmong women completing high school and college, respectively. Indeed, these dramatic differences in educational attainment have led researchers to characterize APIA populations as possessing a "bimodal" distribution in socioeconomic status (Lin-Fu, 1988; Tanjasiri, Wallace, & Shibata, 1995).

Similarly, income data on APIA women and their families paint different pictures at different levels of granularity. In aggregate, Asian Americans enjoy nearly as high a level of income as the national average. In 1989, the Asian American per capita income was $13,806 compared with the national average of $14,143 (U.S. Bureau of the Census, 1993b). By ethnic group, Japanese ($19,373) and Asian Indians ($17,777) possessed per capita incomes that exceeded that of the nation as a whole. However, many Asian ethnic groups also possessed some of the nation's lowest levels of income, such as Laotians ($5,597) and Hmong ($2,692). Pacific Islanders have incomes that are lower than Asians, with a per capita income of only $10,342 (U.S. Bureau of the Census, 1993a). Poverty among Pacific Islander Americans is also a large concern, as 25.8% and 23.1%, respectively, of Samoans and Tongans fall at or below the poverty line, compared with the national average of 13%.

Overall, considering the differences for specific ethnic groups and age groups of APIA women, abortion and family planning researchers must use caution when studying the health needs of these populations. Indeed, selective use of statistics on APIA populations, such as mean income and higher education levels, masks "the misery of those at the other end who are truly in need, but poorly visible and barely audible in a society that views them as all highly successful" (Lin-Fu, 1988 p. 27). Thus, glaring disparities in health and welfare exist for particular groups of API immigrants (Chen & Hawks, 1995; Zane, Takeuchi, & Young, 1994).

ABORTION IN ASIA AND THE PACIFIC ISLANDS

Because of the foreign-born status and recency of immigration for a majority of APIA women, their abortion attitudes and practices in the United States are undoubtedly shaped by the knowledge, attitudes, and behaviors adopted from their countries of birth. In the following section, we highlight research on abortion policies and practices for API women abroad as a foundation for understanding the practices of API Americans, albeit primarily foreign born, in the United States.

According to Sachdev (1988), although Asian countries vary in the degree to which abortion is available and accessible, legalization of abortion has not been as controversial an issue as in the Americas and Europe. All of the major countries from which large numbers of APIA women immigrate either possess policies that legalize abortions (e.g., China, India, and Singapore) or have lenient enforcement of bans that allow abortions to be performed seemingly uninhibited (e.g., Japan and South Korea). Only in a few instances are there countries that continue to actively enforce the illegal status of abortion (e.g., Sri Lanka and Philippines). Abortion services in the Pacific Islands are generally illegal or highly restricted and are often only performed to save the life of the woman (e.g., Tonga and Solomon Islands).

Although the demographic characteristics of women who seek abortions vary by Asian country, some generalizations based on available data can be made. First, reported cases of abortions in Asia generally occur among married women with children. For instance, in South Korea, by 1982 approximately one half of married South Korean women had experienced an induced abortion (Sachdev, 1988). Reported statistics indicate women seeking abortions in Asia are generally older (between 20 and 34 years of age) compared with abortion seekers in Western countries such as the United States. This is probably because pregnancy and abortion among adolescents tend to be less documented in Asian countries such as Japan, India, Singapore, and South Korea. However, with the relaxation of many strict Asian cultural norms against premarital sexual conduct, and the influence of Western values such as independence, more Asian women are engaging in sex at earlier ages. Thus, the proportions of adolescent and unmarried women seeking abortions are already on the rise in several Asian countries.

Of course, for every generalization that can be made, qualifications must also be considered if a fuller understanding of the range of abortion attitudes and practices in the United States is to be gained. First, countries in Asia vary by the level that abortion is socially accepted. For instance, according to Tuan (1988) induced abortions have long been socially accepted among the Chinese, who traditionally view abortion as a private family affair not decided by law (Tuan, 1988). Conversely, Sri Lankan law allows abortion only to save the life of a mother, and traditional citizens believe aborting a fertilized ovum to be analogous to taking a life (Kodagoda & Senanayake, 1988). The frequency of abortion use by women (i.e., the rate of repeat abortions) also varies by country. For example, in India medical termination of pregnancy (MTP) services have been slow to be implemented; consequently, the women seeking repeat abortions constitute a small proportion (from 5% to 15%) of all abortion seekers (Ramachandran, 1988). In comparison, South Korea has one of the highest rates of repeat abortions: Repeat abortions were obtained by between 24.2% (in rural areas) to 34.5% (in large cities) of married South Korean women (Hong, 1988).

Attitudes toward the role abortion plays in family planning also vary. The high rates of repeat abortions among South Korean women have been attributed to their attitudes toward abortion as a primary rather than a backup method of contraception (Sachdev, 1988). In contrast, whereas the proportion of repeat abortions are increasing in Singapore, the use of abortion appears to be associated more with contraceptive failure (perhaps due to higher rates of condom use) than to the primacy of abortion as a family planning method itself (Chen, Emmanuel, Ling, & Kwa, 1985).

Given the diversity of abortion policies found in Pacific Rim countries, we highlight three countries—China, Vietnam, and the Philippines—as examples of the ways in which women from these countries may differ in their use and acceptance of abortion on migrating to the United States.

China

Historically, induced abortion has existed in medical practice for centuries, justified primarily on grounds of practicality (Tuan, 1988). According to Lieh-Mak, Tam, and Ng (1981), no specific tenets in China exist against abortion. In the 1950s, the Chinese government introduced and supported contraception and abortion to control population growth. During this time, abortion was used as a back-up measure in cases of contraceptive failure.

The Chinese government's intervention concerning fertility is summarized in the slogan "wan, xi, shao," which promotes later age at marriage, longer intervals between births, and fewer total births (Li et al., 1990). Because of strict governmental controls, China has achieved dramatic declines in fertility over the past 30 years. The most common contraceptive methods have been female sterilization and intrauterine devices (IUDs). According to the State Family Planning Commission statistics of 1990, in 1989 41.1% of contracepting women used IUDs and 36.6% had tubal ligations, compared to 11.6% vasectomies, 5.4% oral pills, 3.8% condoms, and 0.8% spermicides (Center for Reproductive Law and Policy, 1995).

Whereas abortion has a long history in China, it has played an important role in meeting governmental birth quotas since the inception of the one-child policy in 1979. Abortion services are free of charge and permitted on request, and between 14 and 30 days of paid sick leave are given to women having first- or second-trimester abortions, respectively. The number of reported abortions per 100 known pregnancies rose from 12 in 1971 to 33 in 1980 and reached a peak of more than 14 million total abortions in 1983 (Ping & Smith, 1995). Although the official position continues to stress voluntary abortion only in the event of contraceptive failure, several observers persist in their claims that women are frequently coerced into having abortions (Hardee-Cleaveland & Banister, 1988; Huang, 1989).

The degree to which Chinese women's high use of abortion in China translates to the United States remains unknown. In some cases, it appears that governmental policies have negatively influenced individual women's acceptance of, and desire for, abortion services (Hardee-Cleaveland & Banister, 1988). For instance, in areas where governmental surveillance and controls are weak, couples disregard contraceptive ordinances in order to have several babies. Evidence also continues to exist of family planning programs pressuring couples to undergo sterilization, and of the government criminalizing the removal of IUDs without official permission, to meet family planning targets set by the state and provinces (Hardee-Cleaveland & Banister, 1988; Huang, 1989). The one-child policy may also exacerbate gender preferences that place greater value on boys than girls, leading to practices of female infanticide (Hardee-Cleaveland & Banister, 1988). However, the extent of this practice is clouded by the underreporting and lack of registration of girl births. By the time Chinese children register to enter schools at age five, the male-to-female sex ratio is much less skewed, which tends to support the practice of non-registration over infanticide for girls (Conly & Camp, 1992). Ultimately, further research is needed to understand the impact of coerced abortions and gender preferences on the abortion practices of Chinese women migrating to the United States.

Vietnam

Since unification of North and South Vietnam, the Socialist Republic of Vietnam has stressed population growth and family planning alongside economic and social development efforts (Allman, Nhan, Thang, San, & Man, 1991). Basic health care services are readily available, with nearly all of Vietnam's 8,000 communes possessing a health center. In 1988, the Ministers' Council of Vietnam promulgated the Decree on Population and Family Planning Policies, with the goal of reducing population growth and ensuring adequate availability of family planning methods (Allman et al., 1991). This decree encouraged later marriages, birth spacing of at least 3 to 4 years, and fewer births to women 35 and older. Though individuals remain free to select the desired method of family planning, Vietnamese governmental policies help shape the availability and promotion of specific approaches (Allman et al., 1991).

Abortion was legalized in Vietnam in 1963 and constitutes an important component of Vietnam's fertility regulation policies. Abortion statistics collected by the Ministry of Health include two procedures: menstrual regulation (i.e., suction removal of a fetus performed within 5 weeks of pregnancy) and surgical abortion (Goodkind, 1994). Rates of reported abortions have increased steadily since the mid-1980s and numbered 1.37 million in 1993. The total abortion rate for Vietnam in 1992 was 2.5 abortions per woman's reproductive lifetime, which is high considering the total fertility rate of 3.7 (Goodkind, 1994). According to a study conducted in 1989 by the United Nations Population Fund (UNFPA, 1991), the specific induced abortion rates per 1,000 were 87.3 for women aged 20 to 24 years old, 119.6 for women aged 25 to 29, 103.4 for women aged 30 to

34, and 85.1 for women aged 35 to 39. No significant differences in abortion rates exist for women in rural compared with urban areas (Thang, Swenson, Man, & Trinh, 1992). Whereas the majority of abortions are provided through public facilities, abortions from private providers are increasingly common due in part to the availability of government subsidies since 1991 (Goodkind, 1994).

With regard to family planning, according to 1988 Demographic and Health Survey of Vietnam data, about 95% of currently married women know of at least one modern birth control method. However, the only widely available modern method is the IUD. According to the survey, 53% of married women of reproductive age were using a contraceptive method, with 62% using IUDs (Anh, 1995). Small percentages of users relied on modern methods such as female sterilization (5%), the condom (2%), the pill, or vasectomy (fewer than 1% each). Unfortunately, researchers point out that the contraceptive method mix in Vietnam is poor and the supply of modern contraceptives has been scarce and erratic especially in rural areas (Allman et al., 1991; Goodkind, 1994). Poor contraceptive availability combined with financial disincentives for higher parity childbearing have resulted in women's high reliance on readily-available pregnancy termination and menstrual regulation procedures throughout the country.

Philippines

In stark contrast to China and Vietnam, abortion in the Philippines remains completely illegal. In 1930, criminalization of abortion was contained in the penal code, which had been introduced during Spanish colonization. According to the code, penalties for abortion ranged from 2 to 20 years in prison, with the practice of safe abortion punishable by the maximum penalty (Tadiar, 1989). Although trends in current international abortion laws have been moving toward decriminalization and legalization (Cook, 1989), Tadiar (1989) noted that the Philippines has seen the reverse. Within only the past 10 years, the constitutional provision supporting population control policies has been deleted and abortion has been constitutionally banned in the country. Specifically, the new 1987 constitution provides for the protection of the life of the unborn from conception, thereby preempting the future passage of any permissive abortion laws (de Castro, 1990). Throughout the century the Roman Catholic Church has played a primary role in restricting abortion in the Philippines, most recently securing a controlling majority in the Commission established to write the new constitution, thereby ensuring the permanent and irreversible prohibition of abortion for the entire country.

Although discussion of abortion is virtually taboo due to legal, religious, and cultural restraints, Potts, Diggory, and Peel (1977) have theorized that abortion played a significant role in past fertility declines. Indeed, some studies point to the acceptance of abortion for fertility control among Filipino women. According to a study in Laguna reported by Flavier and Chen (1980), 30% of reproductive-aged women who had ever been married had at least one abortion in their reproductive history. In their own research in Cavite, 13% of the women aged 15 to 49 reported one past abortion; 4% reported two or more abortions.

Given the severe punishments for providers of abortion, abortion practitioners have no modern medical training. The major sources for abortion services are *hilots* (traditional healers), midwives, and herbs collected and taken by women themselves. Although the government does not officially collect data on abortions, it is estimated that between 155,000 to 750,000 induced abortions are performed annually (Tadiar, 1989). Given the illegal nature of these abortions, women who receive these services face an inordinately high risk of death from infection or hemorrhage, infertility, or other chronic health problems. A survey conducted by the Department of Health found that the fourth leading cause of maternal death was abortion, exceeded only by hemorrhaging and internal bleeding during childbirth, hypertension, and pregnancy-related complications during labor and delivery (Health Action Information Network, 1994).

Because 85% of Filipinos are Roman Catholic, family planning programs have been hindered. More than a quarter of married women in the country would like to practice family planning and are not currently using any form of contraception. The total fertility rate in the Philippines is about 4.0, but fertility levels would be nearly 30% lower if Filipino women had only the births that they wanted. Only 40% of married Filipino women use contraception; the most popular methods are female sterilization (12%), oral contraceptives (9%), natural family planning (7%), and withdrawal (7%; Macro International, 1993). Unfortunately, method problems appear to be high, with 40% of contraceptive users quitting in the past 5 years due to method failure and another 18% due to health problems (Alan Guttmacher Institute, 1995). Whereas it is anticipated that religion constitutes an important influence on Filipino American women's abortion attitudes and practices, it is unknown how acculturation moderates women's views on immigration to the United States.

Summary

In this section we discuss major themes of abortion use and policies in Asia and the Pacific Islands. Clearly, wide differences exist in access to, and use of, safe and legal abortion in many Asian Pacific countries. The abortion and family planning policies abroad no doubt hold different implications for recently immigrated APIA women in the United States. For instance, Chinese and Vietnamese women, who are accustomed to relying on abortion as a family planning option in their countries of origin, may more easily turn to abortion services even after immigration to the United States. Conversely, governmental and societal prohibition of abortion in the Philippines may result in lower use among Filipino American immigrants. An associated issue is to what degree Asian immigrant women, especially those who experience few contraceptive options in Asian countries, will remain infrequent contraceptive users in the United States. More research is clearly needed, especially research that explores the migratory and acculturation processes of API women. In the following sections, we further explore the factors contributing to family planning and abortion practices among APIA.

PREGNANCY AND ABORTION AMONG APIAs IN THE UNITED STATES

Very little information exists on the use of, and perceptions toward, abortion among APIA women in the United States. Unfortunately, APIAs are categorized in the racial group "Other" when reporting abortion data by states to the Centers for Disease Control and Prevention (L. Koonin, personal communication, January 26, 1996), rendering comparisons with other racial groups in currently available reports impossible (Henshaw, 1992; Henshaw, Binkin, & Smith, 1985). More generally, problems continue to exist in nationally collected data on natality, mortality, fetal deaths, and induced births, including use of API ethnic group identifiers for only selected vital registration areas, racial/ethnic misclassifications for API groups, and lack of adequate sampling of APIs in current surveys (Yu & Liu, 1992). Finally, APIAs still suffer from the "model minority" myth, perpetuating the fallacy that they are a healthier people, requiring less health care research and fewer services (Chen & Hawks, 1995; Lin-Fu, 1993).

Despite these limitations, various community-based abortion data and literature are available from which emerges at least an initial portrait of abortion practices and perceptions among APIAs. In the following section we discuss available data on the rates of pregnancy and abortion and attitudes toward abortion among APIA women in the United States.

Fertility Patterns Among APIA Women

Current birth characteristics for APIAs may shed important light on the potential need for, and role of, abortion among women of reproductive age. The year 1995 marked the first time that a report was published on the demographic and health characteristics of women with live births among APIAs, using data from the National Center for Health Statistics (Martin, 1995). As expected, wide differences exist between the maternal characteristics of different APIA ethnic groups. Chinese and Japanese American births tend to occur most often among mothers aged 25 to 34 years, whereas among Filipino, Vietnamese, Asian Indians, and Koreans the birth rate is highest for mothers aged 25 to 29 years. Among Hawaiians, Samoans, and Guamanians it is highest for mothers aged 20 to 24 years. Parity of APIA mothers also varies considerably by specific ethnic group. Fourth-order and higher parity births tend to be greatest for Pacific Islander Americans (26.5% for Samoans, 16.6% Guamanians, and 15.3% Hawaiians) compared with Asians (7.0% Filipinos, 3.5% Asian Indians, 2.9% Chinese, and 2.2% Koreans; Martin, 1995).

These maternal data point to areas of potential abortion use among APIA women. For instance, the greater number of high-order births, combined with the younger ages of mothers, suggests that Pacific Islander Americans may have less desire to limit family size and, consequently, lower need for and use of abortion services compared with Asian Americans. Conversely, Martin (1995) suggested that higher levels of later-age childbearing among Japanese and Korean American women may be related to their desire to become more educated. For instance, 98.7% of Japanese and 95.8% of Korean mothers possessed 12 years of education or more, compared with 86.1% of Samoan American mothers. Thus, the desire to time, delay, or limit childbearing may be related to greater use of family planning and abortion services among these ethnic groups. Unfortunately, no specific information exists on the prevalence of unwanted pregnancies and resulting abortions among APIAs (Brown & Eisenbery, 1995).

In particular, Hawaiian Americans appear to be holding on to cultural beliefs and practices that promote childbearing rather than abortion for women of all ages. Of infants born to native Hawaiian women in 1992, 47% of those births were to unmarried women (Martin, 1995). The abortion rate for native Hawaiians was one half of the Hawaii average, an indication that pregnancy termination was not prevalent among this group (Hawaii Department of Health, 1990). In 1990, 45% of births in Hawaii to women under age 20 were accounted for by native Hawaiian mothers, although native Hawaiians accounted for only 24% of total births in Hawaii. Specifically, native Hawaiian adolescents accounted for 49% of all births to women aged 15 to 17 and 46% of all births by women under age 15. Hawaiian adolescents may more likely carry pregnancies through to birth due to enduring Hawaiian cultural beliefs. Hawaiians traditionally accept and welcome infants into family life, regardless of the age or marital status of the mother (Takenaka, 1995).

Nativity differences between first generation (foreign-born) and second or third generation (U.S.-born) women create significant variations in adolescent fertility rates of APIAs. Few births currently occur for Asian American adolescents under age 20. According to Martin (1995), adolescent mothers accounted for only 1% of Chinese and Korean American, 1.5% of Asian Indian American, and 2.6% of Japanese American births in 1992. However, a larger number of adolescent births occurred among Pacific Islander Americans. Births to mothers under 20 years of age accounted for 18.8% of all births among Hawaiians and 17.3% among Guamanians, compared with only 5.6% among Filipinos and 0.7% among Chinese (Martin, 1995). Nativity of the mother is strongly associated with the rate of teenage births: API mothers born in the United States were three times as likely to have a teenage birth as were mothers born abroad.

The succeeding generations of APIAs in the United States are less likely to hold on to traditional cultural values. According to Martin (1995), births to mothers under 20 years of age rose for all APIA women born in the United States compared with those born abroad. Specifically, births to mothers under 20 years old were 5.9, 8.5, and 16 times more likely among U.S.-born Filipino, Korean, and Asian Indian mothers, respectively, compared with those born abroad. These same three ethnic groups also had the highest percentages among APIAs of births to unmarried mothers born in the United States. Socially, second and third generation APIA adolescents assimilate quickly into mainstream American culture, often in conflict with the desires of their parents to maintain traditional values and practices. According to the High-Risk Youth Survey administered in 1991 among multi-ethnic populations (Sasao, 1991), Korean teens exhibited one of the highest scores on the Problem Behavior index regarding such issues as personal knowledge of a pregnant teenager, compared with Filipino, Chinese, and Japanese youth. It is anticipated that in the case of American-born API adolescents, greater sexual freedom may lead to higher future rates of abortion, unless timely and culturally appropriate contraceptive education is provided.

Abortions Among APIA Women

Although we found no published reports on national comparative rates of abortion among APIAs, two regional studies suggest relatively high abortion use for specific APIA ethnic groups (National Institute of Child Health and Human Development, 1996; Tanjasiri, 1995). Due to the small sizes and the geographic specificity of the studies, caution should be used when generalizing to the greater APIA populations. Although the following data analyses are not population based, they can shed some light on potentially important differences in parity and abortion among selected segments of the APIA populations.

In a study by the National Institute of Child Health and Human

Development,[1] 1,534 women recruited from clinics in New York were surveyed to assess information such as basic demographics, health attitudes, beliefs and behaviors, parity, and number of past abortions. Whites had the lowest income levels, with 80% falling under 100% of the poverty line, compared with 48% Chinese, 41.4% African Americans, 35.8% Puerto Ricans, 31.1% Dominicans, and 30.2% Mexicans. Chinese women were generally older than other minority women in the sample, with only 5.3% under 21 years of age, compared with 25.8% of Puerto Ricans, 20.7% of Mexicans, 19.2% of African Americans, and 13.9% of Dominicans. Chinese women were also most likely to ever be married and foreign born than all other groups in the sample. Multivariate analyses indicate that the number of abortions a woman had in the past did not differ by ethnicity when controlling for marital status and gravidity. These results suggest that Chinese clinic patients do not differ from Whites, African Americans, or Hispanics in their use of abortion services.

In a comparative study of Chinese, Korean, and Thai women conducted by Tanjasiri (1995), data were extracted from client charts at three clinics[2] in Los Angeles to determine the rates of prior abortions and demographic characteristics of selected APIA women seeking family planning services. The average age of the women in this study was relatively older (more than 34 years of age) but approximately the same across all three APIA ethnic groups. Similarly, the percentages of foreign-born and non-English speaking women were high across all ethnic groups and indicated that the women were relatively recent immigrants to the United States. Although the majority of women in all three ethnic groups were married, the Thai sample also had a large proportion (37.5%) of never-married women. Among only ever-married women (see Table 2), no differences were found among the three ethnic groups regarding proportions of pregnancies and live births. As expected, given the older ages of the samples, the majority of all women had two or more pregnancies and live births. However, interesting differences were found regarding abortions among Koreans compared with Chinese and Thai women. Chinese and Thai women did not differ in the proportion who had at least one abortion. On the other hand, Korean women were more likely to have had two or more abortions than the other two ethnic groups. No comparisons were made with non-APIA women.

The implications of these data for understanding abortions among

---

[1]The clinic sample consisted of 470 African American, 190 White, 152 Chinese, 217 Mexican, 252 Dominican, and 190 Puerto Rican women.
[2]All three family planning clinics—Chinatown Service Center, Koryo Health Foundation, and The Clinic/Asian Health Project—are located in areas with large populations of APIAs. None of the clinics perform abortion services. However, all three collect information on the number of pregnancies, live births, and abortions of their clients. A total of 220 patient charts were randomly selected and reviewed on 69 Korean, 70 Chinese, and 81 Thai American clients visiting the clinics within the past 4 years.

TABLE 2
Proportion of Ever-Married Female Korean,
Chinese, and Thai Patients, Age 18 to 50,
Reporting 0, 1, and 2 or More Pregnancies, Live
Births, and Abortions From Three Clinics in Los
Angeles: 1995

Measure	Korean ($n = 64$)	Chinese ($n = 69$)	Thai ($n = 50$)
Pregnancies			
0	9.5	8.7	14.0
1	17.5	18.8	16.0
2+	73.0	72.5	70.0
Live births			
0	14.1	11.6	24.0
1	23.4	23.2	16.0
2+	62.5	65.2	60.0
Abortions[a]			
0	43.8	71.0	71.4
1	18.8	20.3	18.4
2+	37.5	8.7	10.2

Note. Table from "Prior Abortions Among Clients of Family Planning
Clinics in Los Angeles: Chinese, Korean, and Thai Americans," 1995.
Unpublished manuscript by S. P. Tanjasiri.
[a]chi square analyses significant at $p = .05$ level.

APIA women are twofold. First, APIA women clearly use abortion services in this country. Second, given the similarities in demographics among especially Chinese and Korean women in this sample, the variations in abortion rates may point to interethnic differences among APIA populations in the United States.

Attitudes Toward Abortion

Even less is known about the knowledge and attitudes toward abortions held by APIA women and men in the United States. However, we expect some of the attitudes and beliefs among Asian women to persist even after immigration to this country. Initial information gleaned from selected surveys and community data support the expectation that APIAs vary widely in their views toward abortion. Given the large number of immigrants from countries such as China, Hong Kong, Japan, and Korea with permissive abortion policies and attitudes, it is expected that the majority of APIA women will continue to view abortion as an acceptable component of family planning. On the other hand, immigrants from the Philippines and Pacific Islanders are more likely to be opposed to abortion in the United States. For example, in a study conducted by Asians and

Pacific Islanders for Reproductive Health,[3] results suggest that Chinese, Japanese, and Korean American respondents appeared to be more supportive of abortion, either conditionally or completely, compared with all other ethnic groups. According to the authors, 63% of Korean respondents supported the right to choose abortion during early pregnancy, as opposed to only 50% of Pacific Islanders and 53% of Filipinos. Unfortunately, it is not clear whether support for abortion among Chinese and Japanese Americans is due more to generational differences or to ethnic/cultural influences.

Acculturation appears to be clearly related to positive abortion attitudes: 80% to 81% of second and third generation API respondents supported the right to choose abortion, compared with 58% of first generation respondents. Whereas recently arriving immigrant women are expected to closely mirror the attitudes of their homelands, more acculturated APIAs will undoubtedly be influenced by attitudes held in the United States. According to the 1995 National Asian American Sex Survey (Gan, 1995),[4] there is an overwhelming acceptance of abortion among Asian Americans today. Specifically, 71.2% of respondents stated that abortion was somewhat or completely acceptable, whereas only 12.1% registered disapproval. Unlike women in Asia, these positive attitudes are not necessarily associated with having had an abortion: Only 12% of male and female respondents reported that they or a partner had an abortion, 3% of whom reported more than one abortion. Although results were not separated by ethnic group, the high proportion of Chinese and Korean respondents (62% of the total) may have contributed to the majority of positive attitudes. However, given that only 12.1% of respondents found abortion either somewhat or completely unacceptable, these results more likely reflect a generation of individuals whose views about abortion are influenced by American culture and their American peers.

Unfortunately, many limitations exist in interpreting data from surveys of community and convenience samples. First and foremost, results should be attributed only to those APIAs with the same sample characteristics (e.g., age, education, language ability, and nativity) as individual survey respondents. Second, the data examined here primarily reflect APIAs who reside in large cities, such as Los Angeles, San Francisco, and New York. To the extent that APIAs of different ethnic groups and immigration and settlement patterns reside in rural areas of the Midwest, the results are similarly ungeneralizable. Thus, all observations and conclusions

---

[3]A total of 1,215 APIA men and women were surveyed from seven groups (Chinese, Japanese, Filipino, Korean, Southeast Asian, Pacific Islander, and other API) through convenience samples from community-based organizations in Los Angeles, Sacramento, and San Francisco.
[4]A total of 604 APIA men and women completed a written, English-language only survey published by A. *Magazine*. Demographic results show respondents to be primarily young (mean age was 25.6 years), educated (attending college or graduate school), single, English-speaking and American born.

EXHIBIT 1
Structural and Cultural Barriers to Abortion and Other Reproductive Health Care for Asian and Pacific Islander Women

- Lack of power in relationship to choose contraceptive methods
- Stringent gender and family roles discouraging abortion practices
- Cultural reluctance to openly discuss sexual and reproductive health issues
- Misperceptions about contraceptive methods
- Lack of knowledge of available services
- Lack of health insurance coverage
- Lack of geographically accessible services
- Communication barriers between providers and clients
- Lack of culturally appropriate services and educational materials

made should be interpreted as providing only initial information for future research.

CULTURAL FACTORS ASSOCIATED WITH ABORTION

As described in previous sections of this chapter, numerous variations in demographics and abortion-specific practices and perceptions exist among APIAs from different ethnic and cultural groups. Indeed, the wide variety of views combined with the complexity of surveying multiple ethnic groups undoubtedly raises significant barriers to conducting further such research. In this final section, we take a closer look at cultural factors—attitudes regarding sexual health, contraceptive use, gender and family roles, and barriers to care—that shape the potential abortion use of APIA women in the United States (see Exhibit 1). Given the dearth of published information on APIA women, key informant interviews (Tanjasiri & Aibe, 1995) with APIA providers in the reproductive health care field in California provide supportive information on the factors associated with abortion use.

Sexual Health

Asian Pacific Islander women face strong cultural barriers against their open discussion of sex and reproductive health. Traditional Asian cultures place primary importance on the virginity of women, expecting women to remain "pure" until marriage. After marriage, sex continues to be a taboo subject for open discussion. For example, according to a study by Ho (1992), Chinese culture places a higher premium on modesty and obedience than on the free expression of reproductive health concerns. Such views are based on Confucian thought, which is pervasive in Korean and Japanese cultures.

Consequently, APIA women are often reluctant to bring up questions about sexual and reproductive health. According to results from community discussions conducted by Asians and Pacific Islanders for Reproductive Health (APIRH, 1995), sexuality was an extremely difficult topic for foreign-born APIA women to discuss with family members, spouses, and partners. This notion was reinforced by a key informant who reported that APIA women are extremely reticent about discussing sex, even in the context of a medical examination (Tanjasiri & Aibe, 1995). For women who are pregnant, it is often the medical provider who first brings up questions about sexual activity.

Cultural barriers to sexual health information continue to exist for American-born API men and women. According to the A. *Magazine* National Asian American Sex Survey (Gan, 1995), 85.7% of all respondents reported little or no discussion of sex with parents. Among women surveyed, the primary sources of information on sex were friends (76.5%), books and magazines (66.8%), and movies (61.8%). Statements made by Chinese and Tongan participants in the APIRH (1995) report support the notion of a cultural silence surrounding issues of sexual health and women's health, including abortion.

Contraceptive Practices

Ethnicity and generation also influence the rate of contraceptive use. Among a sample of Asian Americans in California, approximately 47% of male respondents and 42% of female respondents were current contraceptive users (APIRH, 1992). These proportions vary by ethnic group: Whereas 64% of Pacific Islanders reported current use, this was true for only 41% of Filipinos. Contraceptive use also increased by generation. Whereas only 40% of first and second generation APIA respondents reported current contraceptive use, the proportion increased to 54% for third generation APIAs. Similar findings were reported in the A. *Magazine* survey (Gan, 1995), with approximately 48.7% of all respondents reporting regular contraceptive use. Because these respondents were generally young and unmarried, this relatively high rate of nonuse suggests a large risk for unplanned pregnancies and abortion.

Very little is known about the contraceptive preferences among APIAs. According to results from the A. *Magazine* survey (Gan, 1995), the majority of respondents (58.3%) reported using condoms, with 21.2% preferring birth control pills. Evidence for the high rate of condom use was corroborated by an obstetrician/gynecologist key informant in Northern California, who stated that condoms without spermicide were extremely popular among recent Chinese immigrants (Tanjasiri & Aibe, 1995). A second key informant from Southern California concurred, stating that condoms were preferred by women prior to having any children, with the preference changing to sterilization when they get older. Finally, a third key informant reported that obtaining any contraceptives, including condoms, is culturally embarrassing for APIA women, and women who come for condoms often end up getting pregnant because they run out and are too embarrassed to get more.

Negative past experiences also influence the desirability of other contraceptive methods among APIA women. One key informant observed that female methods requiring insertion were unappealing to APIA clients because they did not like to place their hands in their vaginas. IUDs are generally more acceptable to women, especially among immigrants from China and Taiwan, the majority of whom use IUDs as their primary method. Hormonal methods, such as oral contraceptives and injections, are unpopular among some—especially first generation—women because of fears of side effects. A key informant reported that many APIA women believe oral contraceptives cause acne, infertility, and cancer. For other women, they or their mothers have had negative experiences with high dose oral contraceptives, including weight gain, nausea, and bleeding. Although those women believe that multiple abortions may lead to infertility, their fear of hormonal contraceptives causing sterility is far greater (Tanjasiri & Aibe, 1995). Overall, information regarding the acceptability of contraceptive methods among APIA immigrants must be carefully interpreted given the selective availability and promotion of methods by foreign governments.

Negative cultural beliefs regarding sexuality and many contraceptives may also be brought over from the country of birth. For instance, oral contraceptives have a negative image among some Japanese women not only because of health effects but also because of the fear that women using pills will be regarded as "sukimono" (sex maniacs; Jitsukawa & Djerassi, 1994). Similarly, condom use in Thailand has been associated with the prostitution industry, which may have impeded its use by recent Thai American immigrants (Brown & Eisenbery, 1995).

Other cultural fears exist surrounding abortions and sterilizations, as identified by key informant interviews (Tanjasiri & Aibe, 1995). For instance, one informant observed that Mien women believe they must always keep the first child because a first abortion will cause sterility. Another informant reported that sterilization is believed by Chinese women to cause arthritis and early aging. Vasectomy is not popular among APIA men because it is believed to decrease physical strength and the libido. Finally, Thai women were observed to oppose vasectomy, but for the opposite reason—that it may render their husbands more sexually promiscuous because they no longer have to worry about pregnancy.

Gender and Family Roles

Traditionally, a major role for all API women is one of bearing children, particularly sons in patriarchal societies like China and Korea. According to Ho (1992), a Chinese woman is expected to be "sam sing" (thrice obeying), answering first to her father, then to her husband, then to her son (Ho, 1992). More generally, Ho explained that in Confucian teaching, Chinese women are expected to always be passive and obedient. Consequently, APIA women are taught from an early age to value devotion and responsibility to their husbands and families, respect for parents and elders, and ties to extended families.

The reproductive health of APIA women is intimately tied to the relationships they have with their partners and families. Most Asian and Pacific Island countries are patriarchal societies wherein males control the major decisions for the family. Within APIA immigrant families, men continue to hold greater power in decision making by way of, for example, better language ability and immigration status (i.e., being the sponsor for the family or holding the work visa). Thus, men play an important role in the contraceptive decision making of Asian couples, often restricting the options APIA women are able to choose (APIRH, 1995). For example, Korean American participants in the APIRH report stated difficulties in discussing condoms with their partners, many of whom complain about discomfort in its use. Relatedly, these participants reported that sterilization (tubal ligation) was relatively easier to talk about with husbands, primarily because it only affects the physical health of women. More generally, APIA women described their relative lack of power to refuse unsafe sex or to change their contraceptive practices. In the words of one woman, "(my) life is forced . . . no choice . . . no contraceptives" (APIRH, 1995, p. 16).

Similar difficulties exist for APIA women with regard to abortion. In a survey conducted by the National Council of Negro Women (NCNW, 1991),[5] the primary person Asian respondents reported speaking to about abortion or family planning was a husband or male friend. The proportion of Asian women citing husband/male friend (73%) was higher than the proportion of Native Americans (43%), Latinas (27%), and African Americans (15%) in the study. The primary importance of husbands in APIA women's decisions regarding abortion undoubtedly contributes to the feeling that "sexuality is a controlled and forced practice dictated by her role in the family and community, as a wife, mother and bearer of children" (APIRH, 1995, p. 16). One key informant also suggested that mothers-in-

---

[5]Between May and August 1991, 1,157 women aged 18 years and older throughout the United States were surveyed from four racial groups: African American (n = 314), Latina (n = 321), Asian (n = 304), and Native American (n = 212). African Americans, Latinas, and Asians were selected by random and surveyed by telephone, whereas Native Americans were recruited from health clinics and surveyed by mail.

law have considerable influence over married women's decisions about abortion. Family disapproval may present one of the most formidable barriers to abortion use for APIA women: In the NCNW survey, 26% of Asians reported difficulty in getting an abortion because their family would not approve (compared with only 4% of African Americans and 3% of Latinas citing this reason; NCNW, 1991). The importance of family ties underscores the need to address APIA women's many potentially conflicting values and to involve family members, in reproductive health education and services.

Barriers to Reproductive Health Care Services

Several barriers exist to the procurement of timely, quality abortion and other health care services for APIA women. Lack of knowledge among APIA women about where to get services presents a primary barrier. According to the NCNW survey, 32% of Asian women reported that it would be difficult to get an abortion because they did not know where to get one (compared with only 7% of African Americans and 2% of Latinas citing this reason; NCNW, 1991). The problem of access to health care is not limited to abortion services, but also applies to reproductive and primary health care services. According to the APIRH survey (1992), 21% of all respondents reported no regular source of reproductive health care. The proportion of respondents without care did not vary greatly by ethnic group (19% Japanese, 21% Filipino, 22% Chinese, 24% South East Asian, and 26% Korean), but differences were great by generation (26% for first generation, 24% for second generation, compared with only 14% for third generation). Access to medical care for these populations was slightly better, with only 5% of Japanese and Chinese, 6% of South East Asians, 7% of Filipinos, and 10% of Koreans reporting no source of regular medical care. Finally, in a report by the Commonwealth Fund (1995), Asians had the highest proportion of respondents who reported a "major problem" with accessing specialty care (25%) compared with Whites (8%), Blacks (16%), and Hispanics (22%). In addition to specific cultural barriers to abortion, APIAs (especially recent immigrants) face significant barriers to health care services overall.

In the United States, access to reproductive and other health care services is intimately tied to the cost of care. A primary barrier is lack of health insurance: It has been estimated that 23% of Asian adults nationally are uninsured, which is higher than 14% of Whites but lower than 26% of African Americans and 38% of Hispanics (The Commonwealth Fund, 1995). Many women are fundamentally ignorant about what kind of health facility can best provide which kinds of reproductive health services and whether they can afford those services even with some health insurance coverage. Immigrant women may seek types of services that are similar to what they were used to in their native countries, without realizing the relative advantages and disadvantages of different modes of health services that exist in this country (National Asian Women's Health Organization, 1995).

Language presents another formidable barrier to quality abortion and reproductive health care for APIA women. Issues often mentioned include the lack of available linguistically and culturally appropriate information and counseling about birth control, pregnancy, sexually transmitted diseases, and abortion (APIRH, 1995). APIAs speak a wide variety of languages and dialects, even those who have emigrated from the same country. For example, the dominant Chinese dialect spoken in this country is Cantonese, as many of the first generation as well as recent immigrants come from Southern China's Guangdong Province and from Hong Kong. Nevertheless, Mandarin is the official language in mainland China and Taiwan and is also widely spoken in this country. Whereas the written language is common to all Chinese, verbal health education must be specific in an individual's dialect to be understood. This is especially true for immigrants illiterate in their own native languages. For Filipinos, the misperception exists that immigrants do not require translated materials and that they can fully express themselves in English, because English is an official language in the Philippines. However, not every Filipino is fluent in English, and Filipino-English is not necessarily understood in this country because of accents and mispronunciations by immigrants taught English abroad (Santos, 1983).

A major problem related to language stems from the common practice of direct translation of English language health education materials into Asian languages (APIRH, 1995). Consequently, information is often presented in culturally insensitive contexts, with illustrations that do not include nor apply to APIA women. According to the Commonwealth Fund survey (1995), approximately half of Asian American adults seek care from Asian American physicians. For APIA women, receiving reproductive health care from non-APIA providers may not ensure quality due to the many cultural barriers mentioned earlier. Furthermore, for many APIA ethnic groups, such as for many South East Asians and Pacific Islanders, ethnic-specific providers are not available.

CONCLUSION

In this chapter, we have used available data and literature to construct a portrait of abortion practice and its many associated factors among Asian and Pacific Islander American women. APIAs are the fastest growing racial group in the United States, with its population predicted to exceed 10 million by the year 2000 (Gardner, Robey, & Smith, 1985). Unfortunately, abortion and reproductive health research that focuses on or includes APIA women is extremely rare. Because of the limited data available on APIA women, this review should be considered as only a first step toward more systematic, population-based research.

Overall, a culturally appropriate approach to understanding reproductive health and abortion among recently immigrated APIA women and their daughters must be molded from a combination of medical, cultural, and sociopolitical influences. As presented in this review, it is crucial that researchers and service providers understand the demographic, cultural, and immigration characteristics of APIA populations to develop culturally specific and sensitive reproductive health care approaches. For foreign-born APIAs, who represent 74% of the entire APIA population, the heterogeneous nature of APIA cultures and populations mandates the identification of ethnic-specific factors, including the sociopolitical factors from their country of birth. For American-born, second, and third generation APIAs, issues concerning acculturation and intergenerational conflict may more greatly influence their sexual activity and abortion practices.

Ultimately, much more research is necessary both to understand and address the abortion needs of APIAs. Recommendations for future exploration include understanding the following issues: What is the rate of unplanned pregnancies among APIAs? What is the relative importance of cultural factors in the decision to obtain an abortion among specific APIA ethnic groups? What are the decision-making processes used by APIA women, and whom do APIA women turn to for support? How do they find out about abortion services? How do they obtain quality reproductive health care, including abortion services and counseling? What are the differential influences of nativity, education, income and language on specific APIA ethnic groups' needs for, and use of, contraceptive and abortion services? It is clear that abortion services are an integral part of the continuum of reproductive health care required by APIA women. What remains as a major challenge for researchers and health care professionals is how to develop and secure culturally appropriate and quality reproductive health care, including readily available and accessible abortion services and educational information, for all American women.

REFERENCES

Alan Guttmacher Institute. (1995). *Hopes and realities: Closing the gap between women's aspirations and their reproductive experiences.* New York: Author.

Allman, J., Nhan, V. Q., Thang, N. M., San, P. B., & Man, V. D. (1994). Fertility and family planning in Vietnam. *Studies in Family Planning, 22,* 308–317.

Anh, D. (1995). Differentials in contraceptive use and method choice in Vietnam. *International Family Planning Perspectives, 21,* 2–5.

Asians and Pacific Islanders for Reproductive Health. (1992). *The Asian/Pacific Islander reproductive health survey, 1991–92.* Los Angeles: Author.

Asians and Pacific Islanders for Reproductive Health. (1995). *The health and well-being of Asian and Pacific Islander American women.* Oakland: Author.

Bisignani, J. D. (1994). *The big island of Hawaii, Moon Travel handbook.* Honolulu: Moon Publications.

Brown, S., & Eisenberg, L. (1995). *The best intentions: Unintended pregnancy and the well-being of children and families.* Washington, DC: National Academy Press.

Center for Reproductive Law and Policy. (1995). *Women of the world: Formal laws and policies affecting their reproductive lives.* New York: Author.

Chen, A. J., Emmanuel, S. C., Ling, S. L., & Kwa, S. B. (1985). Legalized abortion: The Singapore experience. *Studies in Family Planning, 16,* 170–178.

Chen, M. S., & Hawks, B. (1995). A debunking of the myth of healthy Asian Americans and Pacific Islanders. *American Journal of Health Promotion, 9,* 261–268.

Chuong, C. H. (1994). Vietnamese students. *Changing patterns, changing needs.* Zellerbach Family Fund.

The Commonwealth Fund. (1995). Minority Americans are shortchanged on health care. *The Commonwealth Fund Quarterly, 1,* 1–2.

Conly, S. R., & Camp, S. L. (1992). *China Family Planning Program: Challenging the myths.* The Population Crisis Committee.

Cook, R. J. (1989). Abortion laws and policies: Challenges and opportunities. *International Journal of Gynecology and Obstetrics, 3*(Supplement), 61–87.

de Castro, L. (1990). The Phillippines: A public awakening. *Hastings Center Report, 20,* 27–28.

Flavier, J. M., & Chen, C. H. C. (1980). Induced abortion in rural villages of Cavite, the Philippines: Knowledge, attitudes and practice. *Studies in Family Planning, 11,* 65–71.

Gan, D. (1995, August/September). The 1995 National Asian American sex survey. *A. Magazine,* pp. 23–31, 47, 69–70.

Gardner, R. W., Robey, B., & Smith, P. C. (1985). Asian Americans: Growth, changes, and diversity. *Population Bulletin* (Vol. 40). Washington, DC: Population Reference Bureau.

Goodkind, D. (1994). Abortion in Vietnam: Measurements, puzzles and concerns. *Studies in Family Planning, 25,* 342–352.

Hardee-Cleaveland, K., & Banister, J. (1988). Fertility policy and implementation in China, 1986–88. *Population Development Review, 14,* 245–286.

Hawaii Department of Health. (1990). *Annual report: A statistical supplement.* Honolulu, HI: Author.

Health Action Information Network. (1991). *A brief history of the Philippines from a Filipino perspective* (Health Alert Special Issue No. 116–117). Quezon City: Author.

Health Action Information Network. (1994). Hemorrhage behind material deaths.

Henshaw, S. K. (1992). Abortion trends in 1987 and 1988: Age and race. *Family Planning Perspectives, 24*(2), 85–86, 96.

Henshaw, S. K., Binkin, E. B., & Smith, J. C. (1985). A portrait of American women who obtain abortions. *Family Planning Perspectives, 17*(2), 90–96.

Ho, B. (1992). Modesty, sexuality and breast health in Chinese American women. *Western Journal of Medicine, 157,* 260–264.

Hong, S. (1988). South Korea. In P. Sachdev (Ed.), *International handbook on abortion* (pp. 302–316). New York: Greenwood Press.

Huang, S. M. (1989). *The spiral road: Change in a Chinese village through the eyes of a Communist party leader.* Boulder, CO: Westview Press.

Jensen, J. M. (1988). *Passage from India: Asian Indian immigrants in North America.* New Haven, CT: Yale University Press.

Jitsukawa, M., & Djerassi, C. (1994). Birth control in Japan: Realities and prognosis. *Science, 265,* 1048–1051.

Kodagoda, N., & Senanayake, P. (1988). Sri Lanka. In P. Sachdev (Ed.), *International handbook on abortion* (pp. 425–436). New York: Greenwood Press.

Li, V. C., Wong, G. C., Qiu, S.-H., Cao, F. M., Li, P. Q., & Sun, J. H. (1990). Characteristics of women having abortion in China. *Social Science and Medicine, 31*(4), 445–453.

Lieh-Mak, F., Tam, Y. K., & Ng, S. (1981). Hong Kong married abortion applicants: A comparison with married women who elect to complete their pregnancies. *Journal of Biosocial Science, 13*(1), 71–80.

Lin-Fu, J. S. (1988). Population characteristics and health care needs of Asian Pacific Americans. *Public Health Reports, 103*(1), 18–27.

Lin-Fu, J. S. (1993). Asians and Pacific Islander Americans: An overview of demographic characteristics and health care issues. *Asian American and Pacific Islander Journal of Health, 1*(1), 20–36.

Macro International. (1993). *Philippines National Demographic Survey 1993: Summary report.* Calverton, MD: Author.

Martin, J. A. (1995). Birth characteristics for Asian or Pacific Islander subgroups, 1992. *Monthly Vital Statistics Report, 43*(Supplement), 1–9.

Melendy, H. B. (1981). *Asians in America: Filipinos, Koreans and East Indians.* New York: Hippocrene Books.

Muecke, M. A. (1983). In search of healers: Southeast Asian refugees in the American health care system. *Western Journal of Medicine, 139*(6), 835–840.

National Asian Women's Health Organization. (1995). *Pathways to wellness: A California statewide resource handbook for Asian women and girls.* San Francisco: Author.

National Council of Negro Women. (1991). *Women of color reproductive health poll.* New York: Author.

National Institute of Child Health and Human Development (1996). Women's life-styles during pregnancy study. Joint study by the NICHD, Center for the Future of Chidren, and Bureau of Maternal and Child Health.

Ong, P., & Hee, S. (1993). The growth of the Asian Pacific American population: Twenty million in 2020. *The state of Asian Pacific America: Policy Issues to the Year 2020.* Los Angeles: LEAP Asian Pacific Public Policy Institute and the UCLA Asian American Studies Center.

Ping, T., & Smith, H. L. (1995). Determinants of induced abortion and their policy implications in four counties in North China. *Studies in Family Planning, 26*(5), 278–286.

Potts, M., Diggory, P., & Peel, J. (1977). *Abortion.* Cambridge, England: Cambridge University Press.

Ramachandran, P. (1988). India. In P. Sachdev (Ed.), *International handbook on abortion* (pp. 235–250). New York: Greenwood Press.

Sachdev, P. I. P. S. (1988). Abortion trends: An international review. In P. Sachdev (Ed.), *International handbook on abortion* (pp. 1–21). New York: Greenwood Press.

Santos, R. A. (1983). The social and emotional development of Filipino-American children. In G. T. Powell (Ed.), *The psychosocial development of minority group children.* New York: Brunner Mazel.

Sasao, T. (1991). [*High-risk youth survey: Preliminary findings.*] Unpublished raw data.

Tadiar, A. F. (1989). Commentary on the law and abortion in the Philippines. *International Journal of Gynecology and Obstetrics, 3*(Supplement 3), 89–92.

Takenaka, C. (1995). *A perspective on Hawaiians.* Hawaii Community Foundation Diversity Project.

Tanjasiri, S. P. (1995). *Prior abortions among clients of family planning clinics in Los Angeles: Chinese, Korean, and Thai Americans.* Unpublished manuscript.

Tanjasiri, S. P., & Aibe, S. (1995). [Asian Pacific Islander Americans and abortion: Key informant interviews with six health care providers in California.] Unpublished raw data.

Tanjasiri, S. P., Wallace, S. P., & Shibata, K. (1995). Picture imperfect: Hidden problems among Asian Pacific Islander elderly. *The Gerontologist, 35*(6), 753–760.

Thang, N. M., Swenson, I. E., Man, V. D., & Trinh, P. (1992). Contraceptive use in Vietnam: The effect of individual and community characteristics. *Contraception, 45,* 409–427.

Tuan, C. (1988). China. In P. Sachdev (Ed.), *International handbook on abortion* (pp. 98–111). New York: Greenwood Press.

Uba, L. (1994). Supply of health care professionals. In N. W. S. Zane, D. T. Takeuchi, & K. N. J. Young (Eds.), *Confronting critical health issues of Asian and Pacific Islander Americans.* Newbury Park, CA: Sage.

United Nations Population Fund. (1991). *Programme review and strategy development report: Vietnam.* New York: Author.

U.S. Bureau of the Census. (1993a). *We the American ... Pacific Islanders*. Washington, DC: U.S. Department of Commerce, Economics and Statistics Administration, Bureau of the Census.

U.S. Bureau of the Census. (1993b). *We the American ... Asians*. Washington, DC: U.S. Department of Commerce, Economics and Statistics Administration, Bureau of the Census.

U.S. Immigration and Naturalization Service. (1981). *1980 Statistical Yearbook of the Immigration and Naturalization Service*. Washington, DC: U.S. Government Printing Office.

U.S. Immigration and Naturalization Service. (1991). *1990 Statistical Yearbook of the Immigration and Naturalization Service*. Washington, DC: U.S. Government Printing Office.

Wang, L. C. (1991). Roots and changing identity of the Chinese in the United States. *Daedalus: Journal of the American Academy of Arts and Sciences, 120*(2), 181–206.

Yu, E. S. H., & Liu, W. T. (1992). U.S. national health data on Asian Americans and Pacific Islanders: A research agenda for the 1990s. *American Journal of Public Health, 82*(12), 1645–1652.

Zane, N. W. S., Takeuchi, D. T., & Young, K. N. J. (1994). *Confronting critical health issues of Asian and Pacific Islander Americans*. Newbury Park, CA: Sage.

III

INTRAPERSONAL AND INTERPERSONAL CONTEXTS OF ABORTION

8

THE ACCEPTABILITY OF MEDICAL ABORTION TO WOMEN

LINDA J. BECKMAN AND S. MARIE HARVEY

Since the Supreme Court decision to legalize abortion in 1973 the only form of legal abortion available to American women has been surgical abortion. Many women express fear and serious concern about surgical procedures, even minor ones. Moreover, in the United States the types and geographic distribution of facilities providing surgical abortion are limited and the number of physicians who provide this service is decreasing (see Henshaw, chap. 3, this volume). Therefore, the enthusiasm generated for the introduction of mifepristone (more commonly known as RU-486 or the abortion pill) among pro-choice advocates in the United States and American women is not surprising. The purpose of this chapter is to (a) describe the characteristics and history of medical abortion and mifepristone in particular, (b) examine international and national research on the acceptability of medical versus surgical abortion, and (c) discuss our own work on the acceptability of mifepristone to American women and the information needed by these women to make educated decisions about choice of abortion methods.

Over 95% of the abortions in the United States currently are performed using the vacuum aspiration method of surgical abortion. This method requires the insertion of a tube through the cervix into the uterus that sucks out the products of conception from the uterus. Although an extremely safe procedure, several of the possible complications of vacuum aspiration are related to its surgical nature and include infection and perforation of the uterine wall. In addition, although use of a general anesthetic is not typical, some facilities and many women prefer to have a surgical abortion performed with general anesthetic, subjecting the women to the additional risks inherent in its use. Finally, surgical abortions in the United States are provided primarily in free-standing abortion clinics that often have been subjected to picketing, harassment, and, in some cases, violence against clinic personnel and particularly the physicians who perform surgical abortions.

In contrast to surgical abortion, medical abortion is induced by a drug or a combination of drugs that usually can be administered orally and cause the uterus to expel the conceptus. RU-486, now called mifepristone in its generic form, was the first method of medical abortion to become available commercially. It belongs to a class of synthetic agents known as antiprogestins that block the action of the natural hormone, progesterone, by binding with progesterone receptors in the lining of the uterus. This action causes a breakdown of the uterine lining and the occurrence of bleeding as in menstruation and the stimulation of uterine contractions (Grimes, 1993). Clinical trials of mifepristone have recently been completed in the United States, and final Food and Drug Administration (FDA) approval of mifepristone for use as an abortifacient in the United States is currently being sought.

However, because antiprogestins like mifepristone are not currently available in the United States, medical researchers have recently begun to examine the use of another drug, methotrexate, to induce medical abortion. This drug has been available in the United States since 1953 and is currently marketed for other uses such as the treatment of rheumatoid arthritis, cancer and severe psoriasis. In combination with misoprostol, methotrexate has been found to produce a successful early first-trimester abortion in most women (Creinin, 1993, 1994; Creinin & Darney, 1993; Creinin & Vittinghoff, 1994; Hausknecht, 1995; Schaff, Eisinger, Franks, & Kim, 1995). Methotrexate, a folic acid antagonist, causes an early abortion by blocking the folic acid from fetal cells so that they cannot divide. It may also affect the attachment of the embryo to the uterine wall. The use of methotrexate/misoprostol for the termination of early pregnancy makes it all the more certain that medical abortion will become an alternative method for women in the United States. In addition, other drugs have been proposed as early abortifacients and their efficacy is likely to be tested in future international and national clinical trials.

CHARACTERISTICS AND HISTORY OF MIFEPRISTONE

Mifepristone was originally developed in France in 1981 by researchers for the pharmaceutical firm of Roussel Uclaf. After several years of clinical studies, mifepristone with a prostaglandin was initially approved for use as an abortifacient in France in 1988. Since that time this drug has been approved for use in Britain, Sweden, and China and tested in over 20 other countries with nearly 200,000 women (Reproductive Health Technologies Project [RHTP], n.d.).

Despite its international acceptance, the intense politics surrounding abortion have delayed the introduction of mifepristone for use in the United States. During George Bush's presidency, Roussel Uclaf neither applied for FDA approval of mifepristone nor granted patent rights to another organization to do so. The rationale for withholding U.S. distribution of the drug apparently was based on the intense political controversy about abortion in the United States, the political opposition of the Bush administration to release of the drug, and concern about product liability. First, in response to political and economic pressures Roussel Uclaf identified criteria that needed to be present before the company would introduce mifepristone into a new country. One of these was that the political climate must be accepting of abortion.

Thus, the battle between pro-choice and pro-life forces and the Bush administration's fervent opposition to abortion led the decision makers at Roussel Uclaf to conclude that the political climate was not appropriate for the introduction of mifepristone. Second, the company appeared to fear the economic repercussions of actions by antiabortion groups such as the National Right to Life Committee, which threatened to initiate wide-scale boycotts of any company that attempted to get FDA approval for mifepristone (RHTP, n.d.). It is important to note that Roussel is controlled by the German company Hoechst AG, the management of which has been accused of being even more conservative than that of Roussel and generally antiabortion. Because Hoechst has a major American subsidiary and U.S. yearly sales of 6 to 7 billion dollars, the refusal also was strongly influenced by concerns about decreasing profits. Finally, potential product liability issues were a legitimate concern given the history of litigation associated with the Dalkon Shield and some other contraceptive devices and the tendency of American juries to be sympathetic to the injured party (Bass, 1994).

The change that led Roussel and Hoechst to modify their decision was a political one. The new administration elected in 1992 was strongly supportive of women's reproductive rights. When President William J. Clinton first took office in January 1993 he requested that the Department of Health and Human Services review the mifepristone situation and identify means of making it available in the United States (Bass, 1994). After a laborious 13-month negotiation process, in May 1994 Roussel Uclaf gave all of the U.S. patent rights, free of charge, to manufacture and market mifepristone to the Population Council, a nonprofit contraceptive research and reproductive health organization. This extraordinary result came about in part because of political pressure and support of the Clinton Administration and pro-choice members of Congress.

From October 1994 to September 1995 the Population Council conducted a clinical trial of mifepristone with 2,100 women at several sites around the United States. On March 31, 1996, the council announced that it had submitted a New Drug Application (NDA) to the U.S. FDA for mifepristone to be used as a medical abortifacient. In addition, the Council had granted Advances in Health Technology, Inc., a nonprofit organization set up to market and distribute mifepristone (see "RU 486 Transforming the Abortion Debate," 1996), exclusive legal rights to coordinate the manufacture and distribution of mifepristone in the United States (Population Council, 1996). In July 1996 the FDA Committee on Reproductive Health Drugs recommended that the FDA approve the Population Council's NDA for mifepristone to be used as a method of early abortion in the United States. The FDA issued a letter in September 1996 indicating that the agency had determined that clinical data demonstrated that mifepristone was safe and effective when used under close medical supervision, but it needed additional information on manufacturing and labeling before a final approval decision could be made. Although it appeared that mifepristone would be introduced into the U.S. market sometime in 1997, lawsuits filed in November 1996 against a businessman who allegedly used his association with Advances in Health Technology for an illegal money-making scheme may have delayed the introduction of the drug in the United States. Although legal issues are being resolved, as of this publication there still is no manufacturer for mifepristone in the United States.

Mifepristone is among the most effective of the antiprogestins, and it has proven to be the one with the fewest serious side effects (RHTP, n.d.). It is most effective if used early in pregnancy (the first 8 weeks) before the placenta begins to produce increasing amounts of progesterone on its own, which are too great to be overwhelmed by the mifepristone. A series of studies in France and other countries suggests the drug is extremely safe and relatively effective. However, when used alone, its success rate is generally no higher than 65% to 80%, a level that is not acceptable to women and their physicians (RHTP, n.d.). Therefore, researchers have explored the combination of mifepristone with other drugs to heighten effective rates. The best combination to date was identified by a Swedish research group. It involves a dosage of mifepristone followed by a small amount of a prostaglandin (misoprostol) 48 hours later. Mifepristone leads to the sloughing off of the uterine lining, whereas the prostaglandin enhances uterine contractions leading to expulsion of the conceptus, usually within

4 hours. This combination of drugs is believed to be about 96% effective in inducing abortion.

INFLUENCE ON THE ACCEPTABILITY OF ABORTION METHODS

The acceptability of an abortion method depends on the mutable and immutable characteristics of the method itself and the circumstances of a woman's life, that is, the situational context in which she lives. First, just as the attitudes and beliefs of consumers are known to play a critical role in the choice of contraceptive methods (Beckman, Harvey, & Murray, 1992), so too do they influence choice and acceptability of abortion methods. Both the value (i.e., importance) of abortion characteristics to the individual and the person's beliefs about whether a specific method possesses these characteristics should influence the acceptability of the method to the individual and, thus, method choice. Many characteristics of abortion (and contraceptive) methods are inherent in the method (e.g., effectiveness, whether it involves surgery, amount of bleeding) and generally immutable, whereas others are determined in part by the service delivery system (e.g., number of visits to the provider, degree of privacy provided; Winikoff, 1995). Acceptability depends on a woman's perception of both mutable and immutable characteristics of methods.

Moreover, the situational context is likely to influence a woman's attitudes toward medical abortion and will be instrumental in her decision to use or not use a particular abortion method. A woman's perceptions and choice of an abortion method are grounded in the circumstances of her life, and multiple factors enter into the decision-making process. We believe that contextual factors (e.g., where she lives, her social support, cultural background, religion, ambivalence toward having an abortion, whether she is employed outside the household or going to school) interact with method-specific attributes to determine choice.

Although the abortion pill has been heralded as the new magic bullet for women seeking to terminate a pregnancy, the use of the mifepristone –misoprostol combination is a relatively complex process that is more time-consuming than surgical abortion. It is not a simple procedure of taking a pill and currently requires a minimum of three visits to a service provider.

The protocol used for the U.S. clinical trials requires a woman to first have a pregnancy test to confirm pregnancy and an ultrasound to determine length of gestation. She then is counseled about her options. If she is early enough in the pregnancy, has no counterindications for use of the drugs, and voluntarily consents to a medical abortion, she receives two tablets of mifepristone that she consumes in the presence of clinic staff. Then she is asked to wait at the clinic for about an hour to ensure she does not have a negative reaction to the mifepristone. She then returns to the clinic 48 hours later to receive a small dosage of misoprostol. After she is given the misoprostol she remains at the clinic for at least 4 hours. The majority of women complete their abortion within this time and most others complete the abortion within the next day. However, if the abortion is incomplete or does not occur, the woman must undergo a vacuum aspiration abortion. Finally, the woman is requested to return to the clinic 2 weeks later for a follow-up visit. Whether a woman finds this relatively complex and time-consuming procedure acceptable and, in particular, more acceptable than vacuum aspiration abortion depends on her attitudes and perceptions about the procedure and the interpersonal, cultural, and sociopolitical context of her life.

INTERNATIONAL RESEARCH ON ACCEPTABILITY

Several studies in other countries have involved clinical trials that randomly assigned participants to medical and surgical abortion groups, others assess women who chose among methods, whereas still others study only women who chose medical abortion. Despite the diversity of research designs of the 11 published studies (summarized in Winikoff, 1995) that have examined the acceptability of first-trimester medical abortion, the findings are quite consistent. Anxiety about surgery and fear of general anesthesia consistently were identified in these studies as reasons women chose medical abortion. In addition, women in these studies stated that they chose medical abortion because it seemed more "natural" and "like a premeditated miscarriage" (Berer, 1992; Tang, 1991; Thong, Dwar, & Baird, 1992). Greater privacy during treatment also was seen as a benefit of medical abortion by some women (Grimes, Mishell, & David, 1992), but the greater length of time and inconvenience (Bachelot, Cludy, & Spira, 1992; Tang, 1991; Tang, Lau, & Yip, 1993) and the greater pain and bleeding experienced (Rosen, Von Knorring, & Bygdeman, 1984; Tang et al., 1993) were mentioned as disadvantages of medical abortion as compared with surgical abortion. Winikoff (1995) concluded that "virtually all the work accessing acceptability shows a strong preference for medical methods . . . among women seeking an abortion" (p. 148). Yet, despite very high satisfaction levels medical abortion also is associated with somewhat higher dissatisfaction, presumably because of unrealistic expectations about its convenience or lack of appropriate counseling regarding the characteristics of the options available (Winikoff, 1995).

ACCEPTABILITY OF MEDICAL ABORTION
IN THE UNITED STATES

Findings from the international studies provide some information by which to gauge the acceptability of mifepristone to American women. Yet in many ways the political situation and current provision of abortion services in the United States is unique, as is the demographic mix of women seeking abortions. First, the intense controversy over abortion that exists in the American political scene is not characteristic of most Western European countries where abortion is less controversial even though it may be considered unacceptable by major religious groups. The American controversy may be both an antecedent and a consequence of the deep set ambivalence most Americans have about the act of having an abortion. This ambivalence appears to exist to a lesser degree in most other Western industrialized countries. Second, the manner in which the service delivery system in America provides abortion is different from that of many countries. The concentration of most abortion services in free-standing abortion or family-planning clinics in major urban areas has created barriers to access for many women. Part of the attraction of medical abortion for pro-choice forces is that it could increase the number of abortion providers; protect the anonymity and, therefore, safety of women seeking abortions; and improve access, especially for poor, young, and rural women. Finally, women seeking abortion in the United States have a diverse ethnic/racial background. Most other countries in which mifepristone has been investigated do not have the ethnic diversity of the United States nor do they have large groups of women of Hispanic, African American, and Asian heritage.

Other than our own work only two studies on the acceptability of medical abortion in the United States have been completed (Creinin & Park, 1995; David, 1992; Grimes et al., 1992). Using a very small sample of 16 women 18 years and older Grimes and his colleagues randomly assigned women whose menses were no more than 10 days late to one of two groups: single 600-mg dose of mifepristone or placebo group. Participants completed a pre-intervention questionnaire and a follow-up instrument 4 weeks later. The women in both groups perceived mifepristone positively both pre- and postintervention. Among the positive attributes identified were convenience, noninvasiveness, the privacy of not having to go to an identified abortion clinic, the absence of side effects, and effectiveness. Those who completed the follow-up questionnaire reported that they would prefer a medical abortion and would recommend this method. This study examined mifepristone as a method of emergency contraception rather than as an abortifacient and is limited by its very small sample and loss of participants to follow-up (only 56% of the women completed the 4-week follow-up questionnaire). Thus, results are not generalizable to the conditions under which medical abortion is likely to be available in the United States.

As part of a clinical trial to assess the efficacy of methotrexate and misoprostol for early abortion, Creinin and Park (1995) included an acceptability evaluation of this new method of medical abortion. The study sample included 85 women who were interviewed before they received methotrexate and after they completed the abortion. The most frequently cited reason for choosing a medical abortion among this sample of women was to avoid a surgical procedure. Over three fourths (79%) of the participants stated that medical abortion was a "good experience," and 89% would choose this method of medical abortion again over surgical abortion.

OUR CURRENT RESEARCH ON ACCEPTABILITY OF MIFEPRISTONE

Our own research on the acceptability of medical abortion to American women, although limited, has a number of advantages over previous research. It is specific to American women and uses larger and more ethnically diverse samples than previous American studies. Most important, we either incorporated the actual protocol used to provide mifepristone–misoprostol abortions in the United States or asked women about a similar service provision scenario (Beckman & Harvey, 1997; Castle, Harvey, Beckman, Coeytaux, & Garrity, 1995). Our major objectives were to (a) examine the perceived benefits and costs of this method as compared with surgical abortion, (b) determine what additional information women in the United States need about mifepristone to choose between abortion methods, and (c) examine U.S. women's experiences and satisfaction with medical abortion. To date, we have conducted two studies on the acceptability of mifepristone. The first study collected data in eight focus group interviews with a demographically diverse sample of women who were potential users of mifepristone (Castle et al., 1995; Harvey, Beckman, Castle, & Coeytaux, 1995). The second examined attitudes and beliefs about mifepristone and surgical abortion among a sample of women who were participants in the national clinical trial of the drug conducted during 1994 to 1995 (Beckman & Harvey, 1997).

Focus Group Study

We examined the knowledge of women in the United States concerning mifepristone, perceived advantages and disadvantages of the medical abortion compared with surgical abortion, and women's preferences between methods (Castle et al., 1995; Harvey et al., 1995). The study was limited to women who were sexually active and not pregnant, were between the ages of 18 to 34, would consider having an abortion at some time in their life, and had not had an abortion within the past 2 months. Women were recruited from family planning clinics in three cities (Los Angeles, New York, and Portland). The participants had a mean age of

25.8, and their mean number of years of education was 13.4. Sixty-three percent had been pregnant and close to half (45%) reported a previous abortion; over three quarters of the women were single. The 73 participants were divided among three racial/ethnic groups: non-Hispanic White (three focus groups, $n = 30$), African American (three groups, $n = 27$), and Latina (two groups, $n = 16$).

We chose focus groups as the methodology for this initial exploratory study because these group discussions offer concentrated insight into participants' thinking and understanding of specific topics. Prior to the focus group each woman completed a brief questionnaire that assessed demographic information and reproductive health history and whether they had ever heard of "the abortion pill." After the focus group discussion, participants completed a poststudy questionnaire that asked them what method of abortion they would choose and the reasons for their choice. (For a more complete description of the poststudy questionnaire see Harvey et al., 1995.)

Each focus group was conducted by a female moderator of the same racial/ethnic group as the group participants. The moderator followed a semistructured topical guide to stimulate discussion during the sessions that averaged 2 hours in length. Members of the research team read transcripts of each session and individually listed themes in the discussion that addressed three topics: (a) knowledge and awareness of mifepristone and medical abortion, (b) gaps in knowledge of mifepristone, and (c) perceived advantages and disadvantages of this method. The team discussed their findings and reached a consensus on which themes were most frequently mentioned and were most salient to the women.

Knowledge About Mifepristone

Nearly two thirds (63%) of the women reported that they had heard about mifepristone, but very few could accurately describe the drug and procedure for its administration. This finding was surprising because during the data collection period in May 1994 the media provided extensive coverage of the unusual transfer of U.S. patent rights from Roussel Uclaf to the Population Council and the imminent clinical testing of the drug in the United States. Many women indicated that they needed more information about mifepristone before they could make an informed decision about this abortion method. The four main areas in which additional information was needed were the current status of medical abortion in the United States, the composition of the two pills and procedures for administering them, a more detailed description of the medical abortion process and procedures (e.g., the number of hours the second visit will entail, what the expelled material will look like), and the potential side effects and complications (e.g., the consequences to woman and the fetus if the second pill is not taken, the amount of pain that should be expected, whether any pain relievers will be given).

Advantages and Disadvantages of Medical Abortion

Women cited a number of advantages and disadvantages of medical abortion compared with surgical abortion. The most frequently mentioned advantages and disadvantages are listed in Exhibit 1. The perceived advantages included fewer major complications, a nonsurgical procedure, a more natural and noninvasive method, and its availability for use early in pregnancy. Fear of surgery, its complications, and, in particular, general anesthetic was evident among these women. One woman said, "The disadvantage (of vacuum aspiration) is general anesthesia. Any time you use general anesthesia, you run the risk of death." Also, women were particularly impressed with the less invasive nature of mifepristone, which they perceived as a natural process in which the body expels the fetus. For instance, one woman stated, "It seems it would be more holistic, more natural. Like it's all taking place from within your body and there's not instruments or human error involved." Finally, the availability of mifepristone early in pregnancy is perceived as an advantage because many women believe that having an early abortion is both physically and psychologically easier for them.

The major perceived disadvantages were number of visits associated with the procedure, the unknown aspects of a new technology, concerns surrounding the expulsion of the fertilized egg, and the concern that the medical abortion procedure was too "easy" and might be abused by some women. The number of visits was a major concern both because of inconvenience and loss of time ("It's time-consuming if you're working or something like that. With vacuum aspiration, you're in, you're out, and that's it") and the psychological trauma associated with the longer experience ("That will be a long two days. You get a lot of questions in your head—

EXHIBIT 1
Perceived Advantages and Disadvantages of Mifepristone Among a
Sample of Potential Users

Advantages
  Fewer major complications and no risk of perforation of the wall of the uterus
  Nonsurgical procedure and does not require anesthesia
  Natural/noninvasive
  Available for use early in pregnancy
Disadvantages
  Number of visits and 2-day wait between the first and second pills
  Mifepristone is an unknown and unfamiliar technology
  Unknowns surrounding the expulsion of the conceptus
  Perceived potential that mifepristone would make having an abortion too
    "easy" and would be used in place of birth control

oh my God, maybe I shouldn't be doing this."). Not only were some women uncomfortable with the new technology, but also many women expressed concern that the abortion might be completed after leaving the clinic (e.g., "That means that it could come out on your way home, at home, watching TV, on the bus, the train or while you're stuck in traffic."). The final disadvantage, that is, mifepristone would be too easy for other women to use (e.g., "People are really irresponsible. With that [mifepristone] available they would be less responsible than they are now.") may be yet another reflection of the general ambivalence toward abortion in the United States.

Choice of Method

In general, women's perceptions of medical abortion were relatively positive. Almost two fifths of women (38%) said they would choose this method, whereas about 35% selected vacuum aspiration and about 25% of the sample remained undecided. These results are congruent with Rosen's (1990) findings from Sweden that nonpatient groups are fairly equally divided about which method to choose, whereas women in clinical studies that ask about acceptability appear to strongly prefer medical abortion (Winikoff, 1995). In our focus group study 78% of the women who chose mifepristone stated they would select this method to avoid surgery and anesthesia. In contrast, women selected vacuum aspiration because of its familiarity and proven effectiveness (60%) and because they thought it more convenient and quicker than mifepristone (48%).

U.S. Women's Experience With Mifepristone

This study examined the characteristics of women who chose to have a medical abortion, the reasons why they chose mifepristone over surgical abortion, their expectations of the method and whether these expectations were met, and their satisfaction with medical abortion (Beckman & Harvey, 1997). The 262 participants were women enrolled in a national clinical trial of the mifepristone–misoprostol method of medical abortion at one of three clinics located in Portland, Oregon; Seattle, Washington; and Burlington, Vermont. All women were between the ages of 18 and 44, had a positive pregnancy test, and had an ultrasound scan to estimate gestational age. Sample characteristics are presented in Table 1. The average age was 27.0 years, with 35.9% in the 18 to 24 age group, 34.7% in the 25 to 29 age group, and 29.3% 30 or older. The sample was largely non-Hispanic White (82.6%), 5.0% were Asian American, 3.9% Hispanic/Latina, 2.3% African American, and 6.0% self-identified as "Other." All but 12.0% of the sample had been born in the United States. The women generally were highly educated, with a mean number of years of education

TABLE 1
Distribution of Sociodemographic and Reproductive Characteristics of the Sample

Characteristic	Percentage	M	SD
Age (in years)		27.01	5.84
18–24	35.9		
25–29	34.7		
30 and older	29.3		
Ethnicity			
Non-Hispanic White	82.6		
Asian	5.0		
Latina	3.9		
African American	2.3		
Other	6.0		
Country of birth			
United States	88.0		
Other	12.0		
Level of education (in years)		13.79	2.58
Less than high school	9.8		
High school graduate	23.5		
Some college	39.2		
College graduate	27.4		
Days amenorrhea[a]		52.02	8.83
Estimated gestational age (in days)[b]		49.50	8.30
Prior pregnancy	71.9		
Prior live birth	39.7		
Prior abortion	51.1		
More than 1 prior abortion	20.3		
Prior miscarriage	32.5		

[a]Based on self-reports.
[b]Estimated from ultrasound.

of 13.8. Only 9.8% had less than a high school education; the majority (66.6%) had at least some college, and 27.4% were college graduates.

The clinical trials protocol required that all women be less than 63 days amenorrheic (days since last menstrual period). The ultrasound used to determine eligibility resulted in an estimated gestational age of 49.5 (ranging from 28 to 66 days). The majority of the women (71.9%) had had a previous pregnancy, almost 40% had delivered at least one child, and one third (32.5%) had a prior miscarriage. Over half (51.1%) admitted they had experienced a previous abortion and 20.3% had two or more previous abortions.

Data were collected at two stages using pretested, self-administered questionnaires. Women completed an initial questionnaire at their first visit for the medical abortion and a second questionnaire approximately 2 weeks later during their follow-up visit. The women whose medical abortion was unsuccessful and who, therefore, had to have a surgical abortion (vacuum aspiration) completed the second survey during their follow-up visit approximately 2 weeks after their surgical abortion. All but 22 of the original 262 participants completed the follow-up questionnaire.

Items from the initial questionnaire that are examined here include reasons for the participant's choice of method; preferences regarding whom they would prefer, if anyone, to wait with for the abortion to occur; expectations of the abortion experience; and demographic characteristics. Analyses of the initial questionnaire data include all participants who completed this survey except in cases in which initial and follow-up responses are compared. Items from the follow-up questionnaire relate to the participants' experience with medical abortion and their satisfaction with this method.

Reasons for Choosing Medical Abortion

When women were asked about their general reasons for terminating their pregnancy 74.3% stated they did not want a child now, 44.8% cited lack of money or resources, and 43.3% indicated other priorities. Between 10% and 30% of the sample also gave the following reasons: "don't want to be a single parent" (27.6%), "my age" (21.5%), and "relationship problems" (19.2%).

Women were asked to indicate from a list of closed-ended responses their three top reasons for choosing a medical abortion (see Table 2). The reasons most frequently chosen (those mentioned by more than 20% of participants) were "I want to avoid surgery" (62.8%); "I think this method is safer (less invasive) than surgical abortion" (56.3%); "I think this is a more 'natural' method" (40.5%); "I want a method that has the least risk of infection or damage to the uterus" (35.1%); and "I can use this method as soon as I know that I am pregnant, sooner than surgical abortion"

TABLE 2
Reasons for Choosing Medical Abortion (*N* = 262)

Reason	No.	%
Avoid surgery	164	62.8
Medical abortion is safer (less invasive) than surgical abortion	147	56.3
Medical abortion is a more natural method	106	40.5
Medical abortion has the least risk of infection or damage to the uterus	92	35.1
Medical abortion can be used as soon as I know I am pregnant, sooner than surgical abortion	71	27.2
Medical abortion will have the least discomfort	51	19.5
During the clinical trials, medical abortion was the least expensive method	47	17.9
Negative experience with prior surgical abortion	38	14.5
Desire to try a new and different method	32	12.2
Bleed less with medical abortion	3	1.1

Note. Women were asked to check the top three reasons they chose medical abortion.

(27.2%). The most important reasons for choosing medical abortion involve its "natural," noninvasive characteristics. Women chose medical abortion because they specifically wanted to avoid the surgical procedure and medical risks they perceived as associated with vacuum aspiration. Because risks of surgical abortion are extremely low, as compared with other medical and surgical procedures and with carrying a pregnancy to term, it appears that these women may have a fear of surgery and medical procedures that leads them to overemphasize the risks involved in surgical abortion. Alternatively they may be highly health conscious and want to minimize any potential risks to their health.

Next, we examined whether reasons for choosing a medical abortion were similar or different for women who varied in age, educational level, prior abortion experience, and prior miscarriage experience. For each of 10 reasons for having a medical abortion, four separate chi-squares were run, one for each demographic or reproductive history variable. We present only significant results ($\alpha < .01$).

Women who had experienced one or more previous abortions were more likely than women who had not experienced an abortion to mention "I want to try this new, different method" as a reason for obtaining a medical abortion (22.6% vs. 6.1%), $\chi^2(1, N = 261) = 9.26$, $p < .01$. Younger and older women differed in the likelihood of reporting one item. Women 24 and under were less likely than older women to mention that they had not liked surgical abortion (15.1% vs. 31.3%), $\chi^2(2, N = 259) = 10.6$, $p < .01$, presumably because they were less likely to have had a prior abortion. The likelihood of mentioning that medical abortion was safer (less invasive) than surgical abortion differed by educational level. More educated women were more likely to mention this as one of their top three reasons for obtaining a medical abortion (63.5% of women with some college or more vs. 41.2% of women who had no more than a high school education), $\chi^2(2, N = 255) = 11.27$, $p < .01$.

Other Aspects of the Abortion Experience

Women were asked who if anyone influenced them to choose medical abortion and whether they would prefer to be alone; sit in a group with other women; or be with their partner, friends, or family members while waiting at the clinic for the abortion to occur. For both questions, percentages total more than 100% because participants checked all applicable options. Over two thirds (67.2%) of the women reported that they made the decision to have a medical abortion alone. However, in those situations in which a woman was influenced by others, the most frequent sources were sexual partner (16.0% of the time), physician or other health professional (13.0 %), friend (8.0%), and family member (6.1%).

Almost half of the abortion patients (49.8%) preferred to wait with partner, friend, or family member for the abortion to occur; nearly one third (30.6%) preferred to be by themselves. Only 17.6% preferred to wait with other women undergoing the same procedure. The remainder of the sample either had no preference (13.0%) or reported they did not care (14.2%). When asked why they preferred their choice of social contact, those who chose to wait with partner, friend, or family most often mentioned comfort and wanting to share the experience with someone else. For instance one woman stated, "It's a personal decision for me and I would prefer not to share it with strangers even though they're waiting for the same thing. I would like someone who I know to be there with me." Another stated, "This is a personal experience that I would want to share with a partner." Similarly, those who preferred to wait with other women mentioned the importance of sharing the experience. For example, one woman expressed, "Everyone is on the same level, experiencing similar things. I would feel very supported." In contrast, those who preferred to be alone most frequently mentioned the need for privacy. Comments of those who preferred to be alone included "I can deal with it in my own way. Not feel I have to close up because other women are around" and "I don't want anyone around. It's not a pleasant thing to see."

Expectations About Abortion Versus the Experience

On the initial questionnaire women were asked about their expectations of four specific aspects of the medical abortion: discomfort, anxiety, amount of bleeding, and length of bleeding. Approximately 2 weeks later, as part of the follow-up questionnaire, they were asked about their actual experience with regard to these four characteristics. Each item consisted of a 5-point Likert scale. For the first three characteristics, scale points ranged from *none* to *extreme*; for the fourth item concerning length of bleeding, the scale was as follows: 1 = 1 to 3 days, 2 = 4 to 6 days, 3 = 7 to 9 days, 4 = 10 to 12 days, and 5 = 13+ days. Identical scale points were used for expectations and experience, but the wording of the item was changed (e.g., "How much discomfort do you expect to experience?" vs. "How much discomfort have you had?"). One sample t tests revealed significant differences between expectations and experience for discomfort ($p < .001$) and length of bleeding ($p < .001$) and differences of borderline significance ($p < .10$) for anxiety and amount of bleeding (Table 3). Women in the sample expected more discomfort (M = 3.23) than they actually experienced (M = 2.99, with 3 indicating moderate discomfort). They also tended to expect more anxiety and a greater amount of bleeding than they actually experienced. Interestingly, women underestimated the length of time they would bleed. Actual days of bleeding (M = 3.84) were greater than they had expected them to be (M = 3.22).

TABLE 3
Expectations and Experiences of Medical Abortion (*N* = 222)

Characteristic	Expectation		Experience		*t* test of differences
	M	*SD*	*M*	*SD*	
Discomfort[a]	3.23	0.58	2.99	0.96	3.71***
Anxiety[a]	2.83	0.78	2.72	0.90	1.87
Amount of bleeding[a]	3.51	0.57	3.42	0.72	1.77
Length of bleeding[b]	3.22	0.93	3.84	1.24	−7.38***

[a]Mean score with 1 = *none*, 2 = *slight*, 3 = *moderate*, 4 = *high*, and 5 = *extreme*.
[b]Mean score with 1 = 1 to 3 days, 2 = 4 to 6 days, 3 = 7 to 9 days, 4 = 10 to 12 days, and 5 = 13+ days.
***$p < .001$.

Satisfaction With Medical Abortion

Overall the women who participated in the clinical trial at the three clinics were very satisfied with their experience of medical abortion (72.8%). Another 15.5% were somewhat satisfied. Ninety-four percent said they would recommend a medical abortion to a friend and 87% stated that they would select a medical abortion if they had to terminate another pregnancy.

Very satisfied women (*n* = 174) were compared with other women (*n* = 65) using *t* tests ($p < .01$ because of multiple tests involved) to examine variables that distinguished between the two groups (Table 4). The variables that consistently differed between the two groups involved experience with medical abortion. Demographic characteristics (age, education) and reproductive history (prior abortion status, miscarriage status, days amenorrhea) did not differ for the two satisfaction groups, and differences between expectations and experience were of borderline significance. The less satisfied group reported experiencing significantly higher levels of discomfort ($p < .001$) and anxiety ($p < .001$) than the very satisfied group.

RECOMMENDATIONS AND CONCLUSION

Our findings lead to recommendations concerning educational materials and counseling for women and the provision of abortion services sensitive to women's perceptions and needs. The implementation of such recommendations can help to ensure the optimal conditions for the general introduction of mifepristone and other methods of medical abortion in the United States.

Several of our findings regarding reasons for choice of mifepristone and its perceived advantages and disadvantages are congruent with results reported for women in other nations. In particular, women are concerned about the safety of surgical abortion and its complications. They express

TABLE 4
Comparison Between Very Satisfied and Other
Users of Medical Abortion

	Mean score	
Variable	Very satisfied (n = 174)	Other users (n = 65)
Demographics		
Age (years)	27.02	26.51
Education (years)	13.90	13.68
Estimated gestational age* (days)	48.98	50.97
Abortion experience		
Discomfort[a]***	2.88	3.88
Anxiety[a]***	2.61	3.06
Amount of bleeding[a]	3.42	3.48
Length of bleeding[b]	3.90	3.66
Differences between expectations and experiences[c]		
Discomfort*	0.32	0.00
Anxiety	0.17	−0.05
Amount of bleeding	0.07	0.13
Length of bleeding*	−0.73	−0.30

[a]Mean score with 1 = *none*, 2 = *slight*, 3 = *moderate*, 4 = *high*, and 5 = *extreme*.
[b]Mean score with 1 = 1 to 3 days, 2 = 4 to 6 days, 3 = 7 to 9 days, 4 = 10 to 12 days, and 5 = 13+ days.
[c]Differences equals expectations minus experiences.
*$p < .05$. ***$p < .001$.

anxiety about having to experience a surgical procedure. It appears then that women choose mifepristone because they see it as a safer, more natural abortion process and they want to avoid the negative aspects of surgical abortion. American women may overestimate the risks associated with vacuum aspiration abortion, in part, because of the unsubstantiated claims of pro-life groups about the consequences of abortion on women's physical and mental health and the national climate of controversy about abortion.

One finding from our focus group study was unique to the United States. Many women were concerned that mifepristone would make the abortion procedure too "easy" and would allow "other women" to make a decision to have an abortion without giving it proper thought. This finding also may be due, in part, to the political controversy surrounding abortion in the United States, where in contrast to most developed countries, the morality of abortion remains a highly volatile and contentious issue.

In this country women seek abortions in unsupportive and often hostile social and political atmospheres characterized by antiabortion harassment and violence (see Cozzarelli & Major, chap. 4; Russo & Denious, chap. 9; and Henshaw, chap. 3). What is clear from comments of women is that they seek comfort and privacy during this procedure. Being identified and harassed by antiabortion activists would appear to be extremely upsetting to them immediately prior to the abortion procedure.

The biggest obstacle at the moment to medical abortion as a method of choice is lack of knowledge and misconceptions about the procedure among women in the United States. Our findings indicate that women need and want more comprehensive educational materials to assist them in making reasoned decisions about use of mifepristone. They need more information about procedures for taking the pills, their chemical effects, details of the medical abortion process (e.g., time, medical supervision, what the expelled material will look like), and potential side effects and complications. Women who have decided to have a mifepristone abortion require additional information that they may have not received in the recent clinical trial; they need to know how much discomfort and anxiety they are likely to experience and the length and amount of bleeding that is typical. Women who receive, understand, and assimilate such information are likely to be more satisfied users of medical abortion than those who do not.

Women who have had a mifepristone abortion in the United States generally are very satisfied with it. However, only about half of potential abortion patients say they would choose medical abortion. More information is needed about how preference for medical over surgical abortion varies by culture, ethnicity, age, education, socioeconomic status, and prior abortion experience. The composition of our sample suggests that women who chose to obtain mifepristone abortions in the three centers we surveyed were well educated, older than the typical abortion patient, and primarily non-Hispanic White. They were more likely to have experienced one or more surgical abortions than women in their age group nationally. Although this could change with the advent of more general educational messages and media attention, service providers may need to target messages for particular groups (e.g., younger, less educated women, women with no prior abortion) to broaden the acceptability of this pregnancy termination option among a diverse group of women. In designing media messages and educational materials for specific groups, we must remember that different groups of women choose to have a medical rather than surgical abortion for different reasons (e.g., younger women may be more concerned about cost as a factor).

It is essential that consumers are satisfied with the procedure and the health care they receive. Although most women are very satisfied, findings indicate that those with less discomfort and more knowledge about the procedure are likely to be the more satisfied medical abortion users.

Women's comments about certain aspects of mifepristone abortion suggest changes in procedures of service providers that would make this type of abortion more acceptable and comfortable for women. Prime among these are arrangements for waiting for the abortion to occur. The majority of women consider the abortion a very private event that they prefer to experience alone or share only with their partner or a close family member or friend. Only a minority of women (17.6%) find it acceptable to share the experience with others who are also experiencing an abortion. Service providers need to consider women's diverse preferences about this waiting period, maintaining flexible arrangements so that each woman can experience the maximum comfort during this difficult time. Also, a medical abortion procedure that requires fewer visits to the provider and shorter waiting time between initial ingestion of pills and completion of the abortion would be more acceptable to American women, leading to an increase in the numbers who select this abortion option.

Feminist theory suggests that it is important to listen to women's verbal descriptions of their experiences and perceptions (e.g., Miller, 1986; Riger, 1992) because researchers' or experts' conceptual categories may not adequately describe women's experience. Findings from our research highlight the diverse needs, perceptions, and lifestyles of women in the United States. Mifepristone—misoprostol and other methods of medical abortion are not a magic bullet that will solve all problems and resolve issues about abortion in the United States. But medical abortion does have the potential to increase access to abortion for underserved groups of women. To achieve this potential, it is necessary that service providers and reproductive health advocates consider women's perceptions, knowledge, and understanding of this new reproductive technology; be sensitive to women's preferences about procedures associated with the technology; and develop appropriate educational materials to assist women in choosing between abortion methods.

REFERENCES

Bachelot, A., Cludy, L., & Spira, A. (1992). Conditions for choosing between drug-induced and surgical abortions. *Contraception, 45*, 547–549.

Bass, M. (1994). Birth control business. *The Women's Review of Books, 11*(10–11), 20–21.

Beckman, L. J., & Harvey, S. M. (1997). Experience and acceptability of mifepristone and misoprostol among U.S. women. *Women's Health Issues, 7*, 253–262.

Beckman, L. J., Harvey, S. M., & Murray, J. (1992). Development of a multidimensional contraceptive attributes questionnaire (CAQ). *Psychology of Women Quarterly, 16*, 243–259.

Berer, M. (1992). Inducing miscarriage: Women centered perspectives on RU 486/prostaglandin as an early abortion method. *Law, Medicine and Health Care, 20*, 199–208.

Castle, M. A., Harvey, S. M., Beckman, L. J., Coeytaux, F., & Garrity, J. M. (1995).

Listening and learning from women about mifepristone: Implications for counseling and health education. *Women's Health Issues, 5,* 130–138.

Creinin, M. D. (1993). Methotrexate for abortion at <42 days gestation. *Contraception, 48,* 519–525.

Creinin, M. D. (1994). Methotrexate and misoprostol for abortion at 57–63 days gestation. *Contraception, 50,* 511–515.

Creinin, M. D., & Darney, P. D. (1993). Methotrexate and misoprostol for early abortion. *Contraception, 48,* 339–348.

Creinin, M. D., & Park, M. (1995). Acceptability of medical abortion with methotrexate and misoprostol. *Contraception, 52,* 41–44.

Creinin, M. D., & Vittinghoff, E. (1994). Methotrexate and misoprostol vs. misoprostol alone for early abortion. *Journal of the American Medical Society, 272,* 1190–1195.

David, H. P. (1992). Acceptability of mifepristone for early pregnancy interruption. *Law, Medicine and Health Care, 20,* 188–194.

Grimes, D. A. (1993). Mifepristone (RU 486) for induced abortion. *Women's Health Issues, 3,* 171–175.

Grimes, D. A., Mishell, D. R., & David, H. P. (1992). A randomized clinical trial of mifepristone (RU 486) for induction of delayed menses: Efficacy and acceptability. *Contraception, 46,* 1–10.

Harvey, S. M., Beckman, L. J., Castle, M. A., & Coeytaux, F. (1995). Knowledge and perceptions of medical abortion among potential users. *Family Planning Perspectives, 27,* 203–207.

Hausknecht, R. U. (1995). Methotrexate and misoprostol to terminate early pregnancy. *New England Journal of Medicine, 333,* 337–340.

Miller, J. B. (1986). *Toward a new psychology of women* (2nd ed.). Boston, MA: Beacon.

Population Council. (April, 1996). *Status of mifepristone in the United States.* New York: Author.

Reproductive Health Technologies Project. (n.d.). *The case for antiprogestins.* Washington, DC: Author.

Riger, S. (1992). Epidemiological debates, feminist voices: Science, social values, and the study of women. *American Psychologist, 47,* 730–740.

Rosen, A. S. (1990). Acceptability of abortion methods. *Balliere's Clinical Obstetrics and Gynecology, 4,* 375–390.

Rosen, A. S., Von Knorring, K., & Bygdeman, M. (1984). Randomized comparison of prostaglandin treatment in hospital or at home with vacuum aspiration for termination of early pregnancy. *Contraception, 29,* 423–435.

RU 486 transforming the abortion debate. (1996, Sept. 19). *USA Today,* p. 1.

Schaff, E., Eisinger, S. H., Franks, F., & Kim, S. S. (1995). Combined methotrexate and misoprostol for early induced abortion. *Archives of Family Medicine, 4,* 774–779.

Tang, G. W. (1991). A pilot study of acceptability of RU 486 and ONO 802 in a Chinese population. *Contraception, 44,* 523–532.

Tang, G. W., Lau, O. W. K., & Yip, P. (1993). Further acceptability evaluation of RU 486 and ONO 802 as abortifacient agents in a Chinese population. *Contraception, 48,* 267–276.

Thong, K. J., Dwar, M. H., & Baird, D. T. (1992). What do women want during medical abortion? *Contraception, 46,* 435–442.

Winikoff, B. (1995). Acceptability of medical abortion in early pregnancy. *Family Planning Perspectives, 27,* 142–148, 185.

9

UNDERSTANDING THE RELATIONSHIP OF VIOLENCE AGAINST WOMEN TO UNWANTED PREGNANCY AND ITS RESOLUTION

NANCY FELIPE RUSSO AND JEAN E. DENIOUS

Male violence against women takes multiple forms and affects women's lives in multiple ways (Koss et al., 1994). In this chapter we consider the relationship of such violence to unwanted pregnancy and its resolution. We argue that the far-reaching consequences of gendered violence—including physical and sexual abuse, rape, and battering—have important implications for family planning and abortion programs and policies (Goodman, Koss, & Russo, 1993a, 1993b). Women's sexual and reproductive decisions are shaped by the nature of their intimate relationships, and insofar as violence is a means to enforce male dominance and privilege in those relationships, it cannot be ignored by reproductive health professionals. If the assumption that women have control over sexual intercourse is faulty, family planning programs based on that assumption will not be fully effective and, indeed, could even be dangerous for their clients. Programs that assume that contraceptive use can be "negotiated" do not recognize that attempts to negotiate may be seen as a challenge to male power, resulting in violence and threats to social and economic support (Heise, 1993). Broad-based approaches are needed. Such approaches should attack sociocultural factors that absolve males of responsibility for contraception, foster inequalities in power between males and females, and link male sexuality with violence (Heise, 1993, 1995; Russo & Pope, 1993).

Knowledge about male violence against women has direct relevance for current public policy debates about abortion. In some states, rape is directly recognized as a permissible reason for public funding for abortion, but only if the rape is reported—a particularly unrealistic scenario for marital rape in the case of battered wives. Understanding the prevalence and consequences of male violence against women takes on increased importance in the current climate of proposed laws and policies that attempt to limit access to abortion for reasons of psychological health. Arguments for such laws and policies may be based, in part, on a misattribution of the psychological effects of intimate violence in the lives of abortion patients.

This chapter is divided into three parts. First, we summarize the literature on male violence against women, documenting its pervasiveness in women's lives and the severity of its consequences for physical and mental health and social relationships. Second, we focus on linkages between intimate violence and unwanted pregnancy. Third, we document violence in the lives of women who have abortions, providing direct evidence of the need to recognize the impact of violence on such women's lives. We hope this work serves as a catalyst for developing a policy-related research agenda on the causes, consequences, and implications of the links among reproductive health, rape, battering, and other forms of gendered violence. These findings underscore the importance of educating health service providers in family planning and abortion clinics about the dynamics of such violence, so that violence-related issues can be incorporated in pregnancy counseling protocols and be reflected in the design of prevention and intervention programs.

VIOLENCE IS WIDESPREAD AND HAS SEVERE CONSEQUENCES

According to a 1995 report from the Bureau of Justice Statistics based on the National Crime Victimization Survey (Bachman & Saltzman, 1995), from 1992 to 1993 more than one million women experienced some form of victimization from an intimate, compared with 143,000 of such incidents for men. Women experienced seven times the number of incidents of nonfatal violence at the hands of an intimate compared with men, with poor women at highest risk for such violence. Women with family incomes of less than $10,000 per year were four times more likely to experience violence victimization than women with family incomes of $30,000 or more a year. Violence at the hands of intimates was also more likely to cause physical injury than violence at the hands of strangers: 52% of women experiencing a violent incident from an intimate sustained at least one injury, compared with 20% of women experiencing a violent incident from a stranger.

In 1994, there was one rape for every 270 women (Federal Bureau of Investigation, 1995). Estimates that correct for underreporting suggest 700,000 to 1 million women are raped each year (National Victim Center, 1992; Sorenson & Saftlas, 1994). An estimated 1 in 8 women has been the victim of forcible rape, and nearly 40% of those women have experienced more than one rape (National Victim Center, 1992). Approximately 5% of rapes result in unwanted pregnancies—which translates into 35,000 to 50,000 unintended pregnancies annually directly attributable to rape (Holmes, Resnick, & Best, 1996). Women who are 16 to 19 years of age, urban, and low income are at highest risk for sexual assault (Bureau of Justice Statistics, 1997).

High proportions of young girls experience rape and other forms of unwanted sexual contact. Data from the National Women's Study, a longitudinal study based on a national sample of more than 4,000 women, suggests that the majority of rapes occur in childhood and adolescence. Approximately 61% of rapes occur before age 17; 29% occur at under 11 years of age (National Victim Center, 1992). Similarly, data from three states reveal that 44% of police-recorded incidents of rape involve victims younger than 18 years of age (Bureau of Justice Statistics, 1997). One survey of 11 states and the District of Columbia found that 16% of females who reported having been raped were under age 16; half were under 18 (Bureau of Justice Statistics, 1994). In another study, which involved a large sample of 7th-, 9th-, and 11th-grade girls, 21% reported experiencing unwanted sexual contact. For 7th and 9th graders, unwanted sexual intercourse represented 25% to 30% of unwanted sexual contacts; for 11th graders, almost half of the unwanted contacts were sexual intercourse (Small & Kerns, 1993). About 15% of persons imprisoned for rape report that their victims were 12 years old or younger. For those imprisoned for other forms of sexual assault (e.g., statutory rape, forcible sodomy, molestation), the figure is 45% (Bureau of Justice Statistics, 1997). These statistics, which show considerable percentages of women experiencing rape and sexual assault at a young age, become of particular significance when we later consider the consistent linkages of early abuse to revictimization and engagement in high-risk sexual behaviors, unwanted pregnancy, and abortion.

About 25% of women become pregnant by age 18, making factors that lead to early and unprotected sexual intercourse of particular interest to researchers (Alan Guttmacher Institute, 1994). All too often rape is the way young women become introduced to sexual intercourse. A 1987 national survey of men and women aged 18 to 22 found that 13% of White women and 8% of Black women reported that they had experienced non-voluntary sexual intercourse and that experience had a powerful relationship to age of initial intercourse. Almost 7% of White women reported having intercourse before age 14; when the age for first voluntary sexual intercourse was computed, however, the figure dropped to 2.3%. For Black women, the comparable figures were 9% and 6.2% (Moore, Nord, & Peterson, 1989). Similarly, analyses of data from the 1995 National Survey of Family Growth found that the lower the age of first intercourse, the higher the percentage of women whose first intercourse was not voluntary. Among women 15 to 44 years of age who had their first intercourse before age 15, 22.1% reported that experience was not voluntary. In contrast, among women who had their first intercourse at 20 years of age or older, 3.3% reported that intercourse was not voluntary (Abma, Chandra, Mosher, Peterson, & Piccinino, 1997).

In addition, among young women who reported their first sexual experience as voluntary, a high proportion had that sexual experience with an older male. Among women who reported their age at first intercourse to be under 16 years of age, more than one out of three (34.4%) had a first voluntary partner who was aged 18 or older (Abma et al., 1997). Another study found that among teenagers who became mothers by age 17, 53% of the fathers were between the ages of 20 to 29; for those who became mothers by age 15, the figure was 39%. This age discrepancy, and the unequal power balance that accompanies it, suggests that sexual exploitation, if not coercion, is an important contributor to teenage birth rates (Glei, 1994).

Battering and rape go together. An estimated 33% to 59% of battered women report being raped by their partners, and the more violent the man, the more likely he is to rape his wife (Frieze, 1983; Frieze & Browne, 1989; Martins, Holzapfel, & Baker, 1992). Sometimes a battered woman may experience forcible rape several times a month (Browne, 1992).

The health consequences of intimate violence for women who survive it are severe and long lasting. More than a third of rape victims report sustaining serious physical injury, and more than half seek medical treatment (Beebe, 1991). Sexually transmitted diseases are a direct result of rape in an estimated 4% to 30% of victims (Koss & Heslet, 1992). Diagnoses of conditions that are disproportionately found among rape victims are wide ranging and include headaches, chronic pain (including chronic pelvic pain and joint and muscle pain), gastrointestinal disorders, psychogenic seizures, and recurrent vaginal infections (Koss & Heslet, 1992; Koss, Koss, & Woodruff, 1991; Randall, 1990, 1991). Further, wife battering is the single most common cause of injuries to women requiring medical intervention, accounting for more injuries than automobile accidents, muggings, and rapes combined (see Goodman et al., 1993a). From 22% to 35% of women seen in emergency services have symptoms directly linked to battering, regardless of their stated presenting complaint (Stark & Flitcraft, 1996).

The psychological outcomes of intimate violence cross affective, cognitive, and behavioral domains (Browne, 1992; Koss & Harvey, 1991; Neumann, Houskamp, Pollock, & Briere, 1996). A history of sexual assault has been found to lead to higher risk for major depressive episode, substance abuse disorders, and anxiety disorder (Burnam et al., 1988). Common psychological sequelae for rape victims include anxiety and fear, depression, sexual dysfunction, and substance abuse (see Goodman et al., 1993a, 1993b, for a review of this literature). Victims may experience nightmares, catastrophic fantasies, feelings of alienation and isolation, and physical distress (Koss & Harvey, 1991). Feelings of vulnerability, loss of control, and self-blame may persist (Burgess & Holstrom, 1978; Kilpatrick, Veronen, & Best, 1985; Resick & Schnicke, 1991). Sexual dysfunctions experienced include fear of sex, arousal dysfunction, decreased sexual interest, and less pleasure in sexual relations (Becker, Skinner, Able, & Cichon, 1984; Ellis, Atkeson, & Calhoun, 1981; George, Winfield, & Blazer, 1992).

Women are at highest risk for battering in their childbearing years. A national study found that pregnant women were more likely to have experienced violence during the previous year than nonpregnant women (17% vs. 12%). The difference appears to reflect the fact that women are most likely to become pregnant during the time in life when they are at most risk for intimate violence (Gelles, 1988). Other research suggests that likelihood of violence during pregnancy is higher for women who are of lower socioeconomic status, have a history of depression, use alcohol and drugs, receive less emotional support from others for the pregnancy, and are involved with partners who use illicit drugs (Adams, 1985; Amaro, Fried, Cabral, & Zuckerman, 1990).

Battered women are more likely to experience stillbirths and miscarriages and to deliver low-birth-weight infants (Helton, McFarlane, & Anderson, 1987; McFarlane, 1989; McFarlane, Parker, Soeken, & Bullock, 1992; Satin, Hemsell, Stone, Theriot, & Wendel, 1991). Other outcomes include placental separation; premature labor; hemorrhaging; and rupture of membranes, uterus, liver, or spleen (Saltzman, 1990). Given these consequences, it is no wonder that in 1985, the Surgeon General of the United States recommended that routine prenatal assessments include evaluation for battering (Surgeon General's Workshop on Violence, 1985).

In summary, male violence against women is pervasive, with long-lasting effects on physical and mental health, including reproductive health. Its consequences encompass many factors correlated with unintended and unwanted pregnancy, including age, income, education, marital status, self-esteem, and depression (Gazmararian et al., 1995; Koss & Mukai, 1993; Russo & Zierk, 1992), suggesting that gendered violence may play a far greater role in issues related to unwanted pregnancy and abortion than previously recognized.

VIOLENCE IS LINKED TO UNINTENDED AND UNWANTED PREGNANCY

According to the Committee on Unintended Pregnancy of the Institute of Medicine (CUP), nearly 60% of pregnancies are unintended—that is, they are mistimed (wanted later) or not wanted at all, ever (CUP, 1995). Why, despite access to modern techniques of birth control and abortion, does unintended pregnancy continue to be so widespread in contemporary American society? We suggest that one reason is male violence against women.

Many of the risk factors for unwanted pregnancy have been identified as outcomes of violence against women. These common links include low self-esteem, depression, feelings of powerlessness and loss of control, and feelings of alienation and dissociation (Becker-Lausen & Rickel, 1995; Finkelhor, 1987; Wyatt, Guthrie, & Notgrass, 1992). Like violence, unwanted pregnancy is associated with social and economic disadvantage and stressful circumstances (Williams & Pratt, 1990). It is greatest for poor women and women with less than a high school education, particularly if they are a racial minority. In 1988, among women with less than a high school education, 44.5% of births to Black women and 15.5% of births to White women were unwanted (Williams, 1990). Other correlates of unwanted pregnancy include forced marriage, teenage childbearing, single parenthood, larger family sizes, short childbirth intervals, and marital conflict and disruption (see Russo, 1992, for a review of this literature).

Women with lower self-esteem, lower income, and fewer years of education are also at particular risk for repeat unwanted pregnancy. This is true whether the pregnancies are resolved by giving birth or having an abortion. Indeed, women who have unwanted births also have a greater number of abortions than other women (Russo & Zierk, 1992). Thus, women who have abortions and women who bear unwanted children are often the same women.

Women who have larger family sizes (Hillard, 1985) and who are unhappy about being pregnant (Amaro et al., 1990) are more likely to experience violence during pregnancy. Violence against women is particularly high among women with unwanted and mistimed pregnancies (i.e., unintended pregnancies; Fergusson, Horwood, Kershaw, & Shannon, 1986; Gazmararian et al., 1995). A large, population-based study of 12,612 mothers across four states (Alaska, Maine, Oklahoma, and West Virginia) found that 43% of women sampled had an unintended pregnancy (Gazmararian et al., 1995). Among women who reported that their husband or partner had "physically hurt" them during the 12 months before delivery, however, 70% reported having an unintended pregnancy. The state-specific prevalences of violence for women with unwanted or mistimed pregnancies ranged from 36.9% to 46.3%; the comparable figures for women with intended pregnancies ranged from 3.8% to 6.9%.

VIOLENCE IS LINKED TO HIGH-RISK SEXUAL BEHAVIOR

Violence in women's lives has been found to be associated with a wide range of high-risk health behaviors from smoking and alcohol use to failure to use seat belts (Koss, Koss, & Woodruff, 1991; Koss, Woodruff, & Koss, 1991). Most relevant here is research that links victimization with high-risk sexual behaviors, in adolescence and beyond (Koss, Heise, & Russo, 1994), that increase the likelihood of unintended pregnancies.

Sexual abuse appears to be a major predictor of high-risk sexual activity during adolescence for both men and women. Abused girls begin intercourse at an earlier age, an average of 13.8 years for abused teens compared with a national average of 16.2 years (Boyer & Fine, 1992). They are also more likely to engage in unprotected sexual intercourse (Heise, 1993). Only 28% of teens with a history of abuse practiced contraception during their first intercourse, compared with 49% of their nonabused peers. Sexually abused girls are also more likely to experience physical abuse; use alcohol and drugs; have sex on a first date; have sex with a stranger; have group sex; engage in partner swapping; and to trade sex for food, money, shelter, or drugs (Boyer & Fine, 1992; Finkelhor, 1987; Meyerding, 1977; Nagy, Adcock, & Nagy, 1994; Paone, Chavkin, Willets, Friedman, & Des Jarlais, 1992; Roosa, Tein, Reinholtz, & Angelini, 1997; Santelli & Beilenson, 1992; Wyatt et al., 1992).

Given these findings, it should not be surprising that a history of childhood physical and sexual abuse has been linked to risk for teenage childbearing and unwanted pregnancy. In one study of pregnant teenagers less than 18 years of age, 25% of the participants reported incidents of sexual or physical abuse (Berenson, San Miguel, & Wilkinson, 1992). Women experiencing sexual assault in childhood have been found to be three times more likely to become pregnant before age 18 compared with nonvictimized women (Zierler et al., 1991). Another study of adolescent mothers in Washington state found that two thirds had been sexually abused and 44% had been raped. Eleven percent of the mothers who had been raped reported becoming pregnant as a result (Boyer & Fine, 1992). Roosa et al. (1997) found that 50% of women in their sample who reported a teenage pregnancy had experienced childhood sexual abuse compared with 31% of women who did not become pregnant as teenagers.

We have yet to understand the causal relationships of childhood abuse and unintended pregnancy. On the one hand, sexual conflict, inhibition, and avoidance are potential outcomes of childhood sexual abuse, which could potentially lower risk of pregnancy. On the other hand, such abuse can also result in sexual precocity and hyperarousal, which may become reflected in earlier onset of sexual intercourse and heightened risk of unintended pregnancy (Wilsnack, Klassen, Vogeltanz, & Harris, 1994). Given that sexual abuse shares many correlates with unintended pregnancy, it is difficult to ascertain whether violence and abuse lead to high-risk sexual behavior, high-risk sexual behavior puts one at risk for abuse, or other factors lead to both high-risk sexual behavior and abuse. In reality, probably all three things are occurring, but little is known about these interrelationships.

Research by Roosa et al. (1997) suggests that understanding these relationships will require distinguishing among types and severity of abuse. Those researchers found that pregnancy rates of abuse victims varied markedly by severity of abuse: 9% for contact molestation victims, 26% for attempted rape victims, 39% for coercion victims, and 43% for rape victims. In comparison, 21% of the women who did not report a history of abuse had a teenage pregnancy. To what extent these figures might reflect a differential reporting bias for women with different histories is unknown. In any case, the finding is important, for the great variability in pregnancy rates suggests that different mixes of types and levels of abuse would lead to very different pictures of the relationship of abuse to teenage pregnancy. For example, data from a sample heavily weighted with contact molestation victims might lead to finding that women reporting abuse had a lower risk for teenage pregnancy compared with other women, whereas data from a sample weighted with coercion and rape victims would lead to the opposite conclusion.

Roosa et al. (1997) explored interrelationships among sexual abuse, precocity, and teenage pregnancy. They classified the women in their study on the basis of *sexual history pathways*, defined by the nature and timing of the women's histories of sexual abuse and sexual precocity. Women reporting some form of sexual abuse (contact molestation only, coercion, attempted rape, or rape) were classified as victims. Women who reported having voluntary sexual intercourse before the age of 16 were classified as sexually precocious. Thus, five pathways were possible: (a) neither victim nor precocious; (b) victim only, not precocious; (c) victim, then precocious; (d) precocious, then victim; or (e) precocious only, not victim.

Of the 1,284 women who were classified by this system, 33% (n = 422) were initially victims of sexual abuse; of this group, 41% later became sexually precocious. Another 37% (n = 475) of the larger group first became sexually precocious; of this precocious group, 22.5% subsequently became victims. Thus, although sexual abuse did not necessarily lead to precocity (indeed, initial sexual abuse victims were less likely to become precocious than other women in the sample), a high proportion of victims became precocious. The probability of becoming precocious once a victim was almost twice (1.86) the probability of becoming a victim once precocious (Roosa et al., 1997). Empirical investigation of factors that contribute to the development of precociousness in sexual abuse victims is dearly needed.

With regard to the question of the relationship between sexual history pathway and teenage pregnancy, unfortunately, the abuse victims who reported only contact molestation were included in the victim category despite their having a substantially lower rate of pregnancy than all other women, even nonabuse victims. Because they made up 8% of the individuals in the victim category, the relationship of the classification system to pregnancy rates becomes difficult to interpret. We cannot assume that individuals who experienced only contact molestation were evenly distributed over the sexual history pathway categories. In any case, it appears that an important line of future research would be to distinguish between these types of abuse and the different consequences they may engender. For example, perhaps experience of contact molestation more likely results in sexually avoidant behaviors, whereas experience of more severe forms of abuse more often leads to precocity.

Although we are looking at the abuse–pregnancy relationship with a muddy lens, Roosa et al.'s (1997) results are interesting. The rates of pregnancy for women who were victims only and for women who were neither a victim nor precocious were similar (11.2% vs. 12.3%). Because outcomes of sexual abuse include fear of sex, arousal dysfunction, and decreased sexual interest, as described above, that some victims of sexual abuse did not develop sexual precocity or show an elevated pregnancy risk is understandable. It may also be that these women experienced a positive and constructive response when they reported their abuse, thus mitigating potentially damaging effects. More research is needed to examine these relationships.

Pregnancy rates were similar for women who were precocious only and women who were precocious and then became victims (42.1% vs. 42.9%). The most interesting point here is that the women who experienced sexual abuse and then became precocious had the highest pregnancy rates (51.5%). This supports the hypothesis that for some women, sexual abuse may interfere with their ability to plan and control their fertility. Providing effective family planning services to them may require addressing issues raised by their histories of sexual abuse.

These findings differ by ethnicity, however, suggesting that understanding the relationship between childhood sexual abuse and teenage pregnancy will require examining those relationships separately for different ethnic groups. Pregnancy rates were higher for women who experienced victimization before becoming precocious compared with women who became precocious before victimization for the largest population group, non-Hispanic Whites (44% vs. 30%), and also for Mexican Americans (71% vs. 52%). But these findings were reversed for African American women (47% vs. 58%) and did not differ for Native Americans (50% for both groups). Lumping all women together clearly masks important differences in the relationship between sexual history pathway and pregnancy rate (Roosa et al., 1997). It may be that the types of sexual abuse experienced differ across ethnic group. Whether there is an interaction of sexual pathway and type of abuse is unknown and could affect the results.

There are many important issues raised by this study that require further research. In addition to lumping victims of varying abuse experiences into one category, this research did not take into account frequency of abuse, which may covary with severity. Research (Wyatt et al., 1992) suggests that women who have two or more incidents of abuse in both childhood and adulthood are most likely to have unintended and aborted pregnancies. It is also possible that some women who reported being abused following precociousness may not recall abuse that occurred in early childhood, the period of time during which such experiences appear more likely to lead to sexual precocity. Future research is needed to explore these issues.

Engagement in sex frequently or with many partners is often depicted in the clinical literature as a coping response to early abuse (Zierler et al., 1991); victims seek out opportunities to "reenact" the experience in attempts at mastery and to overcome the feelings of powerlessness, guilt, and other negative emotions associated with the abusive experience. But sexual precocity may be especially risky for those who have been previously victimized. Research indicates that some of the psychological outcomes of abuse, such as dissociation and feelings of powerlessness (Becker-Lausen & Rickel, 1995) can increase the likelihood of engaging in spontaneous, unprotected sex. Those with a history of abuse may be less likely to foresee the consequences of their sexual behaviors (Wyatt et al., 1992), less likely to believe they can affect their outcomes, and hence more likely to have unintended pregnancies.

Although being sexually precocious is not necessarily evidence of abuse, inappropriately sexualized behavior has been found to be a reliable indicator of abuse in children as young as 4 to 5 years old (Slusser, 1995). This is consonant with other research that suggests that timing of victimization is important: Sexualization may more frequently occur with preschool victims compared with school-age girls (Friedrich et al., 1992).

It should also be recognized that childhood sexual abuse may increase the risk for unintended and unwanted pregnancy beyond the teenage years. Survivors of early sexual abuse are more likely to experience revictimization (Atkeson, Calhoun, & Morris, 1989; Finkelhor, 1987; White, 1996; Wyatt et al., 1992). Outcomes of child sexual abuse include both sexual and relationship problems that heighten revictimization risk (Gershenson et al.,

1989; Kendall-Tackett & Simon, 1988; Russell, 1986; White, 1996; Wyatt et al., 1992; Wyatt & Newcomb, 1990).

Musick (1993) provided an eloquent portrait of how physical and sexual abuse, particularly under conditions of poverty, may lay the ground for later exploitative and dysfunctional relationships with males. We have yet to learn exactly how and why this happens. The important point here is that such encounters may maintain an abused girl's higher risk for unwanted pregnancy throughout adulthood directly (by exposing her to sexual intercourse) as well as indirectly (by changing her health-related behavior, such as alcohol and drug use, that in turn increases her risk for both violence and unintended pregnancy). Negative social responses to victims play an important role in determining levels of psychological distress after victimization (Carmen & Rieker, 1989; Davis, Brickman, & Baker, 1991; Ullman, 1996). Family planning and abortion counselors have potentially important roles to play in derailing the processes leading to psychological distress and revictimization.

The combination of early childhood experience and revictimization during adolescence has particular implications for prevention programs. White (1996) suggested that not only do earlier victimization experiences predict later ones—the effects of the experiences appear to be cumulative. In her longitudinal study of sexual victimization of college women, she found that women who experienced both childhood and adolescent sexual victimization were more likely to be raped during their first year of college than other women. Women who do not experience sexual revictimization during adolescence do not differ from women with no history of victimization. She concludes that adolescence is a particularly important time for acquiring cultural scripts for intimate relationships and that revictimization during adolescence may have a particularly damaging effect on schemas for those relationships.

In summary, intimate violence—rape, battering, and childhood sexual abuse—has been linked to risk for unintended and unwanted pregnancy. We have much to learn about the causal dynamics that underlie these linkages, but the evidence suggests that the pathways will be reciprocal and both direct and indirect. The outcomes of victimization will be mediated and moderated by the nature, severity, and frequency of the abuse and the response of significant others when learning of it. These factors may all vary by ethnicity in complex ways. For counselors of pregnant teenage girls, the causal dynamics are less important than the fact that they must take into account the possibility of a client history of childhood physical and sexual abuse as well as ongoing violence in the lives of their clients, and adapt their counseling strategies to reflect their clients' realities. Meanwhile, research that elucidates causal dynamics is critically needed for informing the design of effective programs to prevent unintended pregnancy and the need for abortion for women across the life cycle.

VIOLENCE IN THE LIVES OF WOMEN WHO HAVE ABORTIONS

Given that violence is linked to unwanted pregnancy, what are the implications of women's experiences with intimate violence for abortion programs and policies? Some researchers have studied violence in pregnancy among populations obtaining prenatal care or having children, but the nature, extent, and impact of intimate violence and the threat of such violence in the lives of abortion patients have yet to be adequately explored. What are the circumstances facing women who choose to terminate an unwanted pregnancy? Are their realities reflected in the public policies and programs that designate the conditions under which they can receive an abortion? What factors influence women's decisions to have an abortion? Can we understand the mental health of women who have abortions without taking into account the violence in their lives?

Research findings suggest that marital problems play a substantial role in women's decisions to seek abortion, particularly if the women do not yet have children. Slightly more than 28% of nonmothers and 17% of mothers cite partner-related reasons for seeking abortion (Russo, Horn, & Schwartz, 1992).

One study of 249 married abortion patients (Russo & Pope, 1993) suggests that marital rape and battering are a fact of life for a substantial proportion of women who seek abortions: 17% reported that their husbands had forced them to have intercourse (the legal definition of rape) in the past 6 months; 11% also reported that their husbands had made them do things during intercourse that they did not want to do during that time period. When women were asked to rate the level of violence in their marriages from "no battering" to "severe battering," nearly 1 out of 4 (24%) reported at least some battering. Similarly high levels of battering were reported during pregnancy; 20% of women reported such violence. When given a modified form of the Conflict Tactics Scale (Straus, 1979) and asked about the occurrence of specific behaviors associated with battering in the past 6 months, women reported the following:

- 50% reported that their husbands had yelled, swore or screamed at them;
- 26% had husbands who threatened to leave the relationship;
- 18% had husbands who threatened to hit or throw something;
- 14% had something thrown at them;
- 13% had been pushed, grabbed, shoved, or slapped;
- 9% had been punched with fists;
- 5% had been threatened with a weapon (e.g., gun, knife); and
- 23% reported having been afraid of their husbands.

Marital rape, sexual degradation, fear, and marital unhappiness were all linked, suggesting that when a woman says she has an unhappy marriage, it is likely that she means she has a violent or potentially violent marriage. In addition, marital rape was associated with involvement in decision making: The more often the husband forced the woman to have sexual intercourse, the more likely it was the woman herself who made the decision to have the abortion. The various forms of violence were consistently and regularly related to husband's involvement in the decision-making process, particularly in the case of being threatened (whether with being hit or threatened with a weapon).

Because coercion is an important predictor of negative postabortion emotional responses (Adler et al., 1992), we examined whether having a violent husband might be related to satisfaction with the abortion decision. Only 5% of the women in this study expressed dissatisfaction with their decision, suggesting that the abortion screening and counseling process was effective. Interestingly, husband's involvement with the abortion decision was associated with less satisfaction with the decision to have an abortion, but fear, unhappiness, rape, and other violent acts had no relationship to satisfaction. In this context, husband involvement may reflect ambivalence on the part of the woman who turns to her husband for support and guidance in resolving her concerns. Because less satisfaction was also correlated with the husband threatening to leave the relationship, it may also be that feeling insecure in one's relationship to one's husband contributes to ambivalence in the decision-making process.

Fear and marital unhappiness were associated with the woman making the decision herself. Thus, women expressed good reasons for not wanting to involve their husbands in the abortion decision, supporting concerns about policies mandating husband involvement in pregnancy decision making (either through requiring notification or approval). Given that women in nonviolent, happy marriages were more likely to involve their husbands in the pregnancy decision-making process, such policies should have the greatest impact on women in violent relationships. Moreover, recent research on the impact of social conflict on women's postabortion adjustment (Major, Zubek, Cooper, Cozzarelli, & Richards, 1997) showed that the more women perceived their partners as sources of conflict the greater psychological distress they evidenced 1 month after the abortion. If women are required to involve partners in the decision to have an abortion, prevalence of symptoms (e.g., depression, anxiety, and somatization) resulting from relationship conflict may increase and could be mislabeled as posttraumatic response to the abortion. Hence, the quality of the partner relationship needs to be considered when studying pregnancy decision making.

Unfortunately, Russo and Pope (1993) were only able to include married women in their study. Expanding on their work, Russo and Denious

(1996) analyzed data from The Commonwealth Fund's 1993 survey The Health of American Women, conducted by Louis Harris and Associates (Bell et al., 1994). The survey involved telephone interviews with 2,525 female respondents and covered a range of health issues, including questions about demographic characteristics (i.e., income, education, race, and marital status), history of violence and abuse, measures of depression and self-esteem, and whether or not the woman had had at least one abortion. Thus, we were able to examine differences in the nature and extent of violence in the lives of the 324 women who answered yes when asked if they had ever had an abortion (abortion group) compared with other women (nonabortion group). Unfortunately, because of the way the question was asked, we were not able to distinguish women who obtained one abortion from those who had repeat abortions. This is a major limitation, as earlier research has demonstrated that women who experience repeated unwanted pregnancies and abortions are more likely to manifest symptoms of psychological distress (Russo & Zierk, 1992). Consequently, relationships that emerge from these data are likely to be even stronger for women experiencing repeated unwanted pregnancies and abortions.

Even with the relatively insensitive methods used, women in the abortion group reported significantly higher rates of childhood abuse than other women: Nearly 50% of the abortion group reported feeling they were verbally or emotionally, physically, or sexually abused when they were growing up; the comparable figure for the nonabortion group was 26%. Further, the women in the abortion group were more than three times as likely to have experienced all three categories of abuse than other women (15.8% vs. 4.4%). Of women who reported no experience of childhood abuse, 9.2% reported having an abortion; in contrast, of women who reported experiencing all three categories of abuse, 34.7% reported having an abortion.

The relationship of partner violence to abortion was examined in a subsample of 1,426 women who were married or living with their partner who were given a modified version of the Conflict Tactics Scale. Respondents were asked whether, in the past 12 months, their partner had ever displayed any of a list of 11 categories of behaviors. Categories listed included 2 dealing with nonphysical conflict (i.e., insulted or swore at you; stomped out of the room/house/yard) and 9 dealing with physical or threat of physical violence (i.e., threatened to hit you or throw something at you; threw or smashed or hit or kicked something; threw something at you; pushed, grabbed, shoved, or slapped you; kicked, bit, or hit you with a fist or some other object; beat you up; choked you; threatened you with a knife or gun; used a knife on you). Although the categories used were not directly comparable to those used by Russo and Pope (1993), the results support the same basic conclusion: High proportions of women who have abortions experience conflict and violence in their relationships. Women in the abortion group were significantly more likely than other women to have conflict in their relationships; 64.6% reported some form of conflict compared with 44.9% of other women. With regard to nonphysical violence, 62.2% of the abortion group reported such violence compared with 43.2% of other women. Similarly, women in the abortion group were significantly more likely to report physical violence: 20% of women experiencing abortions reported experiencing some form of physical violence compared with 11.4% of other women.

Multivariate analysis of variance revealed that the 165 women in the abortion group in this subsample were significantly more likely to express depressive symptoms. However, when a stepwise multiple regression was used to separate the contributions of child abuse, partner abuse, and abortion to depression symptoms, abortion did not make an independent contribution to level of depression. Both history of child abuse and partner abuse continued to make independent contributions to depressive symptoms, however. These findings are congruent with those of earlier research by Russo and Zierk (1992), who analyzed longitudinal data and found that level of well-being before becoming pregnant was the most important predictor of well-being for women, regardless of whether they had had an abortion (reviews of postabortion response literature can be found in Adler et al., 1992; Russo, 1992).

IMPLICATIONS

Overall, existing research findings suggest that exploring the link between unintended pregnancy and intimate violence, including childhood sexual abuse and partner violence, has important implications for family planning and abortion policies and programs. Clearly, more research is needed, particularly with regard to the causal dynamics whereby victimization leads to increased risk for unintended pregnancy and abortion. What factors mediate and moderate the relationship of victimization experiences to unintended pregnancy? What forms and characteristics of victimization put women at higher risk? Characteristics that need to be examined include age at first and last victimization (particularly when pre- and postpuberty); nature and severity of the experiences; frequency, duration, invasiveness, and injuriousness of the violence; the abuser–victim relationship; the type of persuasion, threat, or force involved; whether the experience was disclosed to others; and the response of significant others as well as health care professionals to learning of the violence.

Despite the limitations of our knowledge base, we can conclude that the goals of eliminating unintended pregnancy and the need for abortion services will not be achieved as long as society continues to tolerate physical and sexual violence and abuse of females in general and especially in the marital relationship. In particular, marital rape and its linkage to battering constitute a major impediment to a woman's ability to plan and control childbearing. Having the right and the means to say no to unwanted and unprotected sexual intercourse—even if the person desiring intercourse is her husband—is a necessary condition for a woman to be able to set and achieve her family planning goals. Family planning and abortion services will never be fully accessible unless women feel free to use them without fear of reprisal.

More attention must be given to the impact of the media and other cultural forces that foster social, political, and economic inequalities between men and women. Male gender role socialization is also of concern. Evidence that suggests aggressive men who associate sex with violence are more likely to rape their wives (Frieze, 1983) indicts male gender role socialization and underscores the need to develop intervention programs that focus on male children and adolescents. It is not enough to teach girls about their bodies, contraceptives, and to "just say no." Boys must learn new definitions of manhood, sexuality, and responsibility if rates of unintended pregnancy and abortion are to be minimized. The fact that most men are neither rapists nor violent toward their intimate partners reminds us that there is no necessary link between violence and sexuality. In the meantime, the prevalence of rape and abuse in childhood and adolescence suggests that both children and adolescents need to be more closely supervised and protected from sexual predators (CUP, 1995).

Attention to male roles is no substitute for programs designed to strengthen women's ability to plan and control their lives and protect themselves from violence, however. Battered women are adaptive and creative in making the best of the choices open to them (Gondolf & Fisher, 1988). The task for health professionals is to design programs to broaden those choices. These include programs that increase the educational and career opportunities of girls and women; provide sources of emotional, social, and economic support; and lessen financial dependence on violent partners.

The high rates of intimate violence in the lives of women who have abortions have special significance in today's political context in which there is a concerted attempt to socially construct a "postabortion syndrome." The idea that abortion has widespread and severe negative mental health effects among abortion patients continues to be advanced, including attempts to promote a postabortion syndrome and to pass informed consent legislation mandating that doctors tell their patients that abortion can cause them to experience depression and other mental health problems. In addition to deterring women from abortion through inappropriate and misleading counseling, these efforts are part of a larger strategy to deny women access to abortion by deterring physicians from performing them because of their fear of malpractice suits. For example, ads by the American Rights

Coalition have asked "Having problems with an abortion?" and distributed a toll-free number that, when called, refer the caller to a medical malpractice lawyer. The Elliot Institute advertises The Jericho Plan as a "comprehensive strategy for making abortionists fully liable for all the physical, psychological, and spiritual injuries they inflict on women," asserting that "when they are finally faced with proper liability, abortion clinics will close" (Elliot Institute, n.d.). The institute also distributes materials that use alleged "risk factors" of abortion and warn therapists to be wary of patients seeking guidance about an abortion decision. For example, they explicitly stated

> If a therapist offers an opinion, he exposes himself to civil liability for improper screening and disclosure. As a licenced (sic) counseling professional, he or she may be presumed responsible for screening for these known risk factors and for fully disclosing relevant risk information to the client. (Reardon, 1997, p. 5)

Correlates of negative postabortion emotional responses are viewed as "predictive risk factors" that are to be used to screen abortion patients. In addition to a history of abuse or unresolved trauma, adolescence or immaturity, emotional or psychological problems, and poorly developed coping skills, the list of risk factors includes moral ambivalence, conflicting maternal desires, therapeutic or eugenic abortion, second- or third-trimester abortion, feeling pressured to abort by others, feeling the decision is not one's own or is one's "only choice," feeling rushed to make a decision, biased preabortion counseling, social isolation, accompanied to abortion by male partner, and a history of prior abortion (Reardon, 1997). The clear message is that if a physican performs an abortion on a woman with any one of these characteristics, he or she should be liable for the physical, psychological, and spiritual damages that will *inevitably* occur as a result. "Abortion practitioners who fail to provide proper screening and counseling should, of course, be held accountable for both malpractice and the violation of their patients' civil rights" (Reardon, 1997, p. 6).

Women who are victimized demonstrate a wide range of physical and mental health problems (Goodman et al., 1993a). Their mental health is not served by attributing their symptoms to the experience of abortion rather than to their history of physical and sexual abuse or the violence they have experienced at the hands of their intimates (Russo, 1996). Labeling an experience (e.g., sexual abuse) a *predictive risk factor* for negative postabortion emotional responses does not mean that the link between that experience and negative emotional responses will be severed if an abortion is denied. Indeed, the same factors that predict negative postabortion responses predict negative responses to relinquishing a child for adoption and to raising an unwanted child (Russo, 1992). Most relevant here is the fact that the data provide no justification for using either a pregnant woman's history of sexual abuse or her relationship with a violent man as a rationale to force her to bear a child purportedly to protect her mental health.

CONCLUSION

Reproductive health professionals have critical roles to play in identifying, treating, and referring victims of violence and in creating a more sophisticated, research-based understanding of effects of violence on women's ability to control pregnancy and childbearing. Women's health has been undermined by tolerance of marital rape and other forms of physical and sexual abuse of females of all ages. Health problems as well as related social and economic problems of women that result from unintended pregnancy, including unwanted childbearing, teenage motherhood, shorter birth intervals, and large family sizes (Russo, 1992), will not be fully ameliorated by family planning programs as long as the effects of male violence on women's reproductive choices are ignored. In addition, understanding the effects of intimate violence in the lives of women who have abortions has special significance in the context of current efforts to construct a postabortion syndrome. Such efforts seek to provide justification for malpractice and civil liability suits that would ultimately deny women access to abortion. Mental health professionals have important roles to play in ensuring that women who have a history of victimization are not manipulated in the service of a political agenda and that women's mental health issues are not misrepresented by any side in the abortion debate.

REFERENCES

Abma, J. C., Chandra, A., Mosher, W. D., Peterson, L., & Piccinino, L. (1997). Fertility, family planning, and women's health: New data from the 1995 National Survey of Family Growth. *Vital Health Statistics 23* (Whole No. 19).

Adler, N. E., David, H. P., Major, B. N., Roth, S. H., Russo, N. F., & Wyatt, G. E. (1992). Psychological factors in abortion: A review. *American Psychologist, 47,* 1194–1204.

Adams, H. P. J. (1985). Physical abuse in pregnancy. *Obstetrics and Gynecology,* 66(2), 185–190.

Alan Guttmacher Institute. (1994). *Sex and America's teenagers.* New York: Author.

Amaro, H., Fried, L. W., Cabral, H., Zuckerman, B. (1990). Violence during pregnancy and substance abuse. *American Journal of Public Health, 80,* 575–579.

Atkeson, B. M., Calhoun, K. S., & Morris, K. T. (1989). Victim resistance to rape: The relationship of previous victimization, demographics, and situational factors. *Archives of Sexual Behavior, 18,* 497–507.

Bachman, R., & Saltzman, L. E. (1995). *Violence against women: Estimates from the redesigned survey* (Publication No. NCJ-154348). Washington, DC: U.S. Department of Justice, Office of Justice Program, Bureau of Justice Statistics.

Becker, J. V., Skinner, L. J., Able, G. G., & Cichon, J. (1984). Sexual problems of sexual assault survivors. *Women & Health, 9*, 5–19.

Becker-Lausen, E., & Rickel, A. U. (1995). Integration of teen pregnancy and child abuse research: Identifying mediator variables for pregnancy outcome. *Journal of Primary Prevention, 16*, 39–53.

Beebe, D. K. (1991). Emergency management of the adult female rape victim. *American Family Physician, 43*, 2041–2046.

Berenson, A. B., San Miguel, V. V., & Wilkinson, G. S. (1992). Prevalence of physical and sexual assault in pregnant adolescents. *Journal of Adolescent Health, 13*, 466–469.

Bell, R., Duncan, M., Eilenberg, J., Fullilove, M., Hein, D., Innes, L., Mellman, L., & Panzer, P. (1994). *Violence against women in the United States: A comprehensive background paper.* New York: The Commonwealth Fund.

Boyer, D., & Fine, D. (1992). Sexual abuse as a factor in adolescent pregnancy and child maltreatment. *Family Planning Perspectives, 24*, 4–10.

Browne, A. (1992). Violence against women: Relevance for medical practitioners. *Journal of the American Medical Association, 267*, 3184–3189.

Bureau of Justice Statistics. (1994). *Child rape victims, 1992* (Publication No. NCJ-147001). Washington, DC: U.S. Department of Justice.

Bureau of Justice Statistics. (1997). *Sex offenses and offenders.* Washington, DC: U.S. Department of Justice.

Burgess, A. W., & Holmstrom, L. L. (1978). Recovery from rape and prior life stress. *Research on Nursing and Health, 1*, 165–174.

Burnam, M. A., Stein, J. A., Golding, J. M., Siegel, J. M., Sorenson, S. B., Forsythe, A. B., & Telles, C. A. (1988). Sexual assault and mental disorders in a community population. *Journal of Consulting and Clinical Psychology, 56*, 843–850.

Carmen, E., & Rieker, P. P. (1989). A psychosocial model of the victim-to-patient process. *Psychiatric Clinics of North America, 12*, 431–443.

Committee on Unintended Pregnancy. (1995). *The best intentions: Unintended pregnancy and the well-being of children and families.* Washington, DC: National Academy Press.

Davis, R. C., Brickman, E., & Baker, T. (1991). Supportive and unsupportive responses of others to rape victims: Effects on concurrent victim adjustment. *American Journal of Community Psychology, 19*, 443–451.

Elliot Institute. (n.d.). Let Us Show You How We Will STOP ABORTION. Advertising flyer, Elliot Institute, P.O. Box 7348, Springfield, IL.

Ellis, E. M., Atkeson, B. M., & Calhoun, K. S. (1981). An assessment of long-term reaction to rape. *Journal of Abnormal Psychology, 90*, 263–266.

Federal Bureau of Investigation. (1995). *Crime in the United States: 1995*. Washington, DC: Federal Bureau of Investigation.

Fergusson, D. M., Horwood, L. J., Kershaw, K. L., & Shannon, F. T. (1986). Factors associated with reports of wife assault in New Zealand. *Journal of Marriage and the Family, 48*, 407–412.

Finkelhor, D. (1987). The sexual abuse of children: Current research reviewed. *Psychiatric Annals, 17*, 233–241.

Friedrich, W. N., Grambsch, P., Damon, L., Hewitt, S. K., Koverola, C., Wolfe, V., Lang, R. A., & Broughton, D. (1992). Child Sexual Behavior Inventory: Normative and clinical comparisons. *Psychology and Assessment, 4*, 303–311.

Frieze, I. H. (1983). Investigating the causes and consequences of marital rape. *Signs: Journal of Women and Culture and Society, 8*, 532–553.

Frieze, I. H., & Browne, A. (1989). Violence in marriage. In L. Ohlin & M. H. Tonrey (Eds.), *Crime and justice—An annual review of research* (pp. 163–218). Chicago: University of Chicago Press.

Gazmararian, J. A., Adams, M. M., Saltzman, L. E., Johnson, C. H., Bruce, F. C., Marks, J. S., & Zahniser, S. C. (1995). The relationship between pregnancy intendedness and physical violence in mothers of newborns. *Obstetrics & Gynecology, 85*, 1031–1038.

Gelles, R. (1988). Violence and pregnancy: Are pregnant women at greater risk for abuse? *Journal of Marriage and the Family, 50*, 841–847.

George, L. K., Winfield, I., & Blazer, D. G. (1992). Sociocultural factors in sexual assault: Comparison of two representative samples of women. *Journal of Social Issues, 48*, 105–125.

Gershenson, H. P., Musick, J. S., Ruch-Ross, H. S., Magee, V., Rubino, K. K., & Rosenberg, D. (1989). The prevalence of coercive sexual experience among teenage mothers. *Journal of Interpersonal Violence, 4*, 204–219.

Glei, D. (1994). Age of mother by age of father, 1988. Unpublished data from Sex and America's Teenagers, 1994, by the Alan Guttmacher Institute; retabulated by Child Trends, Inc., Washington, DC, 1994. Cited in Committee on Unintended Pregnancy (1995). *The best intentions: Unintended pregnancy and the well-being of children and families*. Washington, DC: National Academy Press.

Gondolf, E., & Fisher, E. R. (1988). *Battered women as survivors: An alternative to treating learned helplessness*. Lexington, MA: Lexington Books.

Goodman, L. A., Koss, M. P., & Russo, N. F. (1993a). Violence against women: Physical and mental health effects. Part I: Research findings. *Applied & Preventive Psychology: Current Scientific Perspectives, 2*, 79–89.

Goodman, L. A., Koss, M. P., & Russo, N. F. (1993b). Violence against women: Physical and mental health effects, Part II: Conceptualizing post-traumatic stress. *Applied & Preventive Psychology: Current Scientific Perspectives, 2*, 123–130.

Heise, L. (1993). Reproductive freedom and violence against women: Where are the intersections? *Journal of Law, Medicine, and Ethics, 21*, 206–216.

Heise, L. (1995). Violence, sexuality, and women's lives. In R. G. Parker & J. H. Gagnon (Eds.), *Conceiving sexuality: Approaches to sex research in a post-modern world* (pp. 109–134). New York: Routledge.

Helton, A., McFarlane, J., & Anderson, E. T. (1987). Battered and pregnant: A prevalence study. *American Journal of Public Health, 77,* 1337–1339.

Hillard, P. J. (1985). Physical abuse in pregnancy. *Obstetrics & Gynecology, 66,* 185–190.

Holmes, M. M., Resnick, H. S., & Best, C. L. (1996). Rape-related pregnancy: Estimates and descriptive characteristics from a national sample of women. *American Journal of Obstetrics and Gynecology, 175,* 320–325.

Kendall-Tackett, K., & Simon, A. (1988). Molestation and the onset of puberty: Data from 365 adults molested as children. *Child Abuse and Neglect, 12,* 73–81.

Kilpatrick, D. G., Veronen, L. J., & Best, C. L. (1985). Factors predicting psychological distress among rape victims. In C. R. Figley (Ed.), *Trauma and its wake* (pp. 113–141). New York: Brunner/Mazel.

Koss, M. P., Goodman, L. A., Browne, A., Fitzgerald, L., Keita, G. P., & Russo, N. F. (1994). *No safe haven: Male violence against women at home, at work, and in the community.* Washington, DC: American Psychological Association.

Koss, M. P., & Harvey, M. R. (1991). *The rape victim: Clinical and community interventions.* Newbury Park: Sage.

Koss, M. P., Heise, L., & Russo, N. F. (1994). The health burden of rape viewed from the global perspective. *Psychology of Women Quarterly, 18,* 509–530.

Koss, M. P., & Heslet, L. (1992). Somatic consequences of violence against women. *Archives of Family Medicine, 1,* 53–59.

Koss, M. P., Koss, P. G., & Woodruff, W. J. (1991). Deleterious effects of criminal victimization on women's health and medical utilization. *Archives of Internal Medicine, 151,* 342–357.

Koss, M. P. & Mukai, T. (1993). Recovering ourselves: The frequency, effects, and resolution of rape. In F. L. Denmark & M. A. Paludi (Eds.), *Psychology of women: A handbook of issues and theories* (pp. 477–512). Westport, CN: Greenwood Press.

Koss, M. P., Woodruff, W. J., & Koss, P. G. (1991). Criminal victimization among primary care medical patients: Prevalence, incidence, and physician usage. *Behavioral Sciences and the Law, 9,* 85–96.

Major, B., Zubek, J. M., Cooper, M. L., Cozzarelli, C., & Richards, C. (1997). Mixed messages: Implications of social conflict and social support within close relationships for adjustment to a stressful life event. *Journal of Personality and Social Psychology, 72,* 1349–1363.

Martins, R., Holzapfel, S., & Baker, P. (1992). Wife abuse: Are we detecting it? *Journal of Women's Health, 1,* 77–80.

McFarlane, J. (1989). Battering during pregnancy: Tip of an iceberg revealed. *Women & Health, 15,* 69–84.

McFarlane, J., Parker, B., Soeken, K., & Bullock, L. (1992). Assessing for abuse during pregnancy: Severity and frequency of injuries and associated entry into prenatal care. *Journal of the American Medical Association, 267,* 3176–3178.

Meyerding, J. (1977). Early sexual experience and prostitution. *American Journal of Psychiatry, 134,* 1381–1385.

Moore, K. S., Nord, C. W., & Peterson, J. L. (1989). Nonvoluntary sexual activity among adolescents. *Family Planning Perspectives, 21,* 110–114.

Musick, J. S. (1993). *Young, poor, and pregnant.* New Haven, CT: Yale University Press.

Nagy, S., Adcock, A. G., & Nagy, M. C. (1994). A comparison of risky health behaviors of sexually active, sexually abused, and abstaining adolescents. *Pediatrics, 93,* 570–575.

National Victim Center. (1992). *Rape in America: At a glance.* Arlington, VA: Author.

Neumann, D. A., Houskamp, B. M., Pollock, V. E., & Briere, J. (1996). The long-term sequelae of childhood sexual abuse in women: A meta-analytic review. *Child Maltreatment, 1,* 6–16.

Paone, D., Chavkin, W., Willets, I., Friedman, P., & Des Jarlais, D. (1992). The impact of sexual abuse: Implications for drug treatment. *Journal of Women's Health, 1,* 149–153.

Randall, T. (1990). Domestic violence begets other problems of which physicians must be aware to be effective. *Journal of the American Medical Association, 264,* 940–943.

Randall, T. (1991). Hospital-wide program identifies battered women; offers assistance. *Journal of the American Medical Association, 266,* 1177–1179.

Reardon, D. C. (1997, May). Predictive factors of post-abortion maladjustment: Clinical, legal and ethical implications. Paper presented at the annual meeting of the American Psychiatric Association, San Diego, CA.

Resick, P. A., & Schnicke, M. R. (1991). Treating symptoms in adult victims of sexual assault. *Journal of Interpersonal Violence, 5,* 488–506.

Roosa, M. W., Tein, J., Reinholtz, C., & Angelini, P. J. (1997). The relationship of childhood sexual abuse to teenage pregnancy. *Journal of Marriage and the Family, 59,* 1–12.

Russell, D. (1986). *The secret trauma.* New York: Basic Books.

Russo, N. F. (1992). Psychological aspects of unwanted pregnancy and its resolution. In J. D. Butler & D. F. Walbert (Eds.), *Abortion, medicine and the law* (4th ed., pp. 593–626). New York: Facts on File.

Russo, N. F. (1996, August). *Serving the public interest: Psychology and the abortion debate.* Distinguished Contributions to Psychology in the Public Interest Award address presented at the 103rd Annual Convention of the American Psychological Association, Toronto, Canada.

Russo, N. F., & Denious, J. E. (1996, April). *Violence in the lives of women having abortions.* Poster presented at the annual meeting of the Western Psychological Association, Seattle, WA.

Russo, N. F., Horn, J., & Schwartz, R. (1992). Abortion in context: Characteristics and motivations of women who seek abortion. *Journal of Social Issues, 48,* 182–201.

Russo, N. F., & Pope, L. (1993, May). Implications of violence against women for reproductive health: Focus on abortion services. Paper presented at the "Psychology and Women's Health: Creating a Psychosocial Agenda for the 21st Century" Conference, Washington, DC.

Russo, N. F., & Zierk, K. L. (1992). Abortion, childbearing, and women's well-being. *Professional Psychology: Research and Practice, 23,* 269–280.

Saltzman, L. E. (1990). Battering during pregnancy: A role for physicians. *Atlanta Medicine, 64,* 45–48.

Santelli, J. S., & Beilenson, P. (1992). Risk factors for adolescent sexual behavior, fertility, and sexually transmitted diseases. *Journal of School Health, 62,* 271–279.

Satin, A. J., Hemsell, D. L., Stone, I. C., Theriot, S., & Wendel, G. D. (1991). Sexual assault in pregnancy. *Obstetrics and Gynecology, 77,* 710–714.

Slusser, M. M. (1995). Manifestations of sexual abuse in preschool-aged children. *Issues in Mental Health Nursing, 16,* 481–491.

Small, S. A., & Kerns, D. (1993). Unwanted sexual activity among peers during early and middle adolescence: Incidence and risk factors. *Journal of Marriage and the Family, 55,* 941–952.

Sorenson, S. B., & Saftlas, A. F. (1994). Violence and women's health: The role of epidemiology. *Annals of Epidemiology, 4,* 140–145.

Stark, E., & Flitcraft, A. (1996). *Women at risk.* Thousand Oaks, CA: Sage.

Straus, M. A. (1979). Measuring intrafamily conflict and violence: The Conflict Tactics (CT) Scales. *Journal of Marriage and the Family, 41,* 75–88.

Surgeon General's Workshop on Violence. (1985). *Response, 9,* 19–21.

Ullman, S. E. (1996). Social reactions, coping strategies, and self-blame attributions in adjustment to sexual assault. *Psychology of Women Quarterly, 20,* 505–526.

White, J. (1996, August). *Sexual revictimization: Sexual scripts and dating rituals.* Invited address presented at the 103rd Annual Convention of the American Psychological Association, Toronto, Canada.

Williams, L. B. (1990). Determinants of unintended childbearing among ever-married women in the United States: 1973–1988. *Family Planning Perspectives, 23*(5), 212–221.

Williams, L. B., & Pratt, W. P. (1990). Wanted and unwanted childbearing in the United States: 1973–1988 (Advance data from Vital and Health Statistics, No. 189). Hyattsville, MD: National Center for Health Statistics.

Wilsnack, S. C., Klassen, A. D., Vogeltanz, N. D., & Harris, T. R. (1994, May). Childhood sexual abuse and women's substance abuse: National survey findings. Paper presented at the "Psychological and Behavioral Factors in Women's Health: Creating an Agenda for the 21st Century" Conference, Washington, DC.

Wyatt, G. E., Guthrie, D., & Notgrass, C. M. (1992). Differential effects of women's child sexual abuse and subsequent sexual revictimization. *Journal of Consulting and Clinical Psychology, 60*, 167–172.

Wyatt, G. E., & Newcomb, M. (1990). Internal and external mediators of women's sexual abuse in childhood. *Journal of Consulting and Clinical Psychology, 58*, 758–767.

Zierler, S., Feingold, L., Laufer, D., Velentgas, P., Kantorwitz-Gordon, S. B., & Mayer, K. (1991). Adult survivors of childhood sexual abuse and subsequent risk of HIV infection. *American Journal of Public Health, 81*, 572–575.

10

TESTING A MODEL OF THE PSYCHOLOGICAL CONSEQUENCES OF ABORTION

WARREN B. MILLER, DAVID J. PASTA, AND CATHERINE L. DEAN

The psychological consequences of induced abortion are both complex and incompletely understood. They are complex because of the multiple domains of behavior that are affected—childbearing, sexuality, contraception, health, gender identity, love relationships, and moral development, to mention a few—and because of the variety and intensity of opinions about abortion that exist in most contemporary U.S. communities. They are incompletely understood because insufficient evidence about the psychosocial effects of abortion (Koop, 1989) makes it difficult to draw valid inferences, especially with respect to long-term (2 to 20 years) consequences. Although available evidence is sufficient to suggest that abortion is usually psychologically benign and that severe negative reactions are rare (Adler et al., 1992), there is still a great deal we do not know about the psychological processes that follow abortion.

In this context of complexity and uncertainty, it is not surprising to find in the literature a large number of different theoretical approaches to the study of how induced abortion affects women psychologically. Miller (1992) identified six theoretical approaches commonly used by researchers in their efforts to study and understand the psychological consequences of abortion for an unwanted pregnancy. First, there is the stress approach, which assumes that both the pregnancy and the abortion create stress that continues after the abortion in reaction to the procedure. Second, there is the decision-making approach. It assumes a decision-making process prior to the abortion, with the risk—often increased by the occurrence of unexpected postabortion events—of negative feelings about the decision (i.e., regret) after the procedure.

Third, there are two similar approaches that assume a particular type of preabortion conflict and a related type of postabortion negative affect. In the norm violation approach, there is preabortion conflict over the rightness of having an abortion, followed by postabortion shame and guilt. In the loss approach, there is preabortion conflict over wanting the child, followed by postabortion grief and depression. Closely related to these two approaches is the crisis approach in which there is a preabortion crisis with anxiety about the possibility of having an unwanted child and a postabortion crisis resolution with relief from that anxiety. Finally, there is the learning approach, which assumes that both the negative affects experienced and the self-awareness gained as a result of the unwanted pregnancy and abortion produce new behaviors in the various domains listed earlier.

It should be emphasized that none of these six theoretical approaches denies the existence or even the relevance of components present in the other approaches. Rather, the differences among them are primarily a matter of emphasis. Miller (1994) identified the major components of all six approaches and integrated them into a single, overarching theoretical framework. The advantage to such an integration is that it allows us to hypothesize relationships between the components of these six approaches, test those hypotheses, and determine the relative strength of each component in the context of a general model. In this chapter we test Miller's integrated theoretical framework with data from a sample of 145 women having a medical abortion by means of RU486.

METHODS

Design

The research reported here was conducted during clinical trials of the abortifacient RU486 (Mifepristone), which when used in conjunction with the administration of a prostaglandin (Misoprostol) during the first 5 weeks of pregnancy produces a medical abortion. Women participating in the trials at one location in the Saint Louis area were interviewed immediately before the administration of RU486 (T_0), again 2 weeks later (T_1), and then a third time approximately 6 to 8 months later (T_2).

Sample

The clinical trials of RU486 in the Saint Louis area were conducted by one of the authors (CLD) beginning in April and extending through September 1995. Considerable print and broadcast media publicity was generated at the beginning of this period, informing the public of the free availability of medical abortions to women early in an unwanted pregnancy and providing a telephone number to call. The continued availability of medical abortions through September was then made known by ongoing radio advertising. One hundred and seventy-five women volunteered and were eligible to participate in the clinical trial. Of these, 5 were lost to the first follow-up and an additional 25 were lost to the second follow-up, leaving 145 women (82.9%) who underwent the medical abortion procedure and provided interview data at all three data collection points.

Data Collection

The interview was structured and administered by the same female interviewer throughout the study. Interviewing was conducted in person initially (T_0) and at the first follow-up (T_1), and by telephone at the second follow-up (T_2). Although some parts of the interview were arranged in a self-report format, these were generally read to the patients, item by item, and their responses recorded. Interview content was based on previous research on the psychological consequences of abortion (Miller, 1992) and regret following sterilization (Miller, Shain, & Pasta, 1990, 1991).

Theoretical Framework

Figure 1 shows a simplified version of the theoretical framework for this study, as adapted from Miller (1994). It indicates that the psychological

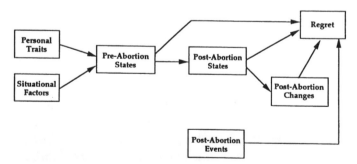

Figure 1. A schematic representation of the theoretical framework used to guide data collection and analysis. From "Reproductive Decisions: How We Make Them and How They Make Us," by W. B. Miller, 1994. In L. J. Severy (Ed.), *Advances in Population: Psychosocial Perspectives*. Copyright 1994 by Kingsley. Adapted with permission.

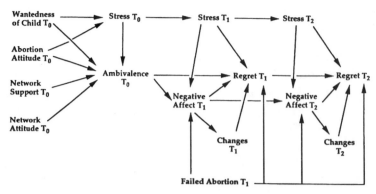

Figure 2. Initial data analytic model showing specific variables and their hypothesized relationships.

states of women who have decided to have an abortion are determined by both personal traits and situational factors. These preabortion states in turn affect postabortion psychological states and the development of regret. The postabortion states also have a direct effect on regret, as well as an indirect effect by producing postabortion changes. Unanticipated postabortion events may also affect the development of regret.

Figure 2 shows the data analytic model that we derived from the theoretical framework shown in Figure 1. It includes the specific variables by which we operationalized the framework. It also takes into account the three interview structure of the study, with variables labeled T_0, T_1, and T_2. Because both the theoretical framework and the data analytic model represent an integration of the six previously discussed theoretical approaches to the psychological consequences of abortion, it will be useful to discuss the variables shown in Figure 2 and their hypothesized connections in terms of the dominant themes of those theoretical approaches. Further, we shall maintain this organizational division during the discussion in subsequent sections.

Stress

Stress, or more accurately the reaction to stress, is both a preabortion and a postabortion state. It occurs in response to the presence of an unwanted pregnancy and the decision to have an abortion. The preponderance of evidence indicates that it is highest just prior to abortion and then drops down immediately afterward, gradually approaching baseline (prepregnancy) levels during subsequent weeks and months (Adler et al., 1992). There are a few investigators, however, who argue that some proportion of women experience a postabortion stress syndrome, including symptoms of avoidance and intrusion, as a manifestation of posttraumatic stress disorder (Speckhard & Rue, 1992).

Decision Making

Ambivalence about the abortion decision is a preabortion state and regret over the decision is a postabortion state. We hypothesized that ambivalence predicts regret and that earlier regret predicts later regret. We also hypothesized that high stress increases both ambivalence and regret. There is considerable evidence that both internal conflict and conflict between the woman and her social network increase preabortion uncertainty and postabortion adjustment difficulties (Major & Cozzarelli, 1992; Miller, 1992) and that support from the social network does just the opposite, hence the four T_0 predictors of ambivalence. Finally, we hypothesized that the most common unanticipated postabortion event occurring in this sample within the time frame of this study, namely a failed medical abortion, predicts postabortion regret. However, there is some uncertainty as to whether this was true at T_1 because this follow-up occurred prior to the surgical abortion made necessary by the failure.

Negative Affect

We grouped the norm violation, loss, and crisis approaches under the term *negative affect*. All three involve a preabortion conflict that leads to some type of postabortion affective state. Disapproval of abortion, whether the source is internal or external, leads to shame and guilt. Wanting the baby leads to feelings of loss and depression. Tension and anxiety about the whole situation lead to relief. We hypothesized that the first two of these act directly through ambivalence and the last acts indirectly through stress at T_0 to produce postabortion affective states that in turn effect regret. When the postabortion affect is predominantly negative, regret will tend to be higher. When it is dominated by feelings of relief, regret will tend to be lower. We also hypothesized that negative affect will be increased by high postabortion levels of stress and by unanticipated postabortion events.

Changes

Freeman (1977) described how the abortion experience changed many women's awareness of themselves, especially with respect to sexuality and contraception, and Miller (1992) found evidence that having an abortion improved contraceptive use and that those with improved use reported less regret. We hypothesized that postabortion changes in the various domains of reproductive behavior will be affected by the level of negative affect and will, in turn, affect regret.

Variable Measurement

Stress

We selected five variables as indicators of a stress response: self-esteem, measured by the Rosenberg's (1965) 10-item subscale; state anxiety, on the basis of a modification of Spielberger, Gorsuch, and Lushene's (1970) State–Trait Anxiety Inventory (STAI); and three variables derived from a modification of Horowitz, Wilner, and Alvarez's (1979) Impact of Event Scale (IES). For our measure of state anxiety, we paired four positive adjectives (*calm* and *secure*, *rested* and *comfortable*) and four negative ones (*tense* and *jittery*, *nervous* and *fearful*) from the STAI, forming two new positive and two new negative items, and asked the women to rate how well these four items applied to them during the last few days on a four-category response scale. Positive items were reverse coded and the four items were summed. This generated a state anxiety measure with an alpha coefficient across the three administrations of .82.

In adapting the IES, we made two types of changes. First, we slightly simplified item wording in several cases for greater comprehension. Second, we added six new items in addition to the original seven Intrusion scale items and the eight Avoidance scale items. These items were more positive in tone and were intended to balance out the generally negative tone of the original items. (The instructions, items, and format of the IES are shown in an appendix to this chapter, together with preabortion response frequencies from our sample.) A cluster analysis of the 21 items (VARCLUS; SAS, 1990) indicated that the original 15 items clustered into the Intrusion and Avoidance scales, just as in Horowitz et al.'s (1979) study. Two new items ("I have day dreamed about it" and "I have had trouble concentrating because of it," where *it* refers to the abortion) also clustered with the 7-item Intrusion scale and were added to it. The four remaining items ("I felt good about it," "I talked about it with someone close," "I wanted to think about it," and "I had positive thoughts about it") formed a third, separate cluster, which we named the Positive Thinking scale. Alpha coefficients across the three administrations during this study were .90, .85, and .61 for Intrusion, Avoidance, and Positive Thinking, respectively.

Decision Making

We selected two variables as indicators of ambivalence. The wording of the two relevant interview questions and their response categories are shown in Table 1. (This and the next three tables also show sample response frequencies, which we discuss in the results section.) The correlation between these two variables was .47. We selected four variables as indicators of regret. A fifth question about whether the abortion had af-

TABLE 1
Interview Questions, Response Categories, and Frequency Distributions of Patient Responses for the Two Indicator Variables That Comprise the Latent Variable Ambivalence at T_0

Interview question and response item	Frequency	%
A. When people make an important decision, they may or may not feel certain about it. We would like to know how certain you feel about your decision to have an abortion. There are four possible descriptions of how women getting an abortion feel. Please pick the one that best describes how you actually feel.		
1. Completely certain. There are no doubts in my mind.	110	75.9
2. Mostly certain. I have a few doubts.	33	22.8
3. Somewhat uncertain. I have some important doubts.	2	1.4
4. Very uncertain. I have a great many doubts.	0	0.0
B. When people make an important decision, it may or may not take them a while to work out any conflicts they have about it. We would like to know how long it took you to work out any conflicts you may have had about getting an abortion. Here are four possible descriptions. Please pick the one that best fits you.		
1. Once I made the decision, I felt no further conflict.	80	55.2
2. At first I had some conflicts, but I quickly overcame them.	45	31.0
3. It took me some time to overcome my conflicts about the decision.	13	9.0
4. I still feel some important conflicts about the decision.	7	4.8

Note. T_0 = immediately before the administration of the abortifacient RU486.

fected the woman's life in any positive ways did not correlate well with the other variables and was therefore omitted from the group of regret indicators. The wording of the four relevant interview questions and their response categories are shown in Table 2. The average correlation between these variables at T_1 and T_2 was .41.

Negative Affect

We selected four variables as indicators of negative affect. A fifth question (asked at the same point in the interview as the other four) about whether the woman had suffered any physical complaints or medical problems since the abortion did not correlate well with the other four and was therefore omitted from the group of negative affect indicators. The interview questions and response categories for the four selected questions are shown in Table 3. These four variables had an average correlation at T_1 and T_2 of .43.

Changes

A single stem question from the interview asked about changes in six reproduction-related domains. The wording of this section of the interview

TABLE 2
Interview Questions, Response Categories, and Frequency
Distributions of Patient Responses for the Four Indicator Variables That
Comprise the Latent Variables Regret at T_1 and Regret at T_2

Interview question and response item	Time 1		Time 2	
	Frequency	%	Frequency	%
A. Since the last interview, how have you felt about your decision to have an abortion?				
1. Only good feelings	53	36.6	35	24.1
2. Mostly good feelings	59	40.7	65	44.8
3. Both good and bad feelings	29	20.0	40	27.6
4. Mostly bad feelings	4	2.8	3	2.1
5. Only bad feelings	0	0.0	2	1.4
B. Since the last interview, have there been some times when you had some doubts about having an abortion?				
1. No, never	113	77.9	101	69.7
2. Yes, a few times	28	19.3	37	25.5
3. Yes, often	4	2.8	7	4.8
C. If you could go back in time, would you make the same decision again?				
1. Yes, I definitely would	93	64.1	102	70.3
2. Yes, I probably would	39	26.9	21	14.5
3. I am not sure	11	7.6	17	11.7
4. No, I would not	2	1.4	5	3.4
D. Has the abortion affected your life in any negative ways?				
1. No	113	77.9	118	81.4
2. Not sure	18	12.4	9	6.2
3. Yes	14	9.7	18	12.4

Note. T_1 = 2 weeks after abortion; T_2 = 6 to 8 months after abortion.

is shown in Table 4. "Don't know" responses were coded as no effect and the coding on each of the domain variables was reversed (i.e., so that a high score indicated the domain state or behavior had "increased a lot"). Although we had planned to use all six of these variables as indicators of postabortion change, their average correlation was only .17. A cluster analysis suggested two primary clusters: A, E, and F and B, C, and D.

Other Variables

The predictors of Stress T_0 and Ambivalence T_0 shown in Figure 2 variously fit into all six of the theoretical approaches we have been discussing and so at this point are considered together. One question formed the basis of the wantedness of child variable. The question describes how women seeking an abortion may have no interest in having a baby at the time, some interest but not enough to seriously consider going through with the pregnancy, or a lot of interest but have too many reasons not to go through with it. The question then asks the women to rate their feelings,

TABLE 3
Interview Questions, Response Categories, and Frequency Distributions of Patient Responses for the Four Indicator Variables That Comprise the Latent Variables Negative Affect at T_1 and Negative Affect at T_2

Interview question and response item	Time 1 Frequency	%	Time 2 Frequency	%
A. How about your state of mind or mood? Have you had any problems with those since the abortion?[a]				
1. No	101	69.7	115	79.3
2. Yes, a little	40	27.6	21	14.5
3. Yes, a lot	4	2.8	9	6.2
B. Some people feel depressed after an abortion. Has that been true of you?				
1. No	92	63.4	93	64.1
2. Yes, a little	49	33.8	41	28.3
3. Yes, a lot	4	2.8	11	7.6
C. Some women feel guilty, as though they had done something wrong by having an abortion. Has that been true of you?				
1. No	102	70.4	93	64.1
2. Yes, a little	38	26.2	43	29.7
3. Yes, a lot	5	3.4	9	6.2
D. Some women feel relieved after an abortion. How much relief did you experience?				
1. A great deal	90	62.1	79	54.5
2. A moderate amount	33	22.8	43	29.7
3. A little	14	9.7	13	9.0
4. None	8	5.5	10	6.9

Note. T_1 = 2 weeks after abortion; T_2 = 6 to 8 weeks after abortion.
[a]This question followed an initial follow-up question that read, "First of all, how have you been feeling? Have you suffered any physical complaints or medical problems since the abortion?"

with the response categories being *no interest, some interest,* and *a lot of interest.*

One question also formed the basis of the abortion attitude variable. The women were asked to look back to the time just before they became pregnant and indicate their attitude toward abortion on a 5-point scale that ranged from *completely approved* to *completely disapproved.*

Two related questions allowed construction of the two network variables. First, each woman was asked to indicate whether or not five specific people knew about her getting an abortion: her husband or partner, her two best female friends, and her mother and father. We formed a composite variable called network support by summing the number of those five people who knew. Second, each woman was asked to indicate how those same five people felt about her getting an abortion, using a 5-point scale from *very much in favor* to *very much against.* Women were asked to guess if they did not know. Those who still said they did not know or who said that

TABLE 4
Interview Questions, Response Categories, and Frequency
Distributions of Patient Responses for the Six Postabortion
Change Variables, as Measured at T_1 and T_2

Interview question and response item	Time 1		Time 2	
	Frequency	%	Frequency	%
Has the abortion affected any of the following areas of your life?				
A. Desire to have another child				
1. Increased a lot	7	4.8	7	4.8
2. Increased a little	11	7.6	17	11.7
3. No effect	113	77.9	107	73.8
4. Decreased a little	5	3.4	3	2.1
5. Decreased a lot	9	6.2	11	7.6
B. Interest in sex				
1. Increased a lot	9	6.2	2	1.4
2. Increased a little	16	11.0	1	0.7
3. No effect	81	55.9	116	80.0
4. Decreased a little	24	16.6	17	11.7
5. Decreased a lot	15	10.3	9	6.2
C. Satisfaction in marriage/relationship				
1. Increased a lot	13	9.0	13	9.0
2. Increased a little	20	13.8	14	9.7
3. No effect	87	60.0	96	66.2
4. Decreased a little	14	9.7	10	6.9
5. Decreased a lot	11	7.6	12	8.3
D. Problems with health				
1. Increased a lot	3	2.1	4	2.8
2. Increased a little	8	5.5	16	11.0
3. No effect	125	86.2	124	85.5
4. Decreased a little	5	3.4	1	0.7
5. Decreased a lot	4	2.8	0	0.0
E. Fear of pregnancy				
1. Increased a lot	35	24.1	38	26.2
2. Increased a little	34	23.4	33	22.8
3. No effect	74	51.1	69	47.6
4. Decreased a little	1	0.7	2	1.4
5. Decreased a lot	1	0.7	3	2.1
F. Regular use of contraception				
1. Increased a lot	90	62.1	90	62.1
2. Increased a little	13	9.0	26	17.9
3. No effect	41	28.3	27	18.6
4. Decreased a little	0	0.0	1	0.7
5. Decreased a lot	1	0.7	1	0.7

Note. T_1 = 2 weeks after abortion; T_2 = 6 to 8 weeks after abortion.

the category was not applicable (e.g., if she only had one good friend) were scored in the middle (neutral) response category. We formed another composite variable called network attitude by averaging the attitude score for all five people.

Finally, whether or not the medical abortion had failed was determined clinically at the T_1 follow-up, in which case the woman was scheduled for a surgical abortion.

Data Analysis

In addition to the correlational and cluster analyses already mentioned, we conducted paired t tests on many of the variables using time as a grouping variable to determine whether—and if so, in what way—variable scores changed across time. The variables that we explored in this way included all the component indicators of the stress variables, the regret variables, and the negative affect variables.

We then tested the model shown in Figure 2 using LISREL, Version 8 (Jöreskog & Sörbom, 1993). All of the variables in Figure 2, with the exception of the four predictors of ambivalence and the failed abortion variable, were specified as latent variables with from two to five indicator variables. In most cases, the indicator variables were based on single interview questions, but in the case of the latent variable Stress T_0, T_1, and T_2, all indicator variables were themselves composites. Having first estimated the model shown in Figure 2, we then proceeded to make changes that would reduce model strain, as suggested by modification indices and normalized residuals. Changes to the measurement model included modifying latent variables and allowing connections between indicators. Both of these types of changes are described later. Changes to the structural equation model generally involved adding paths that we had not hypothesized. By rule, we did not drop non-significant indicators from the measurement model. However, when a hypothesized pathway in the structural equation model was found to be non-significant, we dropped that connection and reestimated the model. With a sample size of 145, t scores of 1.976 and 2.610 have p values of .05 and .01, respectively. We retained no pathways in the structural equation model.

RESULTS

The mean time to first follow-up was 17 days (SD = 8.5, minimum = 9, maximum = 71) and the mean time to second follow-up was 220 days (SD = 42.2, minimum = 153, maximum = 336).

Sample Characteristics

The average age of the 145 women in the sample was 28, with a range of 18 to 44. Fifty-two percent of the women were never married; 22% were currently married; and 26% were separated, divorced, or widowed. Sixty-seven percent were White, 25% were Black, and the remaining

8% were of other races/ethnicities. Most were Protestant (44%) or Roman Catholic (36%) and most were employed full time (56%) or part time (17%). As a whole, the sample had a mean individual income just over $20,000 and a mean household income just over $30,000. The mean level of education was just below 14 years (i.e., 2 years of college). Seventy-eight (54%) of the women reported having a previous surgical abortion.

Individual Variables

Stress

All five components of the Stress scale were based on responses that varied from 1 to 4. This made it possible to calculate individual scores as the average across all items in the component, making all component scores vary between 1 and 4. The average sample value of each of the five stress components at T_0, T_1, and T_2 is plotted in Figure 3. Where the average sample value differed from the previous measurement (paired t test, $p < .05$), the dot representing that value in the figure is circled.

Self-esteem showed essentially no change over time. Positive thinking showed no change from T_0 to T_1 but then dropped significantly at T_3. Anxiety showed an opposite pattern, dropping significantly at T_1 but then

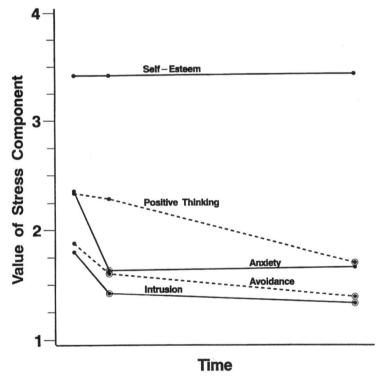

Figure 3. Average value of stress components over time.

showing no further significant change at T_2. Avoidance and intrusion both drop significantly at T_1 and then again at T_2.

Decision Making

Table 1 shows the response distributions for the two components of ambivalence at T_0. Both the certainty and conflict–time components were positively skewed, the certainty component more so. Almost 14% of the sample reported that they did not overcome their conflicts quickly. Table 2 shows the response distribution for the four components of regret at T_1 and T_2. Again, all components were positively skewed, although the modal response in the feel–decision component (Question A) was "mostly good feelings," rather than "only good feelings." When we examined how the four regret components changed from T_1 to T_2, both the feel–decision component and the doubts component (Question B) showed significant increases at T_2 ($ps < .011$ and $< .035$, respectively).

Negative Affect

Table 3 shows the response distributions for the four components of negative affect at T_1 and T_2. Again, all components were positively skewed, with about one third of the women expressing either a little or a lot of depression or guilt and almost one sixth reporting little or no relief. When we examined how these four components changed across time only guilt showed a near significant ($p = .052$) increase at T_2.

Changes

Table 4 shows the response distributions for the change variables. Almost 1 out of 7 women reported the abortion increased their desire for a child, whereas about 10% reported that it decreased that desire. Both increases and decreases were reported in some women's interest in sex and satisfaction in marriage or their relationship. Problems with health tended to increase in a small proportion of women. By way of contrast, fear of pregnancy increased in almost one half of the women and regular use of contraception increased in about three quarters.

Other Variables

At T_0 62.1% of the women expressed no interest in having the baby, 25.5% expressed some interest, and 12.4% expressed a lot of interest. Similarly, 67.6% reported that they completely approved of abortion, 12.4% reported they mostly approved, 12.4% were neutral, and 7.5% reported they mostly or completely disapproved. On average, the women reported that 1.7 of the five social network people we asked about knew of the abortion. The average approval score of those five people was 2.5, half-way between *mostly in favor* (2) and *mixed feelings/neutral* (3), although the average approval score of partners was considerably higher at 1.8. Finally, there were 13 women (9.0%) who experienced a failed medical abortion and required a subsequent surgical abortion.

LISREL Measurement Model

Stress

Very large modification indices in the Lambda-Y matrix indicated that the five components of the three stress variables at T_0, T_1, and T_2 were all strongly associated with each other beyond the associations accommodated by the three variables and their prediction of each other across time. The first step in accommodating this problem was to create a single, across-time latent stress variable, using all 15 stress indicators. This only partly solved the problem because modification indices and p values revealed that this across-time variable needed further modification. Several additional steps led to the best fitting solution, three separate across-time variables, one using state anxiety, intrusion, and avoidance at all three times as indicators, one using self-esteem at all three times as indicators, and one using positive thinking at all three times as indicators.

The names we have given the six latent stress variables require further comment. We decided that the three within-time variables represented acute stress and, therefore, named them acute stress T_0, T_1, and T_2. The standardized weights given them in the measurement model, and the associated t scores of those weights, are shown in Table 5. Intrusion and avoidance are the strongest contributors, followed closely by state anxiety. Self-esteem makes a relatively smaller contribution. Positive thinking was not a significant contribution at T_0 and T_1, but reversed sign and became significant at T_2.

TABLE 5

Measurement Model of the Three Latent Variables Acute Stress at T_0, T_1, and T_2: Standardized Parameter Estimates and t Scores

Indicator variable	Time 0 Estimate	t	Time 1 Estimate	t	Time 2 Estimate	t
State anxiety	.44[a]		.23[a]		.33[a]	
Self-esteem	−.15	−4.46	−.17	−3.74	−.19	−4.52
Intrusion	.62	7.67	.48	4.88	.44	6.31
Avoidance	.46	6.01	.42	4.22	.44	5.68
Positive thinking	−.05	−0.88	−.03	−0.56	.19	3.38

Note. T_0 = immediately before the administration of the abortifacient RU486; T_1 = 2 weeks after abortion; T_2 = 6 to 8 weeks after abortion.
[a]In each latent variable, the parameter estimate of one indicator variable is set at 1.00 before standardization. For that indicator, no t score is estimated.

We decided that the three across-time latent variables represented three aspects of chronic stress. However, as can be seen in Table 6, which shows the standardized weights and associated t scores for each of the across-time variables, the signs of the weights are such that stress is associated with the low end of each scale. Therefore, rather than naming these three scales chronic stress variables, we named them stress coping variables. This is in line with the low chronic stress indicated by high scores and with the trait nature of these across-time variables. As shown in Table 6, each stress coping variable was measured predominantly (exclusively in the case of the second and third) by a positive coping trait: avoidance, self-esteem, and positive thinking. We abbreviated these three and added these abbreviations as suffixes to stress coping to form the latent variable names.

It is noteworthy that high avoidance was associated with low anxiety, intrusion, overall stress in the stress coping–avoidance variable but with high anxiety, intrusion, and overall stress in the acute stress variables. Presumably, what this means is that the trait of avoidance helps prevent anxiety and intrusive thoughts under most circumstances but that under severe stress it tends to be overwhelmed and break down, allowing the experience of anxiety and intrusion, in spite of extra efforts to exert its influence. A related point is the way that positive thinking performed with the two types of stress variables. In stress coping–positive thinking, high positive thinking was associated with low stress, whereas in acute stress at T_2 the opposite was true. Again presumably, this means that under the type of stress that tends to break down defenses, positive thinking is overwhelmed, and high scores tend to reflect the extra effort that is exerted trying to reimpose control over anxiety and intrusive thoughts.

TABLE 6
Measurement Model of the Three Latent Variables Stress Coping
-Av, -Se, and -Pt, Each of Which Is Measured Across T_0, T_1, and T_2:
Standardized Parameter Estimates and t Scores

Latent and indicator variables	Time 0		Time 1		Time 2	
	Estimate	t	Estimate	t	Estimate	t
Stress coping -Av						
State anxiety	−.09	−1.22	−.13	−2.14	−.13	−1.90
Intrusion	−.04	−.66	−.08	−1.79	−.06	1.63
Avoidance	.37[a]		.27	4.06	.17	3.45
Stress coping -Se						
Self-esteem	.38[a]		.29	8.19	.31	8.37
Stress coping -Pt						
Positive thinking	.40[a]		.40	4.35	.31	4.21

Note. T_0 = immediately before the administration of the abortifacient RU486; T_1 = 2 weeks after abortion; T_2 = 6 to 8 weeks after abortion. Av = avoidance; Se = self-esteem; Pt = positive thinking.
[a] In each latent variable, the parameter estimate of one indicator variable is set at 1.00 before standardization. For that indicator, no t score is estimated.

We examined the pattern of the acute-stress latent variables over time by conducting a series of t tests. Because even minor differences in the weights of the five indicators at each time could result in substantial differences in the average value of the latent variable, simple comparison of the computed latent variables over time is potentially misleading. Instead, we performed three sets of paired t tests, comparing T_0 data with T_1 data, T_1 data with T_2 data, and T_0 data with T_2 data. We weighted the five indicator variables in one set using T_0 parameter estimates, in another set using T_1 estimates, and in another set using T_2 estimates. All three sets of weights showed a similar pattern: a large decline in acute stress from T_0 to T_1 ($p < .001$ in all three cases) and a much smaller decline (from .026 to $< .001$) from T_1 to T_2.

Decision Making

Table 7 shows the measurement model for the three variables central to the decision-making approach: Ambivalence at T_0 and Regret at T_1 and T_2. Interestingly, the conflict–time component (Question B, Table 1) made a substantially larger contribution to ambivalence than did the certainty component (Question A, Table 1). For the regret variables, the feel–decision component (Question A, Table 2) was consistently the strongest indicator, although all three of the other indicators made large contributions.

Modification indices revealed two connections with ambivalence at T_0 that were significant in the Psi matrix: one with acute stress at T_1 ($t = -2.19$) and the other with regret at T_2 ($t = 3.26$). These connections

TABLE 7
Measurement Model of the Three Latent Variables Ambivalence, Regret at T_1, and Regret at T_2: Standardized Parameter Estimates and t Scores

Latent and indicator variables[a]	Time 0 Estimate	t	Time 1 Estimate	t	Time 2 Estimate	t
Ambivalence T_0						
Question A: Certainty	.29[b]		—		—	
Question B: Conflict time	.53	6.75	—		—	
Regret T_1 and T_2						
Question A: Feel decision	—		.56[b]		.61[b]	
Question B: Doubts	—		.31	7.05	.46	9.44
Question C: Do again	—		.38	6.17	.54	7.65
Question D: Negative effects	—		.39	6.99	.38	6.46

Note. T_0 = immediately before the administration of the abortifacient RU486; T_1 = 2 weeks after abortion; T_2 = 6 to 8 weeks after abortion.
[a]Word or phrase following question letter identifies key question content. For full question content, see Table 1 for Ambivalence and Table 2 for Regret at T_1 and T_2.
[b]In each latent variable, the parameter estimate of one indicator variable is set at 1.00 before standardization. For that indicator, no t score is estimated.

remained stable regardless of predictive connections that were attempted in the Beta matrix and so were allowed in the Psi matrix.

Modification indices revealed that the four indicators of regret at T_1 were each strongly associated with their corresponding indicator at T_2. Accordingly, we freed up those connections in the Theta Epsilon matrix, where they were all positive and three of four were significant ($t = 2.68$ to 3.65). These connections indicate that three of the individual indicators of regret had across-year residual associations that were independent of the connections between latent variables regret at T_1 and T_2 that appear in the structural equation model. These connections may be viewed as representing the trait aspect of regret in the final model.

We examined whether regret at T_1 was significantly different from regret at T_2 by conducting a series of t tests similar to those described above for acute stress. We compared T_1 data with T_2 data twice, using T_1 weights in one case and T_2 weights in the other. In both cases we found a significant ($ps = .010$ and $.012$) increase in regret from T_1 to T_2.

Negative Affect

Table 8 shows the measurement model for the four indicators of negative affect at T_1 and T_2. Each component contributed about equally to the latent variables at each time point.

Again, modification indices revealed that the four indicators at T_1 were strongly associated with their corresponding indicators at T_2, and the appropriate connections were freed up in the Theta Epsilon matrix. All were positive and significant ($t = 1.72$ to 3.48, the first of these being significant only with a one-tailed test). These connections indicate that all four of the individual indicators of negative affect had across-year residual associations that were independent of the connectors between latent variables negative affect at T_1 and T_2 that appear in the structural equation

TABLE 8
Measurement Model of the Two Latent Variables Negative Affect at T_1
and T_2: Standardized Parameter Estimates and t Scores

Indicator variable[a]	Time 1		Time 2	
	Estimate	t	Estimate	t
Question A: State of mind	.37[b]		.33[b]	
Question B: Depressed	.41	8.12	.47	6.76
Question C: Guilty	.39	7.80	.43	6.55
Question D: Relief	.43	5.96	.54	5.84

Note. T_1 = 2 weeks after abortion; T_2 = 6 to 8 weeks after abortion.
[a]Word or phrase following question letter identifies key question content. For full question content, see Table 3.
[b]In each latent variable, the parameter estimate of one indicator variable is set at 1.00 before standardization. For that indicator, no t score is estimated.

model. Again, these connections may be viewed as representing the trait aspect of negative affect in the final model.

Here too we conducted a series of t tests similar to those described above for acute stress and regret to determine whether negative affect at T_1 was significantly different from negative affect T_2. Although the T_2 variable was higher in both cases, the differences were not significant (ps = .234 and .185).

Changes

The latent variable based on Questions A, E, and F (see Table 4) was not significant in the structural equation model until the two indicators that were not significant (Components E and F) were dropped. Thus, we made Component A into a single indicator η, naming it childbearing desires at T_1 and T_2. Table 9 shows the measurement model for the other change latent variable, which is based on Questions B, C, and D. Because of the far greater contributions of Questions B and C, especially C, we named this latent variable relationship satisfaction at T_1 and T_2. Modification indices revealed that there was a significant association between child desire change at T_1 and relationship change at T_1 and between the same two variables at T_2. Accordingly, we allowed those two connections (t = 2.16 and 2.26) in the Psi matrix.

Other Variables

The four independent variables wantedness of child, abortion attitude, network support, and network attitude were all treated as single variable Ksis and allowed to correlate freely with each other in the Phi matrix. The failed abortion variable was treated as a single variable η. There was a large modification index between it and the relief indicator (Question D, Table 3) at T_1. Accordingly, this connection was freed up in the Theta

TABLE 9
Measurement Model of the Two Latent Variables Relationship
Satisfaction Change at T_1 and T_2: Standardized Parameter
Estimates and t Scores

Indicator variable[a]	Time 1		Time 2	
	Estimate	t	Estimate	t
Question B: Sex	.39[b]		.27[b]	
Question C: Relationship	.88	3.18	.50	3.49
Question D: Health	−.17	−2.96	−.09	−1.82

Note. T_1 = 2 weeks after abortion; T_2 = 6 to 8 weeks after abortion.
[a]Word or phrase following question letter identifies key question content. For full question content, see Table 4.
[b]In each latent variable, the parameter estimate of one indicator variable is set at 1.00 before standardization. For that indicator, no t score is estimated.

Epsilon matrix ($t = 4.66$), indicating that a failed abortion is associated with the experience of little or no relief at T_1.

LISREL Structural Equation Model

Figure 4 shows the final structural equation model, including causal pathways together with their associated standardized estimated coefficients.

Stress

Greater acute stress at T_0 was predicted by a greater wantedness of the child and a more negative attitude toward abortion. Greater acute stress at T_0 predicted greater ambivalence and greater acute stress at T_1. The latter predicted greater regret at T_1 and greater acute stress at T_2, which in turn predicted greater regret at T_2. An unexpected finding is that greater acute stress at T_2 was directly predicted by greater wantedness of the child.

Recall that we hypothesized that greater stress would also predict greater negative affect. Surprisingly, we found that the relationship between acute stress and negative affect was bidirectional at T_1 and was in the opposite direction from that expected at T_2. Another surprise is that greater acute stress at T_1 predicted lesser regret at T_2.

The stress coping variables show some interesting, and in one case surprising, relationships. Higher stress coping by avoidance predicted lower ambivalence as did higher stress coping by positive thinking. The latter also predicted lower regret at T_2. The surprise is that higher stress coping by self-esteem predicted higher regret at T_1.

Decision Making

Greater wantedness of the child, a more negative attitude toward abortion, a lower level of network support, and a more negative attitude toward her having an abortion in the woman's social network all predicted greater ambivalence. Greater ambivalence before the abortion predicted greater regret at T_1 but, surprisingly, regret at T_1 did not have any direct effect on regret at T_2.

Negative Affect

There was no direct connection between the four preabortion independent (Ksi matrix) variables and postabortion negative affect, as might be expected according to the loss, norm violation, and stress approaches discussed in the introduction. The connections were all indirect through acute stress and ambivalence at T_0. Greater ambivalence at T_0 predicted greater negative affect at T_1, which in turn predicted greater regret at T_1. Similarly, greater regret at T_1 predicted greater negative affect at T_2, which in turn predicted greater regret at T_2. As with regret at T_1 not predicting

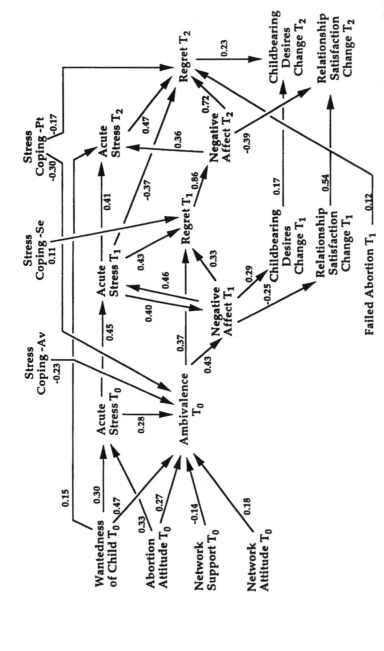

Figure 4. Final structural equation model showing causal pathways with their associated standardized estimated coefficients.

regret at T_2, we were surprised to find that negative affect at T_1 did not predict negative affect at T_2.

Changes

Greater negative affect predicted increased childbearing desires at T_1 and decreased relationship satisfaction at T_1 and T_2. Each of these change variables at T_1 predicted its equivalent at T_2. Contrary to our hypothesis, these change variables did not predict regret at either T_1 or T_2. Instead we found that greater regret at T_2 predicted increased childbearing desires at T_2. A failed medical abortion predicted greater regret at T_2.

Independent Variable Total Effects

A useful way to report the results of a complex estimated model is to examine the total effects of certain key independent variables on certain key dependent variables. Table 10 shows the standardized total effect of eight independent variables on four dependent variables at T_2. Wantedness of the child had the strongest total effects overall. It had a strong effect on acute stress, and abortion attitude had a modest effect. Wantedness of the child also had a strong effect on regret, followed closely by the effect of stress coping based on positive thinking, then followed by a modest effect of abortion attitude. These same three variables had the greatest effects on childbearing desires and relationship satisfaction, but in these cases the effects were weak to modest. The primary effect of failed abortion was on regret.

TABLE 10
Standardized Total Effects of Eight Independent Variables on
Four Key T_2 Dependent Variables

Independent variables	Standardized total effects			
	Acute stress T_2	Regret T_2	Childbearing desires T_2	Relationship satisfaction T_2
Wantedness of child	.41	.36	.10	−.20
Abortion attitude	.21	.21	.06	−.15
Network support	−.04	−.06	−.02	.04
Network attitude	.05	.08	.02	−.05
Stress coping–Avoidance	−.07	−.10	−.03	.07
Stress coping–Self-esteem	.03	.08	.02	−.04
Stress coping–Positive thinking	−.09	−.31	−.08	.09
Failed abortion	.00	.12	.03	.00

Note. T_2 = 6 to 8 weeks after abortion.

LISREL Model Fit

The overall model had a chi-square of 1,302.98, with 930 degrees of freedom. This gives a chi-square ratio of 1.401. The root-mean-square error of approximation (RMSEA) had a value of .053, and the p value for a test of close fit (RMSEA < .05) was .25. In general, these values indicate that the model has a close fit with an acceptable error of approximation in the population.

Once the model had achieved a close fit we did not try to free up the few remaining connections, which modification indices (MI) indicated would be significant. The highest remaining MI was 14.5 in the Lambda-Y. There were four MIs greater than 10.0 in the Lambda-Y and four in the Theta Epsilon. In the Beta matrix, there were only four potentially significant MIs, falling between 4.0 (which suggests a t score of about 2.0 when the connection is freed) and 5.25. Three of these involved predictions that were backward in time and one of them involved a set of relationships we decided not to model (the predictors of the stress coping variables). In the Gamma matrix, there were only four potentially significant MIs falling between 4.16 and 7.28. Two of these involved the unmodeled relationships and two of them did not improve model fit when tested. Finally, there were three MIs in the Psi matrix falling between 4.04 and 4.18, which we decided to ignore.

DISCUSSION OF RESULTS

Before discussing the many interesting findings of this study, we underscore an important caveat about the special nature of the sample, namely that it was relatively small—only 145 women—and was selective—consisting of women who were volunteering for a medical abortion procedure that was being offered for the first time in the United States on a trial basis. Somewhat balancing these threats to the generalizability of our findings is the racial, religious, and marital status diversity of the sample and the relatively small (17.1%) loss to follow-up of those participating. Further, the mean and standard deviation of self-esteem in our sample are extremely close to those reported by Russo and Zierk (1992) for a large probability sample of U.S. women who had sought abortions. Finally, because we were focusing on the psychological processes that come into play in response to abortion, and thus were examining the relationships between variables measured in the sample, some of the characteristics of the sample that are associated with its special nature may be less confounding than if we were trying to generalize from single variables (e.g., degree of regret 6 months after the abortion).

Our findings shed light on all six of the theoretical approaches discussed in the introduction. For this reason, we have organized our discussion around these approaches, continuing to combine the loss, norm violation, and crisis approaches under the label of *negative affect*. In addition, because both the measurement model and the structural equation model provide important insights, we also organized our discussion around these two aspects of our findings.

An interesting finding of this study is the importance of separating measurement of the stress response into its acute and chronic components or, to use a different but closely related terminology, its state and trait aspects. Once this is done we see that the two categories of stress variables have very different structures and functions. Preabortion, acute stress is dominated by high avoidance, intrusion, and anxiety. What appears to be happening is that the women are trying to control their response to the unwanted pregnancy/abortion situation by avoiding thinking about it. However, this strategy is incompletely successful and they find that they are flooded with anxiety and intrusive thoughts. By the second follow-up, 6 to 8 months later, the stress response has diminished considerably and avoidance, intrusion, and anxiety have each been significantly reduced. Although average self-esteem remains unchanged across the three measurement points, it is still a highly significant indicator of acute stress. This means that those women with lower self-esteem tend to manifest the other indications of the acute stress response throughout the pre- and postabortion period. Positive thinking, which is not reflective of the stress response preabortion or immediately postabortion, begins to reflect that response at the second follow-up. In other words, at the peak of the stress positive thinking reflects a coping response. However, when the stressful event is well past, those women who continue to think about it and talk about it with others are manifesting a continuing stress response.

The chronic stress variables, or what we called the stress coping variables because of their reversed signs in the context of the overall LISREL model, present a somewhat different structure. Stress coping by avoidance is characterized by high avoidance and low intrusion and anxiety, indicating that as a trait, avoidance helps to shut down intrusion and anxiety. Considering this variable from the low rather than the high end of its dimension, this means that with high chronic stress, avoidance is low and relatively nonfunctional, whereas intrusion and anxiety are high. Stress coping by self-esteem and positive thinking are both indicated by high scores, with low scores indicating a low level of the respective coping strategies. Note that whereas high positive thinking reflects successful coping, in the acute stress variable at T_2 high positive thinking reflects a failure to contain the stress response.

The connections of the acute stress variables in the structural equation model are generally what we hypothesized, although the several unanticipated connections are interesting and instructive. As implied by the crisis model, internal conflict about either wanting the child or approval of abortion contributed to the level of preabortion stress. Although a case could be made that the network variables should also effect stress, such is not the case in these data, perhaps because a network effect on stress is most likely in a teen sample where parents are likely to be highly involved or in a sample where partners are not supportive of the decision. Neither of these situations apply well in this case. Although the wantedness of the child also predicted acute stress at T_2, it had no direct effect at T_1. This somewhat anomalous T_1 finding suggests that there may have been something unusual about the T_1 period that prevented wantedness of the child from affecting acute stress until a later time. Perhaps T_1 was so close to the abortion itself that the woman was still dominated by her escape from a highly stressful experience and the effect of losing a wanted child had not yet been processed in the same way as, say, 6 to 8 months later. Alternatively, and related to the point we make in the next paragraph, it may be that those women who least wanted a child had a relatively accelerated stress response immediately after the abortion, thereby eliminating the usual covariation between wantedness and stress. This might happen, for example, if they were actually better prepared psychologically to handle the stress.

As expected, acute stress predicted itself across time and, at each point in time, predicted the basic components of the regret model. Its effect on ambivalence may have resulted from disruption of the decision-making process and, on regret, from disruption of the retrospective cognitive appraisal processes, which tend to ameliorate over time any self-criticism for actions taken (Gilovich & Medvee, 1995). Somewhat surprisingly, acute stress at T_1 also predicted low regret at T_2. Again, we believe that this is related to the close proximity of T_1 to T_0. If we assume that different women experience stress, negative affect, and regret in different patterns following an abortion, some letting their reactions emerge almost immediately and some suppressing their reactions for days, weeks, or even months, then it may be that the nonsuppressors had a high-stress response at T_1, but they had dealt with their reaction sufficiently that they actually had less regret by T_2.

We originally hypothesized that the acute stress response would amplify the development of negative affects in response to the abortion, reflecting a weakening of suppressive defenses and other forms of coping under stress. In other words, we expected the stress response to drive the development of negative affect after the abortion. This was true at T_1 (i.e., very soon after the abortion), but not at T_2. However, the final structural equation model indicates that the development of negative affect had a reverse effect, increasing the stress response, both at T_1 and 6 to 8 months later. This temporal pattern suggests that as women get some psychological distance from the abortion experience over time, negative feelings about the experience begin to drive the stress response, rather than the reverse.

The stress coping variables all predicted the main decision-making components. High-stress coping by avoidance reduced only preabortion ambivalence. Positive thinking reduced both preabortion ambivalence and regret at T_2. It had no effect on regret at T_1. On the other hand, stress coping by self-esteem only affected regret at T_1 and in this case the direction of the effect was unexpected: High self-esteem predicted high regret. We interpret this finding again as related to the proximity of T_1 to T_0 and the different temporal patterns women have in experiencing regret. Thus, it may be that high self-esteem women are better able to tolerate the experience of regret, and, therefore, unlike women who tend to suppress their negative reactions to the abortion for longer durations over time, actually experience more regret close in to the abortion. This interpretation is consistent with the view that self-esteem serves to protect the self from regret (Josephs, Larrick, Steele, & Nisbett, 1992; Larrick, 1993).

The various elements of the decision-making approach behave largely as hypothesized. At the measurement level, the main finding of interest is the much greater weight given to the question about conflict time relative to the question about certainty. This suggests that the time it takes people to make a decision may be a better indicator of ambivalence than how certain they are once the decision is made.

At the level of the structural equation model, we found that the four exogenous variables, which we interpreted as representing internal (child wantedness, abortion attitude) and external (network support and attitude) conflict predicted ambivalence and that ambivalence predicted regret at T_1. It is somewhat surprising that the latter did not predict regret at T_2. This may reflect the fact that regret shortly after the abortion has a somewhat different character than it does 6 to 8 months later. We know, for example, that regret at T_1 was significantly lower than it was at T_2 and that both regret variables have distinct connections to the stress coping variables. However, we are not inclined to put too much emphasis on the lack of prediction because regret at T_2 is so completely explained in the model ($R^2 = .96$) and because regret at T_1 had such a powerful indirect effect on regret at T_2 through negative affect, accounting for almost 40% of the regret at T_2 variance.

The final component of the decision-making approach is the experience of increased regret at T_2 by those having an unexpected life event, specifically a failed medical abortion. No such connection occurred at T_1, even though those experiencing a failure by and large knew at that time that they would need an additional, surgical procedure. Knowing that it will be necessary and actually going through the experience of it, however, are not the same, and that difference apparently accounts for the difference at T_1 and T_2 in the prediction of regret by a failed abortion. A related finding is the correlation in the Theta Epsilon matrix between a failed abortion at T_1 and the experience of relief at T_1. This indicates that whereas those women whose medical abortion failed may not have had increased regret 2 weeks after their abortion, they did recognize the failure and did not experience relief to the same degree that other women did. This relationship of a failed medical abortion to less relief and increased subsequent regret is a clinical problem of particular importance for medical as compared with surgical abortions and one that probably will require special vigilance on the part of service providers as the medical abortion procedures gain acceptance and begin to increase in frequency.

The findings derived from the negative affect approach are interesting in several respects. At the measurement model level, although relief makes a somewhat larger contribution than the other three indicators at T_2, the most interesting observation is that all four indicators contributed about equally to the negative affect construct. This suggests that theoretical approaches that emphasize unitary affective responses to abortion, such as the feelings of shame or guilt, loss or depression, and relief, may be missing an important broader picture. To some extent what appears to happen following abortion involves not so much a unitary as a broad, multidimensional affective response.

This conclusion is also supported by the finding in the linear structural equation model that none of the four exogenous predictors at T_0, all of which were selected because of their relevance to norm violation, loss, and crisis, had any direct connections to the negative affect variables (or to their indicators, for that matter). All four predicted negative affect but only through ambivalence and acute stress. However, it should be kept in mind that had we selected a broader range of affects to sample or measured our selected affects with a greater number of items (i.e., more reliably), we might then have found more evidence for the importance of unitary affects. For example, Adler (1975) identified three separate factors accounting for variations in women's postabortion emotions, including one called "positive emotions" (which included relief), one called "socially based negative emotions" (which included guilt), and one called "internally based negative emotions" (which included depression). It is thus not hard to imagine that our broad, multidimensional construct of negative affect could be differentiated into those three affective factors.

It is worth emphasizing that the broad affective response that we did measure was a key variable in our final model. It was closely intertwined with the decision-making variables, being predicted by ambivalence and regret across time periods and in turn predicting regret within time periods. As we have noted, it was also interwined with the acute stress variables, being predicted and predicting within time periods. Finally, it played a dominant role in predicting the two change variables retained in the model. In short, it was, along with the initial motivations and social presses and the ongoing stress responses, one of the three driving forces that determined the psychological consequences of the unwanted pregnancy and abortion decision as they played out over time.

It should be noted that, like the two regret variables, negative affect at T_1 did not predict negative affect at T_2. Again, this may be related to the very high explained variance of negative affect at T_2 ($R^2 = .74$), but another possibility deserves consideration. As mentioned, negative affect and regret were highly intertwined. Negative affect predicted regret within time periods, but only regret predicted across time periods and it only predicted negative affect. Just as negative affect over time comes to drive acute stress, it appears that regret over time comes to drive negative affect. This pattern suggests that the affective response to abortion gets transformed through retrospective appraisal into a cognitive form that then tends to perpetuate those negative affects over time.

The findings derived from the learning (i.e., changes) approach that are embedded in the final structural equation model are somewhat different from what was hypothesized. First of all, fear of pregnancy and regular use of contraception were not significantly associated with any part of the model. In a previous study, Miller (1992) found that an improvement in contraceptive practice was a consequence of abortion and was subsequently associated with low regret, but that latter finding has not been confirmed in this study. Another postabortion change, problems with health, was present in the change latent variable but was only a minor contributor. Thus, in this sample, changes in these three reproduction-related domains were not, or were only weakly, associated with other psychological consequences of abortion.

Second, although changes in childbearing desires and relationship satisfaction were, respectively, positively and negatively predicted by the magnitude of negative affect, they did not predict regret. In fact, at T_2 regret rather than negative affect predicted changes in childbearing desires. This pattern of findings indicates that these two changes occur, so to speak, down stream from the three "back bone" components of our psychological consequences model, namely acute stress, negative affect, and regret. This is not an unreasonable change to our original theoretical framework. Both the negative feelings generated by the unwanted pregnancy/abortion experience and the retrospective cognitive appraisal of its value to the woman can reasonably be expected to affect changes in her behavior.

The results shown in Table 10 clearly indicate those independent variables that had the greatest impact on the four key dependent variables (acute stress, regret, childbearing desires, and relationship satisfaction). The wantedness of the child was clearly the most important factor, having quite substantial effects on acute stress and regret 6 to 8 months after the abortion. Stress coping by positive thinking had a large effect on regret at T_2, reflecting the importance of this form of coping for recovery. Attitude toward abortion also affected stress and regret at T_2 but only about one half that of child wantedness.

RESEARCH, CLINICAL, AND POLICY IMPLICATIONS

There are a number of findings in this study that deserve further exploration. These include the relatively great importance of child wantedness for all postabortion psychological consequences; the central role of ambivalence in the development of postabortion regret; the importance of distinguishing between acute- (state) stress and chronic- (trait) stress coping; the dynamic and changing interactions among stress, affect, and regret; and the effect of all of these factors on postabortion changes in childbearing desires and relationship satisfaction. Some of these findings are confirmatory of the results of previous investigations and some are new. However, taken together as a group and interrelated through the final structural equation model, they convey a coherent picture of many of the important themes affecting the psychological consequences of abortion.

Within this overall picture, there is an intriguing set of findings that deserve special comment. Recall that we observed that high-stress coping by self-esteem predicted high regret at T_1; that high acute stress at T_1 predicted low regret at T_2; that the relationship between acute stress and negative affect was bidirectional at T_1 but not at T_2; that child wantedness did not predict acute stress at T_1, whereas it did at T_0 and T_2; and that regret at T_1 was actually lower than at T_2. We are inclined to view all of these findings as being related to the short interval between the abortion and T_1, generally a week to 10 days. This pattern of findings suggests that during the first few days or weeks following an abortion, many women's reactions are incomplete and not necessarily representative of subsequent reactions and that some women's reactions are either accelerated or delayed relative to others as a result of differences among women in the meaning of the abortion and in their ability to cope with stress.

Previous research into postabortion psychological consequences has varied considerably with respect to when the follow-up data collection occurred. Many studies collected data immediately after the abortion; many others did so in a few weeks, 6 months, or 2 years. Our findings suggest two factors that probably complicate the interpretation and comparability of results obtained through such a nonstandardized procedure. First, there is very likely a time course associated with the coping process that follows abortion and this time course almost certainly does not show a straight line improvement. In other words, the low point following the abortion may not occur for days, weeks, or even months. Second, it is also very likely that different kinds of women follow a different time course. An important research implication of our findings, therefore, is that we need to conduct repeated-measures studies that map this time course, examine its variation across different types of women, and identify the variables that contribute to this variation. In the introduction, we commented about the need for valid studies of the long-term (2 to 20 years) consequences of abortion. Our results now make it clear that we also need more studies that examine the short-term consequences, using sequential "snap shots" so that we can draw inferences about the dynamics of the recovery process.

A related question generated by our findings is whether the unexpected T_1 phenomena result, at least in part, from the women in the study having a medical rather than a surgical abortion. Although there is some evidence that postabortion consequences are no different following a medical abortion compared with a surgical (vacuum aspiration) abortion (Henshaw, Naji, Russell, & Templeton, 1994), it is too early to draw firm conclusions about this issue. We must at least consider the hypothesis that by drawing out the entire abortion experience, the medical procedure may in fact change the way that women respond to the stress of an abortion and process both their affective responses and their retrospective cognitive appraisals. Further, it appears that the occurrence of a failed abortion may contribute to these changes.

The results of this study also have important clinical implications. In the case of preabortion psychotherapeutic efforts to prevent the negative psychological consequences of abortion, our findings suggest several paths that might be pursued. First, the total effects results shown in Table 10 indicate that the wantedness of the child first and foremost, and to a lesser extent both the woman's attitude toward abortion and her coping by positive thinking, deserve focal attention during any early counseling intervention. Second, the length of time it took the woman to make her abortion decision provides a quick read of the degree of her ambivalence and is another important clue about her need for early intervention. Third, a determination of the degree to which her avoidance mechanisms have been overwhelmed by anxiety and intrusive thoughts should also indicate to what extent acute stress is predisposing her to negative postabortion consequences, making her a worthy candidate for counseling.

In the case of psychotherapeutic efforts during postabortion counseling, our findings provide additional clues. The dynamic interaction captured in our model suggests that whereas acute stress compromises preabortion decision making, after the abortion acute stress comes to be driven by negative affects that in turn are driven by the more cognitive factor of regret. This suggests that counseling interventions might best be aimed at working through regret, especially early after the abortion, to better reduce the perpetuation of negative affects over the long-term. Our results also indicate that an increase in the desire for a child (perhaps to replace the one given up) and partner conflict occurring as a result of the abortion are two issues that deserve attention in any postabortion counseling. Although postabortion fear of pregnancy and contraceptive practice are important issues in and of themselves, our findings indicate that there are major positive shifts in both of them after the abortion without regard to stress, negative affects, or regret. This finding would seem to diminish the relative importance of focusing on those issues when counseling for regret. Of course, it almost goes without saying that the occurrence of a failed medical abortion potentially signals the need for a counseling intervention.

Finally, we mention what seems to us to be the most important policy implication of this study: the need for more postabortion longitudinal research. The results of the relatively small study reported here certainly demonstrate the feasibility of elevating our understanding of the patterns and dynamics of postabortion psychology to a new level. This might be accomplished through a set of concerted investigations, each with a repeated-measures design, focusing on some particular postabortion time interval. For example, there might be several studies doing measurements at baseline (at the time of the abortion) and then periodically for up to 6 months. Then, several other studies might begin at baseline and repeat measurements every 6 months for several years. Finally, there might be several studies that conducted truly long-term follow-ups over 5, 10, or even 20 years. If each of these studies used some agreed-on common set of instruments and procedures, each principal investigator could still be free to use additional instruments and procedures to pursue unique special interests. Such a coordinated effort would not only add immensely to our understanding of postabortion psychological consequences but might contribute greatly to important related topics such as decision making under duress, stress and coping, loss and depression, the nature of regret, and the effect of abortion on subsequent reproductive motivation and behavior. Ideally such a set of studies would be initiated and funded through existing mechanisms, such as those available within the National Institutes of Health. However, if the political will to support such a policy could not be generated within the public domain, it might be feasible to conduct a large-scale effort of this type under the leadership and financial support of a group of private foundations.

REFERENCES

Adler, N. E. (1975). Emotional responses of women following therapeutic abortion. *American Journal of Orthopsychiatry, 45*, 446–454.

Adler, N. E., David, H. P., Major, B. N., Roth, S. H., Russo, N. F., & Wyatt, G. E. (1992). Psychological factors in abortion. *American Psychologist, 47*, 1194–1204.

Freeman, E. W. (1977). Influences of personality attributes on abortion experiences. *American Journal of Orthopsychiatry, 4*, 503–513.

Gilovich, T., & Medvee, V. H. (1995). The experience of regret: What, when, and why. *Psychological Review, 102*, 379–395.

Henshaw, R., Naji, S., Russell, I., & Templeton, A. (1994). Psychological responses following medical abortion (using mifepristone and gemeprost) and surgical vacuum aspiration. A patient-centered, partially randomized prospective study. *Acta Obstetrica et Gynecologia Scandinavia, 73*, 812–818.

Horowitz, M., Wilner, N., & Alvarez, W. (1979). Impact of Event Scale: A measure of subjective stress. *Psychosomatic Medicine, 41*, 209–218.

Jöreskog, K. G., & Sörbom, D. (1993). *LISREL 8: Structural equation modeling with Simplis Command Language.* Chicago: Scientific Software.

Josephs, R. A., Larrick, R. P., Steele, C. M., & Nisbett, R. E. (1992). Protecting the self from the negative consequences of risky decisions. *Journal of Personality and Social Psychology, 62*, 26–37.

Koop, C. E. (1989, March 21). Surgeon General's report on abortion. *Congressional Record*, pp. E906-E909.

Larrick, R. P. (1993). Motivational factors in decision theories: The role of self-protection. *Psychological Bulletin, 113*, 440–450.

Major, B., & Cozzarelli, C. (1992). Psychosocial predictors of adjustment to abortion. *Journal of Social Issues, 48*, 121–142.

Miller, W. B. (1992). An empirical study of the psychological antecedents and consequences of induced abortion. *Journal of Social Issues, 48*, 67–93.

Miller, W. B. (1994). Reproductive decisions: How we make them and how they make us. In L. J. Severy (Ed.), *Advances in population: Psychosocial perspectives* (Vol. 2, pp. 1–27). London: Kingsley.

Miller, W. B., Shain, R. N., & Pasta, D. J. (1990). The nature and dynamics of post-sterilization regret in married women. *Journal of Applied Social Psychology, 20*, 506–530.

Miller, W. B., Shain, R. N., & Pasta, D. J. (1991). The pre- and post sterilization predictors of post sterilization regret in husbands and wives. *The Journal of Nervous and Mental Disease, 179*, 602–608.

Rosenberg, M. (1965). *Society and the adolescent self-image:* Princeton, NJ: Princeton University Press.

Russo, N. F., & Zierk, K. (1992). Abortion, childbearing, and women's well-being. *Professional Psychology: Research and Practice, 23*, 269–280.

SAS Institute, Inc. (1990). *SAS/STAT user's guide: Version 6* (4th ed.). Cary, NC: Author.

Speckhard, A. C., & Rue, V. M. (1992). Post abortion syndrome: An emerging public health concern. *Journal of Social Issues, 48*, 95–119.

Spielberger, C. D., Gorsuch, R. L., & Lushene, R. E. (1970). *Manual for the State–Trait Anxiety Inventory.* Palo Alto, CA: Consulting Psychologists Press.

APPENDIX

Format of the Impact of Event Scale as modified from Horowitz, Wilner, and Alvarez (1979). We have deleted the four columns of underlines (for check marking) and replaced them with frequency distributions (%) of preabortion responses. Items labeled (A), (I), and (P) are included in the Avoidance, Intrusion, and Positive Thinking scales, respectively.

IMPACT OF EVENT SCALE

Below on the left is a list of comments that people make about different events in their life. Please read each comment and think about how it applies to you and your getting an abortion. Then, indicate how frequently each comment was true for you DURING THE PAST SEVEN DAYS by placing a check mark in one of the four columns on the right.

| | How Frequently True | | | |
Comment	Not at all	Once or twice	Often but not every day	Every day
1. I thought about it when I didn't mean to. (I)	34 (23.9)	54 (38.0)	26 (18.3)	28 (19.7)
2. I avoided letting myself get upset when I thought about it or was reminded of it. (A)	53 (37.6)	33 (23.4)	38 (27.0)	17 (12.1)
3. I felt good about it. (P)	41 (29.1)	25 (17.7)	36 (25.5)	39 (27.7)
4. I tried to remove it from my thoughts. (A)	50 (35.7)	28 (20.0)	29 (20.7)	33 (23.6)
5. I talked about it with someone close. (P)	29 (20.4)	46 (32.4)	44 (31.0)	23 (16.2)

	How Frequently True			
Comment	Not at all	Once or twice	Often but not every day	Every day
6. Because of it, I had trouble falling asleep or staying asleep. (I)	77 (54.2)	31 (21.8)	20 (14.1)	14 (9.9)
7. I had strong waves of feeling about it. (I)	50 (35.2)	43 (30.3)	31 (21.8)	18 (12.7)
8. I had dreams about it. (I)	113 (79.6)	19 (13.4)	4 (2.8)	6 (4.2)
9. I stayed away from reminders of it. (A)	99 (69.7)	17 (12.0)	17 (12.0)	9 (6.3)
10. I wanted to think about it. (P)	60 (42.3)	35 (24.6)	30 (21.1)	17 (12.0)
11. I felt as though it wasn't really happening or wasn't real. (A)	77 (53.5)	44 (30.6)	10 (6.9)	13 (9.0)
12. I tried not to talk about it. (A)	77 (53.5)	29 (20.1)	20 (13.9)	18 (12.5)
13. Pictures about it popped into my mind. (I)	77 (53.5)	40 (27.8)	16 (11.1)	11 (7.6)
14. Other things kept making me think about it. (I)	73 (50.7)	34 (23.6)	26 (18.1)	11 (7.6)
15. I was aware that I still had a lot of feelings about it but didn't want to deal with them. (A)	84 (58.3)	39 (27.1)	13 (9.0)	8 (5.6)
16. I have day dreamed about it. (I)	89 (61.8)	34 (23.6)	15 (10.4)	6 (4.2)
17. I tried not to think about it. (A)	62 (43.1)	39 (27.1)	24 (16.7)	19 (13.2)
18. Any reminder brought back feelings about it. (I)	73 (50.7)	41 (28.5)	22 (15.3)	8 (5.6)
19. My feelings about it have been kind of numb. (A)	73 (50.7)	37 (25.7)	17 (11.7)	17 (11.7)
20. I had positive thoughts about it. (P)	41 (28.7)	36 (25.2)	35 (24.5)	31 (21.7)
21. I had trouble concentrating because of it. (I)	75 (52.1)	45 (31.3)	13 (9.0)	11 (7.6)

Note. Percentages are in parentheses.

11

MEN AND ABORTION: THE GENDER POLITICS OF PREGNANCY RESOLUTION

WILLIAM MARSIGLIO AND DOUGLAS DIEKOW

A key feature of how abortion is debated and practiced in the United States involves the intersection between the interest group politics and the interpersonal decision-making processes that frame the resolution of pregnancies. At the macrolevel the debate continues to simmer between competing interest groups, most notably, those associated with the pro-life and pro-choice movements (Luker, 1984), and is in some respects fueled by what appears to be a growing gender distrust that is permeating U.S. culture. This debate and the way individuals personally handle the abortion experience is influenced by many factors.

In this chapter, we focus specifically on how gender issues shape the context within which the process of resolving a pregnancy occurs. We consider how individuals' efforts to negotiate and make personal decisions about abortion are structured, in part, by interest group politics played out at the institutional level. Our major objective is to draw attention to a neglected area of research—men's roles in the pregnancy resolution process and abortion. To this end, we examine men's experiences within a larger context by outlining how competing ideologies about family life and relationships, feminist and pro-feminist principles, and the ideology of men's rights groups are related to social policy and law dealing with men and abortion (see Marsiglio, 1998).

The potential struggle between men and women over the abortion issue is shaped largely by these diverse ideologies. These ideologies are significant because they play a role in structuring both the interpersonal context in which abortion is discussed and the institutional context within which abortions are performed. Much can be gained by studying how social institutions—the legal system in particular, structures men's experiences in the reproductive domain. These institutions affect men's involvement or exclusion from the processes surrounding the resolution of a pregnancy, they influence child support policies, and they affect individuals' perceptions of these policies.

HISTORICAL CONTEXT

In 1973 the Supreme Court affirmed in *Roe v. Wade* that women in the United States have a fundamental legal right to make unilateral decisions about aborting or bringing a pregnancy to term. Although the court spoke directly to women's rights, it was silent on fathers' potential rights and responsibilities. In addition, the court did not address the details of how women's right to abortion was to be honored. States therefore assumed the responsibility of regulating the implementation of women's legal access to abortion. This set of circumstances led to a proliferation of state laws requiring women to notify or secure consent from the father of the fetus prior to an abortion.

The Supreme Court revisited the abortion issue in 1976 in *Planned Parenthood of Central Missouri v. Danforth* by considering prospective fathers' rights in the area of abortion. The Court upheld women's right to make unilateral decisions about whether they wished to abort or carry a pregnancy to term. The decision acknowledged the potential conflict between partners and the unique interest of each, but held that "Inasmuch as it is the woman who physically bears the child and who is the [one] more directly and immediately affected by the pregnancy, as between the two, the balance weighs in her favor." The court's ruling in this case effectively denied men the right to have a legal voice in whether a pregnancy was to be brought to term.

This ruling, in conjunction with federal child support enforcement legislation, has in effect placed men in the tenuous position of being held financially accountable for their partners' unilateral decisions. When women choose not to have abortions and to bear and raise their children, the fathers of those children are obligated financially by law to provide for them for at least 18 years, regardless of their level of involvement with them.

Men's standing in the abortion debate has remained essentially unchanged during the past two decades (Shifman, 1990). Some prospective fathers in recent years have been successful in having courts issue restraining orders on their pregnant partners, though all of these women secured abortions anyway (see Axelrod, 1990; Diggins, 1989; Stetson, 1991; Walters, 1989). Today, neither unmarried male partners nor husbands have any legal recourse in terminating or bringing their partners' pregnancy to term, although 10 states have laws that stipulate (but are not enforced) that women must gain consent from or notify their husbands (Lacay, 1992). The U.S. Supreme Court ruled in 1992 in *Planned Parenthood of Southeastern Pennsylvania v. Casey* that the provision in a Pennsylvania law requiring spousal notification prior to abortion was unconstitutional.

The legal rulings during the past few decades have had implications for how conflicts of interest are being expressed on an interpersonal level between sexual partners who disagree about how a pregnancy should be resolved. Put differently, partners' attitudes about the options for resolving a pregnancy, and their strategies for arriving at a decision, occur within a social context that structures the viable options available to individuals and restricts men's ability to negotiate postconception decisions about their potential offspring.

IDEOLOGY AND INTEREST GROUP POLICIES

Abortion, when viewed as a social issue, provides fertile ground for interest group politics. One of the reasons the decision to abort a pregnancy or carry it to term is highly politicized is that it has implications for fathers' potential child support obligations. A decision to abort a pregnancy renders moot the need for child support, whereas a decision to give birth and rear a child accentuates the child support issue.

The politics of abortion are informed by ideologies related to the Christian right, the feminist movement, the pro-feminist movement, and men's rights groups. Each of the ideologies associated with these movements or organizations, particularly the latter three, address abortion issues by explicitly applying a gender lens. The nature of this gender perspective, and its relationship to the four ideologies alluded to above, are connected to two basic philosophies of family life and reproductive issues. These philosophies have been labeled *conservative* and *progressive* (Scanzoni, 1989).

Proponents of the conservative perspective (Bauer, 1986; Bellah, Madsen, Sullivan, Swidler, & Tipton, 1985; Francoeur, 1983), with its religious underpinnings and patriarchal ideals, support social policies and programs that advance a pro-life stance and men's breadwinner role with respect to their partner and children. Those who embrace this type of ideology contend that abortion should be banned, and, at the very least, women should be denied unilateral power in seeking an abortion if it is legal. They believe that prospective fathers should be able to prevent their partners from having an abortion. Finally, when men do become fathers they are expected to support their children financially whether they live with them or not.

Some observers contend that the underlying objectives of the pro-life movement have more to do with gender than religious or moral issues. Luker (1984) argued, for instance, that although pro-life organizations disseminate public messages emphasizing the protection of the child (or fetus) on religious grounds, research shows that their primary concern is to maintain a traditional social organization where men control women's reproductive lives. Although members of the pro-life movement may identify at times with objectives of men's rights groups, they are primarily interested in promoting a traditional "family" ideal.

The ideology of men's rights groups does not neatly parallel either a conventional or progressive perspective. In a sense, these groups incorporate aspects of both the conventional and progressive positions. Men's rights activists have recently increased their efforts to promote policies and draft legal initiatives that would balance men's and women's rights with respect to abortion and child support. Two key considerations are at the crux of their orientation.

Men's rights organizations are most concerned with those single men who do not necessarily wish to assume social fatherhood responsibilities for children because their children's conception was unplanned. Some men may prefer that a fetus be aborted, whereas others favor bringing the pregnancy to term but placing the child up for adoption. In 1992, the National Center for Men (NCM) proposed a specific strategy to avoid the prospects of "forced fatherhood." This organization developed a controversial consent form called the consensual sex contract. This document sets forth the terms under which heterosexual partners might agree to have sexual relations. The document currently has no legal bearing in court although the NCM believes it should. The document's purpose is to encourage partners to be aware of each others' sexual and reproductive expectations. Although most of this document deals with sexuality concerns, one item affords partners the opportunity to agree to the following condition: "We're not ready to be parents now. If an unplanned pregnancy occurs, neither one of us will try to force the other into parenthood." A man can therefore indicate that he is having sexual relations by choice but not consenting to fatherhood responsibilities should his partner get pregnant.

In January 1996, the NCM officially unveiled its document called the reproductive rights affidavit in conjunction with its Reproductive Rights

Project, which is designed to balanced men's and women's rights in this area. This document reads, in part,

> I hereby relinquish all legal rights and responsibilities for the child referred to in this affidavit. I have made no commitment to, and will accept no obligation for this child. I will not recognize the authority of a court to strip me of my constitutional right to reproductive choice and I will challenge any court order that seeks to impose a parental obligation upon me against my will. By filing the affidavit with a court of law I am joining with others in an act of peaceful resistance to unfair and unjust laws.

The NCM's innovative proposals have provoked heated discussions among the limited number of individuals who are familiar with them. One of the major criticisms of these approaches, even from those who are somewhat sympathetic to them, is that the proposals do not address the best interests of children who may be conceived from the sexual liaisons in question (Marsiglio, 1998). For this reason, it is unlikely that this document will ever be formally recognized or supported by the government or courts.

Men's rights advocates also express some informal concern that women are permitted to abort their pregnancies against the wishes of the prospective fathers who are interested in raising the resulting children on their own. Those who support provisions that would enable men to have greater say in this respect are leaning toward a conventional ideology that favors greater male involvement in pregnancy resolution—so long as the men in question oppose abortion. Some scholars argue that these individuals tend to be concerned with reaffirming traditional ideals of manhood; consequently, they differ considerably from those men who align themselves with the pro-feminist men's movement (Kimmel & Kaufman, 1994). Nevertheless, most activists in the men's rights organizations do share pro-feminists' views that abortion should be legal, even though they are interested in enhancing men's legal rights in this area, especially in terms of relinquishing, prior to conception, any potential paternity rights or responsibilities.

The other basic ideology that addresses family life and gender issues, the progressive viewpoint, is closely linked with feminist thinking in that it supports women's reproductive and economic autonomy (Scanzoni, Polonko, Teachman, & Thompson, 1989). Most progressives, feminists,[1] and male pro-feminists, endorse in principle a woman's autonomy over her body. They also recognize that, given comparable incomes, men and women should be equally responsible for the financial support of their children, although there may be some disagreement when specific circumstances are considered.

---

[1]A vocal subset of women have historically identified themselves as both feminists and pro life (MacNair, Derr, & Naranjo-Huebl, 1996). These types of women tend to represent only a small segment of the feminist movement today.

Individuals who associate with the pro-choice movement tend to identify with the progressive perspective and some version of feminism. Male pro-choice activists are likely to hold white collar positions and are committed to more egalitarian views of gender relations. They are supportive of women maintaining control of their bodies and the reproductive decisions affecting them (Luker, 1984). Male pro-feminists acknowledge the dilemma men face in not being able to control whether a pregnancy they are responsible for is brought to term. They also recognize that some men will face financial child support obligations even though they oppose bringing a pregnancy to term. Newman (1987) concluded that men must recognize women's autonomy over their bodies and accept the notion that men's power begins and ends with their ability to control their sexuality. In other words, men are free to make their own decisions about whether to have sex with a woman who may or may not share their views on abortion. According to Newman, if men's views on abortion are inconsistent with those of their female partner, or men simply are not ready to assume fatherhood responsibilities, they can abstain from having vaginal intercourse, thereby avoiding the possible dilemma of being responsible for a child they did not want to sire.

Until recently, much of the public debate about abortion at the macrolevel has focused on who should control women's ability to make decisions about resolving a pregnancy, the government or pregnant women in consultation with their doctors. Concerns about whether men should have the right to influence the decision-making process involving a pregnancy has received far less public scrutiny. In short, the courts have determined, with little public debate, what limitations and responsibilities should apply to men's roles with respect to paternity and abortion. Meanwhile, there has been far more public discussion about fathers' child support responsibilities because the financial well-being of millions of children and their mothers are at stake.

Although there hasn't been much public discussion of men's roles in abortion, there is substantial public support among North American males for greater male authority in making decisions about abortion. Sixty percent of young males aged 15 to 19 in a national survey conducted in 1988 disagreed at least a little that it was "all right" for an unmarried woman to have an abortion when her partner objected (Marsiglio & Shehan, 1993). Unfortunately, the phrasing of the survey item in this case does not explicitly tap men's views on what a woman's legal right should be, rather it appears to capture men's attitudes about the morality of abortion when a partner objects. In another study, only slightly more than one third of Canadian male respondents reported that they would support a law that allowed a woman to have an abortion without her husband's consent (Adebayo, 1990, see also Shostak, McLouth, & Seng, 1984). These findings are consistent with the results from an anonymous classroom survey conducted by William Marsiglio in 1992. Thirty percent of 200 first-year male college students enrolled in an honors course strongly agreed that an unmarried, 20-year-old prospective father "should have the legal right to prevent his partner from having an abortion" if he is "prepared to pay for all of her medical expenses and he intends to raise the child by himself with the help of his family." Only 10% of a comparable sample of female respondents gave a similar response.

Different biological and social aspects of gender have clearly had implications for the interest group politics surrounding the abortion and child support controversies. For example, gender differences in human reproductive physiology have meant, in effect, that ideologies pertaining to men's and women's reproductive rights must take into account the fact that only women gestate and give birth to children. Not surprisingly, the various ideologies differ in how they interpret men's and women's dissimilar reproductive physiologies and abortion rights.

Some feminists are reluctant (DeCrow, 1982), as are members of men's rights groups (NCM, 1996), to assert that men should always be held financially accountable for their children if only women have the power to make abortion decisions. DeCrow (1982), a former president of the National Organization of Women, argued that

> Justice . . . dictates that if a woman makes a unilateral decision to bring [a] pregnancy to term, and the biological father does not, and cannot share in this decision, he should not be liable for 21 years of support. Or, put another way, autonomous women making independent decisions about their lives should not expect men to finance their choice. (p. 108)

Kapp (1982) echoed Decrow's point by noting that

> to saddle a man with at least eighteen years of expensive, exhausting child support liability on the basis of a haphazard vicissitude of life seems to shock the conscience and be arbitrary, capricious, and unreasonable, where childbirth results from the mother's free choice. (p. 376)

Overall, then, the progressive ideology is consistent with social policy and legislation that enables women to retain the ultimate power to make decisions about abortion in consultation with their physician. However, there is disagreement as to whether men should automatically be obligated to pay child support if the mother decides, contrary to the father's expressed wishes, to bring the pregnancy to term and raise the child—especially when the child is born to unmarried parents. For many men, their chief complaint is not about being shut out of the final pregnancy resolution decision. Instead, they are concerned with the notion of "forced fatherhood" and the long-term financial commitment that can be thrust on them if they impregnate a woman who brings the pregnancy to term and keeps the child (Shifman, 1990). Support for this observation can be found in Shostak et al.'s (1984) survey of 1,000 men who accompanied their partners to an abortion clinic in the early 1980s. In this study, 51% of the respondents did not object to women's unilateral right to abortion but, in fact, objected to being held accountable for a decision in which they had no legal right to participate. Some men who experience forced fatherhood will also feel frustrated and bitter because they will be confronted with the reality that they have a biological child who they are unprepared to nurture and care for at this point in their life.

MEN'S PERSONAL AND INTERPERSONAL EXPERIENCES

Unfortunately, little is known about how men think, feel, and act when they are personally dealing with the resolution of a pregnancy and making abortion decisions. Shostak et al.'s (1984) study provides the most extensive data on men's abortion experiences. Other related work has focused on how women's experiences are affected by their male partner's involvement (Barnett, Freudenberg, & Wille, 1992; Major, Cozzarelli, & Testa, 1992). A body of literature also explores the relationship between demographic factors and men's perceptions about abortion in general (Barnett et al., 1992; Figueira-McDonough, 1989; Major et al., 1992; Marsiglio, 1989; Marsiglio & Shehan, 1993; Walzer, 1994). Some of this attitudinal research deals specifically with questions related to social policy and legal issues, for example, men's thoughts about women's legal right to have an abortion.

Research has seldom explored men's emotional reactions and coping styles in response to an abortion (Major et al., 1992; Shostak et al., 1984). This is unfortunate because even though men do not directly experience the physical aspects of the abortion process in the way women do, many have feelings about those pregnancies that their partners terminate (as well as those they wanted their partners to terminate). Understanding men's abortion roles is also important because some research suggests that male partners' coping expectations affect women's adjustment to the abortion process (Major et al., 1992).

Many factors are likely to affect how men experience and feel about resolving a pregnancy. Some of the more important factors include their views about the morality of abortion, their feelings toward their partner, and their attitudes about becoming a father at this point in their life.

Men differ widely in their perceptions of abortion. Whereas many men recognize women's right to choose to have an abortion, some are confronted with moral issues due to their individual experiences and belief systems. Men with pro-choice views are unlikely to experience a great deal of emotional trauma if they feel as though having a child right now would disrupt their daily routine and life plans too dramatically. Those who embrace a pro-life stance, however, are much more likely to feel distressed about an impending (or completed) abortion, especially if they are optimistic about their potential parenting abilities.

It appears that many men respond to an abortion experience by being silent about their own pain and confusion because they believe that discussing these issues would only heighten their partners' concerns (Shostak et al., 1984). This type of reaction is relevant to Major et al.'s (1992) study of 73 couples in which they examined the impact of men's coping expectations on women's postabortion adjustment. They found that men's expectations were not important in situations where women had high coping expectations, but men's coping mechanisms and support were important for women with low coping expectations.

Whereas many men are silent, or at least stoic about their concerns, some men need to express their thoughts and feelings regarding an impending or recent abortion. Shostak et al.'s (1984) study showed that some men are profoundly affected by the abortion experience. Twenty-nine percent of their respondents reported having frequent thoughts about the fetus around the time of the abortion, and some men continued to daydream about the fetus after the abortion. For some men, the sense of loss about experiencing an abortion with their partner tends to linger.

> Sometimes I regret it. I have friends who have young or infant children, and when I go there, I kind of regret it. Maybe you love kids when they're someone else's. . . .

> I personally really love kids, so it was kind of rough for me. . . . So, I kind of always wonder what kind of kid would this have been.

> Now, often, I wonder what the baby might have been like. And for awhile after I thought about asking her if she wanted to try it all over again. We broke up about six months after it. (p. 108)

Although many men are upset by their partner's abortion, at least for a brief period of time, many others are indifferent to their partner's abortion. Some men are simply relieved that they will not have to assume any social or financial responsibilities.

The way men respond emotionally to the process of resolving a pregnancy will be influenced by the extent to which they agree with their partner about the appropriate course of action. Unfortunately, it is not possible to document in a reliable fashion the number of partners who disagree about how a pregnancy should be resolved. However, a significant percentage of couples probably have disputes of one sort or another about this issue.[2] Some evidence that bears on this question can be gleaned from

---

[2]Many of these disputes are likely to involve men who are expected to make child support payments but who would have preferred to have resolved a pregnancy through abortion.

Zelles's (1984) survey of 521 men who accompanied their partner to the Midwest Health Center for Women in Minneapolis, Minnesota in 1982. This study revealed that 93% had discussed the abortion decision with their partner. Overall, 88% of all of the respondents agreed with the abortion decision, 2% disagreed, and 10% did not provide an answer. Given the restricted nature of this sample it was not possible to study those who did not accompany their partner to the health center. It is reasonable to assume though that a higher percentage of men who did not accompany their partners to the clinic, compared with those who did go, disagreed with their partners' decision to have an abortion. One crude estimate based on clinic staffers' impressions from a study of 26 abortion clinics suggests that at least 6% of the men who do not attend a clinic with their partner are absent because they are opposed to their partners' abortion decision, another 4% are too upset to join their partner, and 14% are unaware that their partner is having an abortion (Shostak et al., 1984). In another survey of women who attended a full-service family planning center in Granite City, Illinois, none of the married women in this sample reported that their husband disapproved of the abortion decision (Ryan & Plutzer, 1989).

In the Ryan and Plutzer survey, about 90% of the women reported that they told the co-conceiver of their pregnancy, and roughly 83% indicated that their co-conceiver was aware of their decision to have an abortion (Ryan & Plutzer, 1989). Surprisingly, when compared with single women, married women were no more likely to inform the co-conceiver. However, women who were married and not involved in extramarital affairs, those who were engaged, those living with the co-conceiver, and those who described their relationships as "going steady" were all quite likely to inform their partner of their pregnancy. Over 95% of these women notified their co-conceiver. In those instances where women told their husbands of their pregnancy, 12% reported that their husbands expressed anger and another 6% were described as "upset." Whereas 6% of these couples discussed the possibility of adoption and 42% discussed having the baby, more than half never discussed the idea of whether to terminate the pregnancy. According to these wives, about half of the husbands shared their feelings with them and 47% asked them about their feelings. The authors concluded that they found no evidence to suggest that couples' relationships improved as a result of these disclosures and discussions, contrary to what many proponents of spousal notification laws tend to expect. Moreover, they concluded after examining wives who had mixed feelings about telling their husbands and those who did not that women in intimate relationships were capable of making a fairly reliable guess about how their relationship's harmony would be affected by notification.

A 1985 survey of 577 high school students from a metropolitan city is tangentially related to our discussion of partners' possible disputes about whether a pregnancy should be terminated by abortion (Marsiglio & Menaghan, 1990). Students were presented with a hypothetical vignette wherein they were asked to assume that they had been dating the same person for about a year and the woman was 2 months pregnant. When students were asked to indicate how they would prefer to resolve an unplanned pregnancy if they were confronted with this situation now, about 19% of the young men and 18% of the young women chose abortion as their first preference. Although gender was not a significant predictor of abortion preferences, and these data are not couple data, there are many opportunities for partners within particular couples to disagree.

In addition to men's personal beliefs about the morality of abortion, the type and quality of their relationship with their partner will affect the way men respond to an abortion. In some respects concerns about morality and feelings for one's partner may be linked. Men involved in committed relationships, especially men who are either married or cohabiting, are probably more likely to experience confusion about the morality or validity of their choice. The connection between men's feelings toward abortion and their feelings for their partner are poignantly captured by one of Shostak et al.'s (1984) 28-year-old respondents.

> It's hard for me to talk, but I've got to do it. I'm an emotional guy. There are friends that don't give a shit. It's programmed in them to think like that, but I don't think they love the women they've gotten pregnant.
>
> If I were to get a woman pregnant on a one-night stand, abortion would be right. With my girlfriend, I loved her, I loved what was inside her.
>
> It still bugs me; it's always going to bug me. I had plans to some day marry this girl and have a family. I'm just trying to cope with it. It's hard, really hard. I'll never forget about it, never. Sometimes I feel like a killer, a killer . . . and I could have changed it. (p. 121)

This man was left with a lasting impression from his abortion experience because he felt strongly about his former partner. His abortion attitudes and feelings are clearly interwoven with his loving feelings toward his partner. Although we cannot say for sure how many prospective and new fathers have had these types of feelings, this man is surely not alone.

MEN AND ABORTION: A RESEARCH AGENDA

As our discussion has made clear, little research has examined men who are involved in a pregnancy resolution process that incorporates the abortion option. As a result, there are plenty of opportunities to conduct theoretically informed research as well as applied research that explores men's views on abortion and their personal involvement in the social and psychological aspects of the abortion process.

A critical avenue of research relevant to issues we discussed in this chapter focuses on the potential conflict of interest between male and female sexual partners about abortion decisions. Men's reactions to learning about an unplanned pregnancy can in some instances either directly or indirectly shape women's ultimate decision whether to abort a pregnancy. We should therefore consider why some men are more willing than others to become a father at a given point in time. Researchers also need to study the ways in which men participate in the decision-making process related to the resolution of a pregnancy. What are the circumstances surrounding situations wherein men try to persuade their partner about pregnancy resolution options, particularly abortion? How often, and in what ways do men resort to emotional or physical abuse when confronting their partner on these matters?

Men's responses to their partner's pregnancy are likely to be shaped by both personal and interpersonal factors. Shostak et al.'s (1984) study of men who had accompanied their partner to an abortion clinic during the early 1980s is the last significant study that examined how men think and feel about their own abortion experiences. This study provides us with some valuable insights about a subset of men's views and experiences. However, because this novel study primarily contained men who actually accompanied their partner for an abortion, we know very little about those men who are aware that their partner is having an abortion but who are either asked to stay away or choose not to get involved. Moreover, it is possible that younger cohorts of men may differ from their older counterparts in terms of their abortion views and experiences. Thus, researchers need to examine recent cohorts of young men and make a concerted effort to include specific subsamples of men. It would be useful, for example, to study those men who do not accompany their partner to an abortion clinic and to differentiate those who have no prior experience with abortion from those who do. As noted previously, the nature of men's relationship with a pregnant partner is likely to affect how men view the prospects of their paternal roles. The notion that interpersonal issues will be important is consistent with the literature that underscores men's tendency to view children as part of a "package deal" in which their commitment and bond to their children is linked to their attachment to the children's mother (Furstenberg & Cherlin, 1991). On average, men in committed relationships may be more active in the decision-making process to resolve a pregnancy and will probably be more reluctant to opt for an abortion, although they may be more willing to compromise their views if their partner has a strong preference one way or the other. For example, those men in committed relationships who prefer to abort a pregnancy, but are confronted with a partner whom they love and who is adamantly opposed to having an abortion, are probably more likely to acquiesce to their partner's wishes than would be the case if they had weaker feelings for their partner.

One possible theoretical framework that can inform research dealing with these types of issues is identity theory (Burke & Reitzes, 1991; Stryker, 1980, 1987; Stryker & Serpe, 1982, 1994). Stryker's version of this theory suggests that an individual's "self" is composed of a set of identities that are based on an individual's structured role relationships with others. These negotiated identities are dynamic and therefore subject to change in response to various factors. According to this framework, an individual's identities tend to be ordered in terms of a saliency hierarchy that is determined by each identity's relative likelihood of being used in a given situation or a variety of situations. An identity's degree of "psychological centrality" is another key aspect to Stryker and Serpe's (1994) recent discussion of identity theory and their efforts to predict behavior. Psychological centrality, unlike the identity salience notion, assumes that individuals are aware of how important an identity is for them and that they have at least a somewhat positive view of the identity.

When one considers men's experiences with the resolution of a pregnancy, one would anticipate that men's reactions will be shaped in part by their level of commitment to their partner identity and their need for validation or social acceptance of this position. Other identities may influence how men behave when they experience events surrounding the resolution of a pregnancy. These identities may either reinforce or compete with men's partner identity and will include men's masculine gender identity, prospective or current (if they already have children) paternal identity, and perhaps a religious identity.

Researchers could use identity theory to examine how men view and express their partner identity and associate it with their prospective paternal identity during the prenatal period. Other questions that could be addressed include the following: What types of expectations do men feel their partners have of them in the short- and long-term? How important do men feel it is for them to fulfill these expectations? When do men allow their desires to please their partner to override their personal concerns about becoming a father at the present time?

Another potentially fruitful area of research, and one with policy implications, deals with how men and women think about and discuss their expectations about sexuality and pregnancy prior to initiating a sexual relationship, or at least prior to conception. Under what circumstances are men and women likely to be aware of their partner's preferences for resolving a potential pregnancy prior to its actually occurring? Which couples discuss these matters ahead of time? When if ever do partners make informal agreements about issues germane to how a pregnancy should be resolved, and are these pacts honored when an unplanned pregnancy occurs?

Research needs to identify and evaluate the varied options available to men and their partners for negotiating pregnancy resolution decisions. Men's and women's personal reactions to strategies such as the consensus sex contract or the reproductive rights affidavit developed by NCM, or alternative initiatives, should be examined.[3] Although the prospect for these types of agreements ever being enforced is quite low, especially if children's rights are not taken into account, it would be intriguing to explore what types of individuals would be receptive or opposed to dealing with pregnancy resolution issues in a formal way prior to having sexual intercourse. Moreover, an innovative social experiment *might* be developed that enables individuals to present this document to potential sexual partners in real life situations. This type of applied research would underscore how important it is for men and women, unlike what is typically the case, to confront pregnancy resolution issues prior to entering a sexual relationship. With a bit of ingenuity, this research could also evaluate the effectiveness of sex education courses and promotional campaigns designed to foster more candid discussions about pregnancy resolution preferences among romantic partners prior to having sex. Researchers might consider how these initiatives take into account issues associated with men's and women's relative legal standing in the abortion debate that are due, in part, to their varying reproductive physiologies.

The areas of research we have mentioned are each relevant to understanding how the politics of gender shape men's general and personal reactions to abortion issues. Research of this kind will continue to be relevant so long as *Roe v. Wade* (1973) remains in effect and women are able to make unilateral decisions about having abortions. This avenue of research will also take on added significance as policy makers accelerate their efforts to make fathers more accountable financially to their biological children. As more and more fathers are encouraged to establish paternity for children they did not intend to sire, and then provide financial child support to them for 18 years, the gender dimension to the abortion controversy is likely to become even more prominent than it has been in the past. Researchers can contribute to this ongoing debate by studying men's general perceptions about abortion as well as their personal responses when they are confronted with an unplanned pregnancy.

REFERENCES

Adebayo, A. (1990). Male attitudes toward abortion: An analysis of urban survey data. *Social Indicators Research, 22,* 213–228.

[3]William Marsiglio recently proposed a preliminary outline for a contractual agreement suitable for use by a select group of heterosexual couples wherein the individual partners are economically autonomous (Marsiglio, 1998). The agreement would enable the respective parties to stipulate their concerns and preferences for pregnancy resolution and child support while ensuring that the children's financial needs are addressed.

Axelrod, R. H. (1990). Whose womb is it anyway: Are paternal rights alive and well despite Danforth? *Cardozo Law Review, 11,* 685–711.

Barnett, W., Freudenberg, N., & Wille, R. (1992). Partnership after induced abortion: A prospective controlled study. *Archives of Sexual Behavior, 21,* 443–455.

Bauer, G. L. (Ed.). (1986). *The family: Preserving America's future.* Washington, DC: White House Working Group on the Family.

Bellah, R. N., Madsen, R., Sullivan, W. M., Swidler, A., & Tipton, S. M. (1985). *Habits of the heart: Individualism and commitment in American life.* Berkeley, CA: University of California Press.

Burke, P. J., & Reitzes, D. C. (1991). An identity theory approach to commitment. *Social Psychology Quarterly, 54,* 239–251.

DeCrow, K. (1982, May 9). Letter to the editor. *New York Times Magazine,* p. 108.

Diggins, M. (1989). Paternal interests in the abortion decision: Does the father have a say? *University of Chicago Legal Forum,* pp. 377–398.

Figueira-McDonough, J. (1989). Men and women as interest groups in the abortion debate in the United States. *Women's Studies International Forum, 12,* 539–550.

Francoeur, R. T. (1983). Religious reactions to alternative life styles. In E. D. Macklin & R. H. Rubin (Eds.), *Contemporary families and alternative lifestyles* (pp. 379–399). Beverly Hills, CA: Sage.

Furstenberg, F. F., Jr., & Cherlin, A. I. (1991). *Divided families: What happens to children when parents part?* Cambridge, MA: Harvard University Press.

Kapp, M. B. (1982). The father's (lack of) rights and responsibilities in the abortion decisions: An examination of legal–ethical implications. *Ohio Northern University Law Review, 9,* 369–383.

Kimmel, M. S., & Kaufman, M. (1994). Weekend warriors: The new men's movement. In H. Brod & M. Kaufman (Eds.), *Theorizing masculinities* (pp. 259–288). Thousand Oaks, CA: Sage.

Lacay, R. (1992, May 4). Abortion: The future is already here. *Time,* p. 29.

Luker, K. (1984). *Abortion and the politics of motherhood.* Berkeley, CA: University of California Press.

MacNair, R., Derr, M. K., & Naranjo-Huebl, L. (1996). *Prolife feminism: Yesterday and Today.* New York: Sulzburger & Graham.

Major, B., Cozzarelli, C., & Testa, M. (1992). Male partners' appraisals of undesired pregnancy and abortion: Implications for women's adjustment to abortion. *Journal of Applied Social Psychology, 22,* 599–614.

Marsiglio, W. (1989). Adolescent males' pregnancy resolution preferences and family formation intentions: Does family background make a difference for blacks and whites? *Journal of Adolescent Research, 4,* 214–237.

Marsiglio, W. (1998). *Procreative man.* New York: New York University Press.

Marsiglio, W., & Menaghan, E. (1990). Pregnancy resolution and family formation:

Understanding gender differences in adolescents' preferences and beliefs. *Journal of Family Issues, 11*, 313–333.

Marsiglio, W., & Shehan, C. (1993). Adolescent males' abortion attitudes: Data from a national survey. *Family Planning Perspectives, 25*, 162–169.

National Center for Men. (1992). *Concensual sex contract*. Brooklyn, NY: Author.

National Center for Men. (1996). *Reproductive rights affidavit*. Brooklyn, NY: Author.

Newman, R. (1987). His sexuality, her reproductive rights. *Changing Men, 47*, 2–4.

Planned Parenthood of Central Missouri v. Danforth, 428 U.S. 52 (1976).

Planned Parenthood of Southeastern Pennsylvania v. Casey. 505 U.S. 833, 112 S. Ct. 2791, 120 L. Ed. 2d 674 (1992).

Roe v. Wade, 410 U.S. 113 (1973).

Ryan, B., & Plutzer, E. (1989). When married women have abortions: Spousal notification and marital interaction. *Journal of Marriage and the Family, 51*, 41–50.

Scanzoni, J. (1989). Alternative images for public policy: Family structure versus families struggling. *Policy Studies Review, 8*, 599–609.

Scanzoni, J., Polonko, K., Teachman, J., & Thompson, L. (1989). *The sexual bond: Rethinking families and close relationships*. Beverly Hills, CA: Sage.

Shifman, P. (1990). Involuntary parenthood: Misrepresentation as to the use of contraceptives. *International Journal of Law and the Family, 4*, 279–296.

Shostak, A. B., McLouth, G., & Seng, L. (1984). *Men and abortion. Lessons, losses, and love*. New York: Praeger.

Stetson, D. M. (1991). *Women's rights in the U.S.A.: Policy debates and gender roles*. Pacific Grove, CA: Brooks/Cole.

Stryker, S. (1980). *Symbolic interactionism: A social structural version*. Palo Alto, CA: Benjamin/Cummings.

Stryker, S. (1987). Identity theory: Developments and extensions. In K. Yardley & T. Honess (Eds.), *Self and identity* (pp. 89–104). New York: Wiley.

Stryker, S., & Serpe, R. T. (1982). Commitment, identity salience, and role behavior. In W. Ickes & E. S. Knowles (Eds.), *Personality, roles, and social behavior* (pp. 199–218). New York: Springer-Verlag.

Stryker, S., & Serpe, R. T. (1994). Identity salience and psychological centrality: Equivalent, overlapping, or complementary concepts. *Social Psychology Quarterly, 57*, 16–35.

Walters, M. F. (1989). Who decides? The next abortion issue: A discussion of fathers' rights. *West Virginia Law Review, 91*, 165–191.

Walzer, S. (1994). The role of gender in determining abortion attitudes. *Social Science Quarterly, 75*, 687–693.

Zelles, P. (1984). Feedback from 521 waiting room males. In A. B. Shostak, G. McLouth, & L. Seng (Eds.), *Men and abortion: Lessons, losses, and love* (pp. 299–304). New York: Praeger.

12

ABORTION AMONG ADOLESCENTS

NANCY E. ADLER, LAUREN B. SMITH, AND JEANNE M. TSCHANN

Abortion continues to be a highly politicized issue in the United States. In addition to the issues that are relevant to women in general, specific concerns have been raised about abortion among adolescents. Each year, approximately 1 million adolescents become pregnant; of these, about 20% experience a spontaneous abortion and about equal proportions of the rest terminate their pregnancy or carry to term. It should be noted, however, that adolescents still make up a relatively small proportion of the women who are obtaining abortions (Henshaw, Koonin, & Smith, 1991). Teenagers obtain less than 25% of abortions performed in the United States (Alan Guttmacher Institute, 1996). The vast majority of adolescents who undergo abortions are unmarried and are terminating their first pregnancy (Russo, Horn, & Schwartz, 1992). When asked the reason for seeking an abortion, over 75% say that it is because they are not ready or not sufficiently mature to raise a child (Torres & Forrest, 1988).

In recent years, much of the public debate about abortion has focused on psychological issues. Such debate shifted in the late 1980s from being focused on only moral issues to including possible health consequences of abortion (Wilmoth, 1992). Legislation regarding abortion has included regulations regarding informed consent and the necessity of providing women with information on the psychological and physical health risks of abor-

285

tion. In relation to adolescents, a number of states have passed more restrictive legislation requiring parental consent for an adolescent to have an abortion. A number of these statutes have been reviewed by the Supreme Court, and these reviews have established that "while a minor female, like an adult female, does have the right to an abortion, the minor's right is more restricted" (Pliner & Yates, 1992, p. 204).

Parental consent legislation for minors implicitly or explicitly assumes that protective legislation is necessary because (a) abortion carries with it substantial risk, and (b) adolescents are incapable of making informed decisions regarding these risks. This has prompted debates over the decisionmaking capabilities of adolescents and the psychological repercussions of abortion in this age group. In this chapter, we examine the empirical evidence relevant to these two assumptions.

PSYCHOLOGICAL SEQUELAE

Part of the rationale for restrictive protective legislation regarding adolescent access to abortion without parental consent is that the decision to have an abortion carries with it a substantial risk of adverse outcomes from which adolescents need to be protected. It is clear that the medical risks of abortion are low, particularly risks from first-trimester abortions, which constitute the vast majority of procedures (Koonin, Smith, & Ramick, 1993). In addition, medical risks from legal abortion are far less than from pregnancy. Mortality risks are 20 times greater for pregnancy and childbirth than for abortion for young women 15 to 19 years of age (O'Keeffe & Jones, 1990). Much of the debate on restrictive legislation regarding abortion in general and legislation regarding adolescent abortion in particular has focused on psychological risk and whether there is a substantial danger of psychopathology caused by having an abortion (Speckhard & Rue, 1992). There is little basis for the assertion that abortion leads to severe psychological sequelae among women in the general population. An expert panel assembled by the American Psychological Association (APA) to review the evidence on the psychological risks of abortion concluded that "the weight of the evidence from scientific studies indicates that legal abortion of an unwanted pregnancy in the first trimester does not pose a psychological hazard for most women" (Adler et al., 1992, p. 41).

Although women in general show few adverse effects of abortion, it is possible that adolescents are at increased risk compared with adult women and that their risk is great enough to require added protection. Although few studies compare adolescents and adult women, the available data do not lend support to the view that adolescents are at substantial risk for adverse psychological sequelae. Some early studies, conducted soon after abortion became legal, found that age was correlated with psychological response, with younger women reporting more negative responses (Adler, 1975; Bracken, Hachamovitch, & Grossman, 1974; Osofsky & Osofsky, 1972). However, these findings do not necessarily indicate that adolescents are at increased risk. First, there are other variables that are confounded with age that may affect the relationship. Marital status is associated both with postabortion responses and with age. Unmarried women show more negative responses following abortion than do married women, and younger women are more likely than older women to be unmarried. In addition, two of the studies found the correlation of age and negative responses among women across the whole range of reproductive years, ranging from adolescents to women over age 40. The percentage of legal minors in these samples was probably small, because less than 15% of women seeking abortions are minors (Henshaw et al., 1991). A correlation of age and risk of negative responses across all age groups does not mean that adolescents are at particularly great risk compared with others; instead, it could be that women who are older (in their 30s and 40s) have relatively more positive responses than those in their 20s or younger.

Research directly focused on adolescents does not show them to be particularly vulnerable to serious negative responses following abortion. Hatcher (1976) studied a small group of adolescents within a few weeks of their having had an abortion and again 1 year later, and found no substantial psychological effects. Cvejic, Lipper, Kinch, and Benjamin (1977) found that none of the young women 15 to 25 years of age whom they followed for 2 years post-abortion reported serious negative sequelae, and the majority reported the abortion to have been a positive experience.

Zabin, Hirsch, and Emerson (1989) conducted one of the few investigations of abortion on a sample of adolescents. They studied 334 urban African American adolescents under the age of 17 who sought a pregnancy test. Three groups of adolescents matched for socioeconomic status, age, and marital status were followed for 2 years: Those who had a negative pregnancy test, those who were pregnant and carried to term, and those who were pregnant and had an abortion. Adolescents were interviewed at the time of pregnancy testing but prior to receiving the test results. They were subsequently followed at 6-month intervals for two years. Psychological measures that were administered included the Rosenberg Self-Esteem Scale, the Rotter Locus of Control Scale, and the Spielberger State–Trait Anxiety Index. The researchers also examined the economic and educational status of the adolescents at each time point.

The results of Zabin et al.'s (1989) study indicated that there were very low rates of negative psychological change in all three groups: 4.5% of the abortion group, 5.5% of the childbearing group, and 10% of the negative pregnancy test group had a decline in psychological scores on the three measures at the 1-year follow-up. Of particular interest is the finding that a large proportion of the negative change in both the abortion and the negative test group was related to a subsequent pregnancy during follow-up. The abortion group had the lowest rates of subsequent pregnancy (37%) compared with the childbearers (47%) and the negative test group (58%). Educationally and economically, the abortion group also fared better than the childbearers unless they became pregnant and gave birth subsequent to the abortion. The abortion group also showed a more favorable profile on specific measures. State anxiety, as expected, was high for all adolescents while awaiting the results of their pregnancy tests. Scores on both state and trait anxiety fell over the 2 years of follow-up. At the end of the 2 years, adolescents who had terminated their pregnancies by abortion were significantly lower on trait anxiety than either adolescents who carried to term or those who had a negative pregnancy test. The abortion group also had a higher sense of self-esteem and a more internal locus of control, compared with the other two groups.

In sum, the few studies that have specifically examined adolescents' responses to abortion suggest that adolescents do not seem to be at substantial risk of negative psychological responses up to 2 years following abortion (Hatcher, 1976; Cvejic et al., 1977; Zabin et al., 1989). Moreover, in the sample studied by Zabin et al. (1989), adolescents who had an abortion, compared with adolescents who either were pregnant and carried to term and adolescents who were not pregnant, showed a more favorable psychological profile over time. Data from our own recently completed study, which compared scores on several psychological measures, showed no differences in psychological responses among young women under age 18 compared with those ages 18 to 21. These studies provide no compelling rationale for restrictive legislation for adolescents based on their degree of risk of adverse psychological effects.

Although relatively few adolescents have severe negative responses following abortion, it is useful to determine the characteristics of adolescents that are associated with relatively more negative responses. Knowing those adolescents who are at increased risk would help to target counseling and other resources toward them. Just as there are few studies that have had a sufficient number of adolescents to allow identification of the specific responses of the adolescents postabortion, existing studies have not examined adolescents separately to assess whether different factors are associated with postabortion distress among adolescents than among older women. In samples of women of childbearing age who have had an abortion, several psychological variables predict more negative responses. These include having had more difficulty in deciding about abortion and more serious conflict about abortion, less social support for having an abortion, and more negative coping expectations and effectiveness. Partner support has shown to be particularly important, although for younger adolescents it appears that support from parents may be relatively more important

(Bracken et al., 1974). An important research agenda will be to determine whether these factors play an equally important role in determining post-abortion adjustment in adolescents as in the more general population of abortion patients or whether factors unique to the adolescent also need to be considered.

ADOLESCENT DECISION MAKING

The other key issue in the debate over parental consent is whether adolescents are competent to make autonomous decisions about having an abortion. The question of competence to make an adequately informed decision requires a definition of *competence* and of *informed consent*. *Competence* is defined as the ability to (a) understand the information presented, (b) display reasoning in the decision-making process, (c) make a choice or decision, and (d) appreciate the consequences of the decision (Koocher & DeMaso, 1990). *Informed consent* has similar elements. An informed choice requires (a) access to sufficient information, (b) understanding the information, (c) competence to evaluate potential consequences, (d) freedom to make a choice, and (e) ability to make and express the choice. With adults, the focus has been on providing information in a way that assures informed consent; with children and adolescents, the focus has been on competence to make an informed choice. As Koocher and DeMaso (1990) observed, "Children are often more capable of expressing preferences and participating in making major life decisions than is generally recognized in medical settings or under the law" (p. 68).

General laws governing informed consent apply to children of all ages. The role of the child in the decision-making process has not been legally defined for different ages, and these guidelines apply to infants as well as adolescents up to 18 years of age. For all children, parents or guardians are allowed to act on the behalf of the child (Koocher & DeMaso, 1990). Under the law, minors are assumed to be incompetent unless proven otherwise, whereas adults are assumed to be competent. However, adolescents have been given exceptions to allow them to consent on their own for certain medical services, including contraceptive examinations and treatment for sexually transmitted diseases and substance abuse. Parental consent laws for abortion generally include a provision for judicial bypass. This allows a judge to provide permission in lieu of parental consent if there is compelling reason for why parents cannot be informed or provide consent.

There are no clear standards for determining if adolescents (or, in fact, adults) are capable of making an adequately informed decision. The APA presented amicus briefs in court cases regarding parental consent laws, arguing that adolescent decision making is comparable to that of adults.

In critiquing these briefs, Gardner, Scherer, and Tester (1989) agreed that there is no evidence that adolescents are incompetent in their decision making, but they argued that this is not the same as having evidence showing that adolescents are comparable to adults in their decision-making abilities or process. They believe that the APA briefs went too far in asserting definitive evidence of adolescent competence. Since that critique, there has been additional research showing no substantial differences between adolescent and adult biases in decision making (Adler, Moore, & Tschann, 1997; Ambuel & Rappaport, 1992; Quadrel, Fischoff, & Davis, 1993). The question of when the evidence is sufficient to be used in legal proceedings is a difficult one. What is clear is that, as Gardner et al. (1989) noted, "There is little psychological evidence in support of the Court's view of adolescent incompetence" (p. 896).

In weighing the evidence for adolescent competence to make informed decisions about abortion, one needs to consider not just the general data on adolescent cognitive development but more specific data on domain-specific functioning; one needs to know how well adolescents faced with a decision about an unwanted pregnancy are able to meet the criteria for competence. There is some evidence that older adolescents respond differently to a decision regarding abortion than to other decisions. Finken and Jacobs (1996) examined anticipated patterns of responding to four types of life decisions among predominantly White male and female college students. The researchers asked the students whom they would consult if they were faced with four situations: (a) an abortion decision (resolution of an unintended pregnancy), (b) an interpersonal decision (how to resolve a conflict with a close friend), (c) a medical decision (whether to have chemotherapy for a tumor), and (d) a future-oriented decision (involving a job choice).

The investigators found significant differences in anticipated consultation patterns across these situations. Faced with a decision about abortion, both men and women were most likely to indicate they would consult their partner. Both men and women indicated they would also consult their mothers, but the mother's input was more important for women. The pattern of consultation differed in the other situations. For example, friends were more likely to be consulted in relation to the future-oriented decision than the abortion decision. Professionals were more likely to be consulted for medical decisions. The expected pattern of consultation is consistent with actual patterns regarding abortion (Cicirelli, 1980). This pattern may not hold for younger adolescents; college students may be relatively more likely to consult partners rather than parents, whereas younger adolescents may be more likely to consult their parents, as described below.

Parental consent laws presume that adolescent decision making requires the guidance of adults and that adolescents will not on their own obtain sufficient input. In fact, most pregnant adolescents voluntarily consult with an adult and the majority involve their parents. Zabin, Hirsch, Emerson, and Raymond (1992) found that 91% of adolescents in their study consulted a parent or guardian after receiving a positive pregnancy test. An additional 4% had discussed it with another adult (besides the partner or an elder sibling). Satisfaction with their decision was unrelated to whether or not a parent was involved in the decision. In a study of 184 adolescents undergoing abortion, Resnick, Bearinger, Stark, and Blum (1994) found that all of the adolescents they studied discussed their abortion with at least one other person and 75% discussed it with a parent or other adult.

The likelihood that adolescents will consult with their parents varies as a function of age: The younger the adolescent the more likely it is that she will involve her parents. This finding suggests that those adolescents most in need of guidance will consult with their parents. Zabin et al. (1992) found that younger adolescents were more likely than older adolescents to discuss their pregnancy with a parent. Griffin-Carlson and Mackin (1993) found that whereas only 51% of adolescents 12 to 21 years old informed their parents about their pregnancy, relatively more of the younger than older adolescents confided in their parents. Young women who chose not to tell their parents were more financially independent and more likely to live alone. Adolescents who rated themselves as less mature were more likely to confide in their parents.

Henshaw and Kost (1992) found that of 1,500 adolescents, 75% voluntarily told a parent about the pregnancy, and very few parents (5% of mothers and 6% of fathers) did not support their child's decision to have an abortion. In two thirds of the cases in which one parent did not support the decision, the other parent did. Adolescents who did not tell their parents tended to be older than the ones who did. Further, adolescents who chose not to tell their parents about their pregnancy often had good reason for doing so. Henshaw and Kost reported that 30% of the young women who did not tell their parents had experienced domestic violence, feared it would occur, or were fearful of being forced to leave home.

The figures cited above reveal that most adolescents do seek guidance, which suggests that they have engaged in active reasoning about their decision. Because having an abortion requires taking action, it seems likely that, on average, adolescents who seek to terminate a pregnancy will act in a relatively more deliberative way than those who continue their pregnancy. Many of those who continue their pregnancy may make an active choice to do so, including seeking consultation. For others, however, continuing a pregnancy may be a default choice resulting from inability or unwillingness to confront the reality of an unwanted pregnancy, lack of knowledge about choices, or both.

Adolescents who seek an abortion to terminate an unwanted pregnancy may be relatively more mature than their peers. They may be more oriented toward the future and to perceive that childbearing at that age would be problematic for them and for their child. Phipps-Yonas (1980) found that young women choosing abortion were relatively more likely to come from families with higher socioeconomic status and to have higher educational goals. Moreover, among adolescents seeking abortion, it may be that it is the more mature adolescents who do not notify their parents. As Pliner and Yates (1992) observed,

> Mature minors are more concerned with protecting their privacy and, hence, are less likely to desire parental involvement (Melton, 1983). Immature minors, on the other hand, are often more financially and emotionally dependent on their parents. As a result, they are more inclined to seek their parents' advice and support (Blum, Resnick, & Stark, 1987; Clary, 1982; Torres, Forrest, & Eisman, 1980). (p. 208)

There are substantial individual differences among adolescents in their ability to reason; therefore, any age-dependent restrictions may be inadequate. There are conflicting findings concerning whether younger adolescents are less capable than older adolescents of competent reasoning in general (Lewis, 1981). However, in the specific domain of reasoning about abortion, findings are more consistent and show little evidence that adolescents lack the capacity to reason effectively about this decision. Foster and Sprinthall (1992), administered the Washington University Sentence Completion Test to young adolescents (12–14 years) and older adolescents (17–19 years) and found developmental differences in moral reasoning; however, these differences were not found in reasoning tasks directly assessing the abortion decision. Lewis (1980) did not find significant differences between adolescents and adults in their hypothetical reasoning about abortion. Importantly, Ambuel and Rappaport (1992) found no differences in reasoning when they conducted assessments of legal competence. Because this study is so salient, we describe it in more detail below.

Ambuel and Rappaport (1992) studied women at a clinic for pregnancy testing. The women were separated into four groups: 15 years or younger, 16 to 18 years of age, legal adults aged 18 to 21 years, and adults over age 21. The women were interviewed regarding their thinking about their pregnancy, including the difficulty of the decision regarding continuation or termination of the pregnancy, the pros and cons of parenthood and abortion, the effect it could have on other people in their lives, and the implications of the decision for personal educational goals. The interviews were then rated on decision conflict, social support, and competence. The competence variable included volition, global quality and consequences, and richness. Because legal competence is not strictly defined, two definitions of *competence* were used for the analyses; one defined legal competence as a single variable encompassing the three components and the other analyzed each of the components individually.

Ambuel and Rappaport (1992) found that adolescents considering abortion in every age group were as competent as the adults. The only group that was found to be less competent than the adults were the adolescents 15 years of age or younger who did not consider abortion; these adolescents were lower on volition and global quality than the adults. This study is of interest not only because of the comparison of adolescent and adult competency, but it also examined factors that predicted competence among adolescents. Social support, decision conflict, knowledge about abortion, cognitive skills, and educational goals predicted each of the criteria of competence. It is interesting to note that affect, and knowledge about adoption, pregnancy, and parenting, were not associated with greater competence.

Issues of adolescent competence and the need for parental consent are important policy issues. The intended effects of parental consent laws are to assure adequate guidance for adolescents and to promote parental involvement. However, there are possible negative consequences as well. Adolescents who fear telling their parents, and who may have a basis for concern about their parents' response, may not feel comfortable in trying to obtain a judicial bypass of consent laws. They may be intimidated by the court system and may not know how to go about obtaining legal approval. This may lead some adolescents to seek illegal abortions, which place them at heightened risk of medical complications and even death. A clear example of this was the case of Becky Bell, an adolescent who died after an illegal abortion she obtained to avoid telling her parents. There appears to be some evidence of a rise in self-induced abortions (Honigman, Davila, & Petersen, 1993), which could reflect this trend.

The need for judicial bypass may also increase risk for adolescents because it delays the time at which their abortion is performed. Later abortions, performed in the second trimester, carry greater risks of both medical and psychological morbidity (Kaltreider, Goldsmith, & Margolis, 1979; Rooks & Cates, 1977). A greater percentage of adolescent than adult women have second-trimester abortions (O'Keeffe & Jones, 1990). Some delay in obtaining an abortion may be due to greater difficulty among adolescents in diagnosing the pregnancy and in accessing services. When the need for judicial bypass is added to this, more adolescents may get pushed into having second-trimester procedures. It may take some adolescents considerable time to negotiate their way through the judicial system. Similarly, if adolescents make arrangements to go out of state to obtain a legal abortion in a state that does not require parental notification or consent, they may also be delayed. In addition to the added risks associated with later abortion, the experience of judicial bypass itself may be stressful and anxiety-provoking for adolescents (O'Keeffe & Jones, 1990). Ironically, judicial bypass appears generally to be unnecessary as virtually all requests for judicial permission have been granted (Pliner & Yates, 1992). For example, 3,500 adolescents petitioned for judicial bypass in Minnesota between 1985 and 1990; of those requests only 9 were denied (Rodman, 1991).

There is mixed evidence on the effects of parental consent laws. Pierson (1995) found an increase in late abortions as well as an increase in abortions sought out of state after enactment of parental consent/notification in Missouri. Within the state, fewer White adolescents chose abortion following enactment of this law. The live birth rate among teens was 60% in 1985, prior to the legislation, and rose to 74% by 1992. Fewer teens who chose to continue their pregnancies were opting for marriage during this time as well. A somewhat different pattern emerged in Minnesota following enactment of its parental notification law (Klitsch, 1991). Pregnancy rates as well as birth and abortion rates fell among the 15 to 17-year-olds in Minnesota following the enactment of the law. There was an increase in the ratio of late to early abortions. This shift could have resulted from a decrease in early abortion because overall pregnancy rates fell, or could have resulted from increases in second-trimester abortion, but information at this level of detail is not available.

CONCLUSION

Apart from a limited number of studies that examine adolescent abortion directly, much of our understanding of the psychological sequelae of abortion and decision making regarding abortion is based on samples of women across the entire reproductive lifespan. These studies have shown that abortion does not result in negative psychological repercussions in the vast majority of women; this is likely to hold for the adolescent as well as the adult participants in these studies. Although some research has shown younger age to be a risk factor for more negative postabortion responses, it is not clear whether the heightened risk is attributable to more adverse response of adolescents or to differences between responses of women in their 20s versus those in their 30s or 40s. In addition, we do not know whether risk is attributable to age per se or to factors, such as marital status, that are confounded with age.

For the small number of women who do suffer postabortion emotional distress, certain risk factors have been identified, including psychological difficulties prior to procedure, ambivalence about the decision, low coping expectancies, and inadequate social support. Younger women with these characteristics may also be at increased risk, although this has not been fully examined. Carefully controlled studies such as the one by Zabin et al. (1989) are needed to expand our knowledge of the experiences of adolescents, and specifically of different age groups within adolescence.

More research is also needed on adolescent competence and decision making. Studies suggest that unintended pregnancy is a unique crisis that may be approached differently from other life decisions. We need to know how adolescents function in relation to this specific situation as well as more about their general capacities relevant to the requirements of being able to make an adequately informed decision. Future research should examine the decision-making process to determine the specific ways the decision about abortion is similar to and differs from other decisions. Legislation and policies based on generalizations from other areas of decision-making research may not pertain to the abortion decision.

Critical evaluation of restrictive policies is needed, because these policies are having adverse effects on the adolescents they are supposed to protect. Consent laws appear to be unnecessary, because the vast majority of adolescents voluntarily consult their parent or an adult. Those adolescents who do not consult a parent appear to have good reason for wanting to avoid doing so; this is reflected in the fact that almost all requests for judicial bypass have been granted. The obstacles created by these laws increase stress for adolescents who have reason to fear informing their parents, and they increase the chance that the adolescent will undergo a second-trimester abortion, or seek an illegal abortion, both of which carry increased risk of medical and psychological sequelae. Some creative alternatives have been used, such as the policy in Connecticut that allows young adolescents (15 and younger) to have an abortion without parental consent if they receive adequate counseling from a professional (O'Keeffe & Jones, 1990).

Although we have focused on the evidence pertinent to the explicit rationale for most parental consent laws, we should note that such laws have other purposes as well. They may be intended to strengthen families and encourage better parent–child communication. However, mandating consultation, particularly in families with a history of abuse or other problems, may not achieve these goals. In addition, as O'Keeffe and Jones (1990) observed, such laws "are not intended to protect adolescents from harm. Their real intent is to make abortion more difficult to obtain" (p. 80). Similarly, Stotland (1996) questioned the rationale for restrictions on adolescent access to abortion on the basis of adolescents' incompetence to consent for the procedure:

> The very young woman who is presumably too immature to decide to have an abortion will, without one, become the mother of a newborn infant, fully responsible for its life and for decisions about its medical and other care. (p. 243)

This observation reminds us that need for a decision about abortion arises only in the context of an unwanted pregnancy. In addition to our extending our efforts to understand the abortion decision, we must also increase our efforts to find ways to prevent the occurrence of unwanted pregnancy. A significant proportion of pregnancies among adolescents are unwanted; of adolescents who get pregnant and do not miscarry, almost half terminate their pregnancy (Henshaw & Van Vort, 1989). Studies of abortion among adolescents are likely to add to the extensive literature indicating a minimal incidence of negative psychological sequelae. Such studies should also shed light on the conditions that lead to optimal adjustment and provide new information on how adolescents decide about resolution of an unwanted pregnancy. These findings may result in useful recommendations for providing counseling and state policies on issues such as parental consent legislation.

REFERENCES

Adler, N. E. (1975). Emotional responses of women following therapeutic abortion. *American Journal of Orthopsychiatry, 45*, 446–454.

Adler, N. E., David, H. P., Major, B. N., Roth, S. H., Russo, N. F., & Wyatt, G. E. (1992). Psychological factors in abortion. *American Psychologist, 47*, 1194–1204.

Adler, N. E., Moore, P. J., & Tschann, J. M. (1997). Planning skills in adolescence: The case of contraceptive use and non-use. In S. L. Friedman & E. K. Scholnick (Eds.), *The developmental psychology of planning. Why, how, and when do we plan?* (pp. 321–336). Mahwah, NJ: Erlbaum.

Alan Guttmacher Institute. (1996). *Facts at a glance: Induced Abortion.* New York: Author.

Ambuel, B., & Rappaport, J. (1992). Developmental trends in adolescents' psychological and legal competence to consent to abortion. *Law and Human Behavior, 16*, 129–153.

Blum, R. W., Resnick, M. D., & Stark, T. (1987). The impact of a parental notification law on adolescent abortion decision-making. *American Journal of Public Health, 77*, 619–620.

Bracken, M. B., Hachamovitch, M., & Grossman, G. (1974). The decision to abort and psychological sequelae. *Journal of Nervous and Mental Disease, 158*, 154–162.

Cicirelli, V. (1980). A comparison of college women's feelings toward their siblings and parents. *Journal of Marriage and the Family, 42(1)*, 111–118.

Clary, F. (1982). Minor women obtaining abortions: A study of parental notification in a metropolitan area. *American Journal of Public Health, 72*, 283–285.

Cvejic, H., Lipper, I., Kinch, R. A., & Benjamin, P. (1977). Follow-up of 50 adolescent girls two years after abortion. *Canadian Medical Association Journal, 116*, 44–46.

Finken, L., & Jacobs, J. (1996). Consultant choice across decision contexts: Are abortion decisions different? *Journal of Adolescent Research, 11(2)*, 235–260.

Foster, V., & Sprinthall, N. A. (1992). Developmental profiles of adolescents and young adults choosing abortion: Stage sequence, decalage, and implications for policy. *Adolescence, 27,* 655–673.

Gardner, W., Scherer, D., & Tester, M. (1989). Cognitive development and adolescent legal rights. *American Psychologist, 44,* 895–902.

Griffin-Carlson, M. S., & Mackin, K. J. (1993). Parental consent: Factors influencing adolescent disclosure regarding abortion. *Adolescence, 28,* 1–11.

Hatcher, S. (1976). Understanding adolescent pregnancy and abortion. *Primary Care, 3,* 407–425.

Henshaw, S. K., Koonin, L. M., & Smith, J. C. (1991). Characteristics of U.S. women having abortions. *Family Planning Perspectives, 23,* 75–81.

Henshaw, S. K., & Kost, K. (1992). Parental involvement in minors' abortion decisions. *Family Planning Perspectives, 24,* 196–207, 213.

Henshaw, S. K., & Van Vort, J. (1989). Teenage abortion, birth and pregnancy statistics: An update. *Family Planning Perspectives, 21,* 85–88.

Honigman, B., Davila, G., & Petersen, J. (1993). Reemergence of self-induced abortions. *Journal of Emergency Medicine, 11,* 105–112.

Kaltreider, N. B., Goldsmith, S., & Margolis, A. (1979). The impact of mid-trimester abortion techniques on patients and staff. *American Journal of Obstetrics and Gynecology, 135,* 235–238.

Klitsch, M. (1991). Teenage abortions fell after Minnesota imposed parental notification law. *Family Planning Perspectives, 23,* 238–239.

Koocher, G. P., & DeMaso, D. R. (1990). Children's competence to consent to medical procedures. *Pediatrician, 17,* 68–73.

Koonin, L. M., Smith, J. C., & Ramick, M. (1993). Abortion surveillance—United States, 1990. *Morbidity and Mortality Weekly Reports, 42,* 29–57.

Lewis, C. C. (1980). A comparison of minors' and adults' pregnancy decisions. *American Journal of Orthopsychiatry, 50,* 446–453.

Lewis, C. C. (1981). How adolescents approach decision: Changes over grades seven to twelve and policy implications. *Child Development, 52,* 538–544.

Melton, G. B. (1983). Minors and privacy: Are legal and psychological concepts compatible? *Nebraska Law Review, 62,* 455–493.

O'Keeffe, J., & Jones, J. M. (1990). Easing restrictions on minors' abortion rights. *Issues in Science and Technology, 7,* 74–80.

Osofsky, J. D., & Osofsky, H. J. (1972). The psychological reaction of patients to legalized abortion. *American Journal of Orthopsychiatry, 42,* 48–60.

Phipps-Yonas, S. (1980). Teenage pregnancy and motherhood: A review of the literature. *American Journal of Orthopsychiatry, 50,* 403–431.

Pierson, V. H. (1995). Missouri's parental consent law and teen pregnancy outcomes. *Women & Health, 22,* 47–58.

Pliner, A. J., & Yates, S. (1992). Psychological and legal issues in minors' rights to abortion. *Journal of Social Issues, 48,* 203–216.

Quadrel, M. J., Fischoff, B., & Davis, W. (1993). Adolescent (in)vulnerability. *American Psychologist, 48,* 102–116.

Resnick, M. D., Bearinger, L. H., Stark, P., & Blum, R. W. (1994). Patterns of consultation among adolescent minors obtaining an abortion. *American Journal of Orthopsychiatry, 64,* 310–316.

Rodman, H. (1991). Should parental involvement be required for minors' abortions? *Family Relations, 40,* 155–160.

Rooks, J., & Cates, W. (1977). Emotional impact of D and E versus instillation. *Family Planning Perspectives, 9,* 276–278.

Russo, N. F., Horn, J. D., & Schwartz, R. (1992). U.S. abortion in context: Selected characteristics and motivations of women seeking abortions. *Journal of Social Issues, 48,* 183–202.

Speckhard, A. C., & Rue, V. M. (1992). Postabortion syndrome: An emerging public health concern. *Journal of Social Issues, 48,* 95–119.

Stotland, N. L. (1996). Conceptions and misconceptions: Decision about pregnancy. *General Hospital Psychiatry, 18,* 238–243.

Torres, A., & Forrest, J. D. (1988). Why do women have abortions? *Family Planning Perspectives, 20,* 169–177.

Torres, A., Forrest, J. D., & Eisman, S. (1980). Telling parents: Clinic policies and adolescents' use of family planning and abortion services. *Family Planning Perspectives, 12,* 284–292.

Wilmoth, G. H. (1992). Abortion, public health policy, and informed consent legislation. *Journal of Social Issues, 48,* 1–17.

Zabin, L., Hirsch, M. B., & Emerson, M. R. (1989). When urban adolescents choose abortion: Effects on education, psychological status and subsequent pregnancy. *Family Planning Perspectives, 21,* 248–255.

Zabin, L. S., Hirsch, M. B., Emerson, M. R., & Raymond, E. (1992). To whom do inner-city minors talk about their pregnancies? Adolescents' communication with parents and parent surrogates. *Family Planning Perspectives, 24,* 148–154, 173.

IV

ABORTION IN THE
CONTEXT OF PRACTICE

13

A COGNITIVE APPROACH TO PATIENT-CENTERED ABORTION CARE

BARBARA FISHER, MARY ANN CASTLE,
AND JOAN MOGUL GARRITY

Mortality and morbidity rates associated with abortion dramatically declined in the United States immediately after the legalization of abortion in 1973 (Atrash et al., 1987; *Roe v. Wade*, 1973). These rates have remained low ever since. Why, then, more than 20 years later do we write about patient-centered abortion care? We do so because abortion remains peripheral to mainstream reproductive health care (Chavkin, 1994). Physicians, including gynecologists, have not been required to learn to perform surgical abortion procedures as a routine part of their graduate medical education (Westhoff, Marks, & Rosenfield, 1993). They also vary in their understanding of women's emotional responses to deciding to have an abortion and in the communication skills necessary to respond sensitively to patients.

For most women, an unplanned pregnancy and the decision about whether to continue it is associated with a wide range of psychological reactions and cognitive and affective responses and stressors. Research indicates that fewer adult women have severe psychological reactions to abortions than is commonly believed (Adler, 1992; Burnell & Norfleet, 1991).

In general, the wide range of emotions expressed by women seeking abortions can be considered normal (Garrity & Castle, 1996). It is important for reproductive health care professionals to understand that, despite the patients' emotional response, most women who want an abortion usually are resilient; whereas while those who succumb to external social pressures may react negatively after the abortion (Romans-Clarkson, 1989). Women who respond with difficulty to short-term stressful events will benefit from support in using problem-solving skills to make the best decision. Poettegen (1988) recommended that, in preabortion sessions, the counselor identify and help resolve social and cultural issues associated with the decision as well as intrapsychic and interpersonal conflicts. This is important because if women believe they can cope with their decision to abort, their post-abortion responses will be positive (Major, Mueller, & Hildebrandt, 1985; Scheirer & Carver, 1987).

The use of the patient-centered approach to abortion care described in this chapter has advantages for clinicians, counselors, other staff, and patients. The patient-centered approach recognizes that the social context in which abortion counseling occurs can profoundly affect the patients' reactions before, during, and after the abortion. By providing patient-centered abortion care to a woman, the counselor can (a) help the patient explore available options regarding her pregnancy and choose the option that is best for her; (b) demonstrate respect for her emotional responses; (c) help her cope psychologically and physically with the entire process; and (d) support, and potentially increase, her ability to take control over reproductive health issues that affect her life.

Using a cognitive framework, providers can recognize and respond to the highly personalized way a woman reacts to an abortion. They can also identify women who are likely to experience negative reactions following the abortion. These issues can be addressed in the counseling session (Gameau, 1993; Speckhard & Rue, 1993), or women can be referred to counselors, if necessary. Even in short-term interactions, in clinic settings, the counselor can help a patient use cognitive reframing to reduce her stress and to make, and then act on, a decision.

This chapter discusses the psychosocial dimensions of abortion that are within the context of counseling patients before, during, and immediately after the procedure. It offers a model of patient-centered care that is based on cognitive theory. The theory is used in the context of pre- and postabortion counseling of women seeking a first-trimester abortion using local anesthesia. It also forms the basis for supportive patient–staff interactions during the abortion procedure. First, the literature on abortion counseling is reviewed, pointing out the dearth of research, most of which is atheoretical and primarily focuses on psychopathology in abortion counseling. The principles underlying the cognitive approach to counseling are described. Second, we present the basic cognitive techniques to be used in the counseling process. Third, using a single case, specific cognitive interventions and techniques appropriate at various stages of the process are illustrated. Finally, strategies for counseling under special circumstances (e.g., women who have been abused or are conflicted because of their religious beliefs) are briefly discussed.

LITERATURE REVIEW

In reviewing the abortion counseling literature, two major issues emerge. First, because biological reproduction has historically been considered the primary focus of women's health, research has focused on the psychopathological reactions to abortion. Second, the literature that exists is primarily descriptive rather than theory based (Adler et al., 1992). Several published articles on counseling issues date from the 1970s, immediately after legalization (see Belsey, 1977; Brashear, 1973; Hildebrand, 1977; Khan-Edrington, 1979; Ness, 1976). After that time the number of published articles diminished. However, from the training manuals and materials used in reproductive health clinics (Baker, 1995; Baker & Clark, 1997; Beresford, 1988; Garrity & Castle, 1996) and a sexuality counseling text (Baker, Garrity, Beresford, & Halvorson-Boyd, in press) counseling approaches can be inferred. Kaminsky and Shecter (1979) are the only authors to discuss abortion counseling as an integral part of comprehensive care.

The literature on the psychology of women indicates that women's health has been marginalized in medicine, reflecting women's subordinate social status (Stanton, Danoff-Burg, Cameron, & Ellis, 1994). Biological reproduction has, historically, been considered as the primary focus of women's health (Johnson & Hoffman, 1993). The request for an abortion is (within this ideology) antithetical to the view that the primary role of women is that of mother. Therefore, the view of abortion as pathological has become a normative approach in the research on women's reproductive health; it is part of a field that has, in general, emphasized psychopathological issues. Moreover, a literature review cites cultural, racial and gender biases in mental health approaches (see Comas-Diaz & Greene, 1994). Comas-Diaz and Greene (1994) indicated that when North American psychotherapy is applied to women's health it tends to reflect a white male, middle-class orientation. Because of their orientation, professionals with traditional training can be insensitive to the special needs and perceptions of a client from a socioeconomic, ethnic, and racial background different from those they usually counsel. They may fail to consider the differences between their client's perception of the "relative power" and their own, which may critically alter the interactions between them. The social context of a woman's experiences may also play a critical role in shaping the way she selects strategies for coping with a stressful situation, such as an unwanted pregnancy (Pinderhughes, 1994; Solomon & Rothblum, 1986). Professional bias, both in the counseling approach and in the perception of the client's responses to it, can contribute to the view that women tend to exhibit dysfunctional coping strategies around issues of abortion.

Loader (1995) discussed the negative effect of unresolved emotions on repeat unintended pregnancy and abortion. She recommended addressing unconscious processes to bring the conflict to closure to break the pattern of repeat unwanted conception. The psychopathological presentation of women's reproductive health has had ramifications for what is studied and how women are treated. Gibb and Millard (1982) demonstrated that counselors and their abortion patients have discordant perceptions about unintended pregnancies. They found that counselors attributed the pregnancy to women's lack of control, whereas women perceived themselves as having substantial control over the situation. The stereotypic attitudes of counselors and the contradictory perceptions between them and their patients can negatively affect patients' emotional state and disrupt the counseling process. It can also bias research (Adler et al., 1992). To address the impact of conflicting patient–counselor perceptions, the National Abortion Federation (1998) has written a guide to assist health professionals who perform abortions and counsel women who seek them. The manual is designed to help professionals examine their values and attitudes about unintended pregnancies and the decision to terminate them.

The atheoretical and psychopathological literature on reproductive health presents a very limited and skewed framework for counseling abortion patients. In the theory-based research that exists, research questions and methodologies are often influenced by the researcher's orientation. For example, authors who derive data from clinical experience tend to present theories that focus on psychopathology. Some researchers have begun to examine resiliency and to identify counseling strategies that support women's ability to handle difficult reproductive health choices (O'Leary & Ichovics, 1995). Compared with counseling alone, interventions that enhance self-efficacy are more effective in lowering women's risk for postabortion depressive symptoms (Mueller & Major, 1989).

The foregoing review demonstrates a dearth of theoretical frameworks other than a biological model in the literature on abortion counseling. Some researchers, however, have begun to identify counseling strategies that support women's ability to handle difficult reproductive health choices (Garrity & Castle, 1996). This chapter describes a cognitive approach to patient-centered counseling that emerges from cognitive social psychological theory. Lewis (1994) recommended a cognitive therapeutic approach to women of color, which can effectively take into account the complex interaction among gender, class, and race. She stated that cognitive therapy can empower women of color to make healthy decisions, manage problems, and promote an idea of options for those with limited external supports and resources. Because the cognitive model provides reproductive health care professionals with an approach and specific interventions and techniques that individualize their interactions, in writing this chapter we assumed that the cognitive model is an effective approach for all women who are deciding whether to terminate a pregnancy. The cognitive model results in a paradigm shift in counseling from a biomedical to a patient-centered approach. The cognitive approach illustrates a framework worthy of consideration in theorizing about, and providing, abortion care.

COGNITIVE REFRAMING

Cognitive theory hypothesizes that people's emotions and behaviors are influenced by their perception of events (J. S. Beck, 1995). Thus, it is not the situation in and of itself that solely determines how a patient feels. The way a patient interprets and thinks about the event also influences emotions and behavior (A. Beck 1964; Ellis, 1962). The approach and techniques of cognitive theory are generalizable. However, the examples provided in this chapter are specific. They are based on staff interactions with patients during first-trimester abortion, using local anesthesia and the vacuum aspiration method of termination.

Women experience a range of feelings related to making a decision about their pregnancy. These feelings may include anxiety, fear, shame, confusion, distress, helplessness, guilt, ambivalence, sadness, and grief. If a woman confronts these emotions, comes to terms with her decision, and takes control over this life crisis, she may feel empowered. Patients express their emotions differently. Some patients openly display their feelings. They may be nervous, cry, or withdraw. Others express their anger, hostility, and fear with sarcasm. In contrast, some patients are calm; some exhibit denial. Extreme behaviors can sometimes occur within a very short span of time.

In addition to the range of patient feelings that counselors may confront, they also respond to emotionally charged, and often difficult, questions by (a) remaining sensitive to both expressed and nonverbal emotions, (b) clarifying and acknowledging the feelings involved, and (c) providing accurate information. One of the most challenging tasks in communicating with the patient is for counselors to identify the latent meanings and concerns expressed in the patient's questions. Using specific communication techniques and modes of inquiry that are based on the cognitive approach, the counselor tests the validity of latent meanings rather than making assumptions about what the patient means. Certain principles that underlie the cognitive approach (J. S. Beck, 1995) have been applied to patient-centered abortion counseling.

PRINCIPLES OF THE PATIENT-CENTERED
COGNITIVE APPROACH

Principle 1: *The patient-centered cognitive approach to counseling is based on the belief that the social psychological elements within the environment (the clinic) need to be managed to ensure the best possible care for the patient.* Within this framework, all of the health care professionals are involved in the clinical process and ideally will build therapeutic alliances with the patient. How the receptionist greets the patient can significantly shape the patient's thoughts and feelings about the situation and how she will respond to the clinical processes and procedures. The sensitivity and responsiveness of the physician to the patient's reactions to the medical procedure is critical to the outcomes as well. Numerous staff interface with the patient; therefore, ideally messages are consistent and interactions are warm, empathetic, and caring. Staff display a genuine concern for the patient.

Principle 2: *Patient-centered cognitive abortion counseling is time limited, goal oriented, and problem focused.* The counselor conceptualizes the patient's reactions in cognitive terms, basing this on information from the intake evaluation and relevant data as it emerges during the session. It should be noted that many patients are not conflicted over the decision to terminate a pregnancy; others, however, do experience conflict. To cognitively conceptualize the process around the decision to have an abortion, the counselor considers (a) the patient's thoughts and beliefs; (b) the reactions (emotional, social, psychological, and behavioral) associated with the factors that may cause conflict; and (c) the experiences contributing to difficulties the patient may have with making, or committing herself to, a decision. The patient is helped to evaluate and formulate more adaptive responses to the issue and problem solve within the limited boundaries of the service provisions. She is counseled before the procedure, when she has (or returns for) the abortion, and then after the abortion procedure. If the patient requires further counseling, a referral is made and followed up to ensure that an appointment has been made.

Principle 3: *Cognitive counseling sessions focus on reframing the way that patients think about their decision.* In the process, counselors are sensitive to behaviors expressed through irrational beliefs (Ellis, 1962), distorted thinking (A. Beck, 1964), or internal dialogues that inhibit the patient from making an optimal decision for herself (Meichenbaum, 1977, 1986). It must be pointed out that the negative nature of a patient's thinking about the decision does not suggest pathology. A life crisis often results in difficulties in clearly thinking through a problem. Using a variety of tools and techniques the counselor can help to reframe the way in which the patient perceives the problem (A. Beck, 1970). For example, the patient may draw a conclusion in the absence of evidence to support it. Patients who are ambivalent about their decision may believe they know what others are thinking and fail to consider other, reasonable explanations. For instance, a patient may exclaim, "My husband is so mad, he won't talk to me. He won't even discuss what he wants to do about the baby." The counselor can help the patient explore alternative explanations for the husband's response. The counselor may ask her what reasons might make him act that way. Sometimes the patient distorts the situation by focusing on a detail taken out of context. She conceptualizes the entire experience on the basis of this one element, ignoring other, more salient features of the situation. This approach takes the form of rigid thinking. The patient views a situation as either "black or white," rather than on a continuum. Another statement may be, "Because I'm having the abortion, I'm a failure." In labeling themselves or others, or predicting future outcomes, the patient may consider the negative aspects and disqualify or discount the positive ones. The patient may also draw a general conclusion from a single incident—for example, when a patient says, "My mother once said she cannot understand how a person can have an abortion. She'll never forgive me." Finally, the patient can distort the situation by magnifying the negative or minimizing the positive (e.g., "If I don't have this baby, I'll never be a mother."). Even in the limited time available in most clinic counseling sessions, the counselor can help the patient restructure the way in which she has conceptualized the social situation from which the decision about the abortion emerges.

Principle 4: *Patient-centered cognitive abortion counseling focuses on the decision to determine the outcome of the pregnancy.* Emphasis is given to the current problem, and resolution involves a realistic appraisal of the situation that will lead to the solution that is best for the patient. If, within the limits of preabortion counseling, the patient is unable to come to a resolution, the counselor must assist her to obtain more extensive help in resolving the conflict. This may mean family counseling or psychotherapy.

Cognitive counseling is one approach that is particularly effective for short-term clinical encounters with patients. Counseling does not have to be a lengthy, complex psychological intervention. Rather in this chapter we describe an approach for counseling that can be effectively conducted in one or two clinic-length (i.e., 20 to 30 minute) sessions. Women are helped to make and carry out decisions regarding unintended pregnancy and helped to reduce their stress. The counseling relationship is collaborative, and the counselor and patient work together to define problems clearly, delineate alternative solutions, and consider those alternatives (Lewis, 1994).

Highly charged emotional reactions to issues come from deep-rooted core beliefs that influence attitudes, expectations, and assumptions, and, ultimately, direct behavior. The counselor who uses the cognitive approach is interested in the level of thinking that shapes the patient's manifest behaviors—how she "really" conceptualizes the problem of an unintended pregnancy. *Core beliefs* make up the most fundamental level of belief. They are ideal states, and because they develop during early childhood, they usually occur at an unconscious level, guiding a person's thoughts and behaviors. They are global, inflexible, and overgeneralized. For example, a patient's core belief may be that "a women's most important life role is procreation." Core beliefs influence *intermediate beliefs*. Intermediate beliefs take the form of attitudes, rules, and expectations. On the basis of the core belief described above, the patient's *attitude* is "I'm a failure if I don't give birth." The *rules* the patient has established for how she is to behave and the *expectations* she has about how she will be viewed by society emerge from her beliefs. They lead her to believe that she "must fulfill her role as a woman." Her *assumption* is that "if I fulfill my role as a woman, I will be respected." Conversely, if she chooses abortion, she may think "How can anyone respect me? I cannot respect myself." While, in this situation, the patient may say, "It's too much. I can't have another child"; she feels sad because she thinks of herself as a failure, someone who will not be respected by others. It is the counselor's task to conceptualize the patient's concerns in cognitive terms and to reduce her ambivalence about the decision. By listening closely to the latent message in what the patient is saying, the counselor may be able to help her think more clearly about the appropriateness of the rules, expectations, and assumptions she holds.

TECHNIQUES FOR COUNSELING

Patients use a variety of strategies (e.g., projection, repression) to cope with their belief systems. The counselor determines what coping mechanisms the patient has and how she views herself, others, her personal world, and her future. Stresses that contribute to the patient's psychological problems or interfere with her ability to make a decision about her pregnancy, or implement one, are also assessed by the counselor. There are many techniques that can be used by counselors to help the patient through the decision-making and adjustment processes (see J. S. Beck, 1995). We describe several techniques, including reverse role playing and imagery. Within each of these techniques the counselor uses interventions, such as *Socratic questioning* (the process of inquiry to evaluate actions), to facilitate the process. Counselors may also ask patients to suspend reality and act "as if" the present situation were different. A variety of communication skills (e.g., using open-ended questions) can enhance communication between counselor and patient.

Framed collaborative questions (Socratic questioning) are used by the counselor to examine the patient's beliefs in the context of specific situations. This makes the meanings of the beliefs more concrete and less intellectual (J. S. Beck, 1995). Socratic questioning can identify the major issues causing the patient emotional pain. To further clarify the problem, the patient is presented with, and asked to hypothesize about, a critical problem. For example, the counselor might suggest that the patient imagine the "worst case scenario" describing, for example, her boyfriend's reactions to her decision to terminate the pregnancy. Then, the counselor sets up a role play with the patient playing the role of her boyfriend and the counselor playing the patient.

Reverse role play is particularly effective because, first, the counselor has a chance to model for the patient the possible language of, and the approaches to, the interaction. Second, the performance pressure of this counseling strategy is on the counselor, who has to come up with effective responses to the "significant other." Third, the patient gets a sense of what it is like to be on the receiving end of the communication, sometimes realizing that the worst outcome is probably unlikely. Fourth, the patient may come to realize that, in her presence, the significant other is not as powerful as she initially thought. By witnessing how the patient plays the other, the counselor learns important information about the perception of the other person that may inform, and even redefine, the understanding of the problem.

Counselors (A. Beck, 1970), as well as researchers (Mathews, 1971), have known that repeated imaginations of fearful scenes lead to reduced insecurity, anxiety, and fear. *Imagery* is a technique to help patients verbalize and bring to the surface concerns that interfere with their decision making, or cause deep emotional distress. Core beliefs may be experienced as mental pictures or images (A. Beck & Emery, 1985). For example, the patient may think that her mother will tell her she is selfish or evil, and, at the same time, she may envision her mother standing over her scowling and looking angry. The counselor tries to help her to recognize the distressing images and intervene effectively in addressing the emotion that the images conjure (J. S. Beck, 1995). The imagery should be followed through to a logical conclusion. Either the patient will work through the crisis and will feel better or she may imagine the ultimate catastrophe, such as being disowned by her mother. The counselor then explores the meaning of the ultimate catastrophe by the *worse case scenario approach*. The counselor helps the patient to induce a coping image and continues until the patient copes with the problem.

Many women come to reproductive health care clinics with their minds made up to have an abortion. Others have difficulty handling their previously made decision. By applying cognitive techniques during the counseling process, patients can learn how to break down big problems into manageable components. They can then generate alternative responses to their problems. One problem-solving technique that helps a patient come to terms with ambivalence is to ask her to *list the advantages and disadvantages of each choice*. Then the counselor helps the patient weigh each possible choice, drawing a conclusion about which option seems best given her current situation (J. S. Beck, 1995).

Acting as if is a technique that is useful in modifying core beliefs. The patient is asked to suspend judgment and to act as if the situation exists (even though it may not). For example, the patient might be asked to act as if she has the baby (e.g., "What would it be like?"). The question provides her with the opportunity to imagine that choice and, with the counselor's help, confront the reality of the situation. In this way, the counselor can help the patient "counterdistort" her, perhaps, poor assessment of social reality (e.g., the feasibility of having another child at this point in her life).

THE ABORTION PROCESS

This section uses a hypothetical case study to illustrate specific cognitive interventions and techniques that are appropriate at various stages of the abortion process.

The Preabortion Counseling Session

Along with a medical and reproductive health history, including a history of contraceptive use, the patient receives an explanation of tests, and test results. She also receives information on specific choices, the advantages and disadvantages of each choice, and the procedures associated with the abortion options presented. The patient's decisions can involve determining whether to continue the pregnancy to term or whether to keep the baby, to consider adoption or foster care placement, or to have an abortion. The preabortion counseling session should include (a) establishing a working level of trust and rapport, (b) explaining the abortion procedures and counseling process to the patient, (c) identifying the patient's issues, and (d) educating the patient about her decision.

If the patient chooses an abortion, then the counselor (a) explains the steps of the surgical procedure; (b) prepares the patient to manage the physical experience of the procedure; and (c) obtains her informed consent, which includes explaining the risks and complications of the procedure and obtaining a signed and witnessed consent form.

Early in the process, the counselor quickly and specifically sets boundaries of the counseling process. The patient is given an explanation of the rationale and goals of the counseling and how the session will proceed to make the process more understandable to her. By describing the parameters of the session, the counselor focuses the discussion on critical issues and encourages the active participation of the patient in a relatively structured process. In this process, the counselor directs the discussion to issues that are of critical importance to the patient. Next the patient's reasons for her decision are explored. Finally, immediately after the abortion procedure, the counselor can begin a discussion with the patient about past contraceptive use and her plans for future use.

In patient-centered abortion counseling, the working assumption is that informed consent extends beyond the point when the patient signs, and has had witnessed, a consent form. Even if a woman agrees to an abortion, she may, at any time, call that decision to question (either directly or indirectly). If she continues to question her decision, staff should check the patient's commitment to the abortion. Testing the patient's commitment may continue until the point beyond which the physician can no longer stop the abortion process. If the patient continues to vacillate about her decision, additional counseling or referral may be needed.

To demonstrate the concepts and processes of the cognitive approach, a single case example is used throughout the following sections. Although the cognitive approach is applicable regardless of the patient's decision, the illustrations in this chapter are of a woman who chooses to have an abortion.

> The case is of "Sonya," a married 25-year-old who has decided to have an abortion. She has two children and has returned to college to finish her degree. Although she is ambivalent, she also feels that she cannot devote the time or make a financial commitment to a third child. The case study follows her through the process.

> Sonya thinks of herself as a failure because she has decided not to take the pregnancy to term. As a reaction to her thoughts she becomes depressed. Therefore, even though she has decided to terminate her pregnancy, she is ambivalent and has feelings of low self-worth. The contrast between Sonya's words and actions makes it important for the counselor to try to perceive the world as Sonya does. To do this, the counselor listens closely to what Sonya says, accurately summarizes her concerns and identifies how Sonya is conceptualizing the problem at a deeper level. In addition, while being positive and supportive, the counselor also helps Sonya test the reality of her reactions to the situation.

Staff need to have the skill to properly assess the patient's affective state. For example, the patient's statement that she feels sad about having the abortion may reflect an inappropriate decision, but more often it is simply an expression of a normal psychological state that results from the present crisis. If the counselor assesses this to be the case, the patient's feelings can be acknowledged as typical, normal responses. An assessment must also be conducted of whether the patient has been coerced into her decision by significant others in her life. This is particularly important for a minor, whose family and partner may be pressuring her to reach a particular decision.

> Sonya: I am never going to be able to face my parents. They told me that they admire me because I cared so much about children.

> Counselor: Sounds like you think that they won't respect you if you have an abortion?

> Sonya: No they won't. They won't understand how I can do that to a child of mine.

This response gives the counselor a clue that Sonya feels guilty about the decision.

> Counselor: And what do you think?

> Sonya: I don't have a choice but I think I'm awful for what I am doing to my baby. I love children.

> Counselor: A lot of women think that choosing an abortion makes it seem like they don't care about children. I think that women often choose abortion because they care so much about children that they only want to have one when they know they are able to care and provide for a child. What do you think?

The purpose of the counselor's follow-up response is to normalize Sonya's feelings. This case continues below.

> Counselor: What was your partner's reaction to your decision to have an aborton?

> Sonya: He says it's up to me. **OR** I haven't told him because he wouldn't be happy.

> Counselor: Will this be a problem for you after the abortion?

> Sonya: No, not really.

> Counselor: What is the most difficult part for you?

> Sonya: [Cries.]

Sonya's affect has clearly changed, presenting the counselor with an opportunity to probe the emotions that are causing her indecision.

> Counselor: Sonya, how about you play your mother, because you certainly know her better than I do—and I'll play you, since I, at least, know you a little bit—and we'll try to have that conversation in which you tell her

	about the abortion. I'll start by telling you that I'm going to have an abortion.
Counselor as Sonya:	Mom, I've made a difficult decision that I want to tell you about. I've decided not to have this baby. I've decided to have an abortion.
Sonya as mother:	How could you do this to your own baby?
Counselor as Sonya:	I wish I didn't have to do this. I wish I had gone to school when I was younger. But I didn't and I had two children when I was too young, one right after the other, and we can hardly support them now. What would life be for them if we have to share our small . . .
Sonya as mother:	Well, I would have babysat for you, if that's what you are worrying about.
Counselor as Sonya:	This isn't about babysitting. It's about my children and our future. I really need to finish my degree so that I can get a better job. I want a career for myself and a better life for Diana and Iris (her two children). I want to be able to send them to college and I'm so close to getting my degree.
Sonya as mother:	You're selfish, you're just selfish. What's wrong with being a full-time mother, anyway? It was good enough for me.
Counselor as Sonya:	It's just not the life I want. I tried that for all these years and it hasn't worked. I want my children to have a whole person for a mother. And I will probably remember this with sadness for a long, long time, but my children and I—my family—will be better off when I have my degree, a better job, and less stress because we can finally afford to take care of them like they deserve.

By modeling communication in this reverse role play, the counselor helps the patient identify major underlying issues and guides her toward a positive resolution of the conflict. Sonya considers what she wants and differentiates it from what she thinks her mother wants. Role playing the situation may increase her confidence in her decision-making ability. The counselor explores the meaning of the ultimate catastrophe by using the worse case scenario approach.

Counselor:	What would be the worst thing that could happen?
Sonya:	My mother would disown me. (Sonya begins to cry again.)
Counselor:	And then what would you do?
Sonya:	Well . . . I would just have to go on and go to school and finish and get a job. Then I would be able to take care of my family.

In this case, the counselor has helped Sonya induce a coping image and continues until the patient copes with the problem. Notwithstanding, the counselor may have to return to Sonya's fear of abandonment. Using Socratic questioning, the counselor proceeds in the following manner:

Counselor:	You've said that you can't face your parents. How do you picture your parents at the moment you would tell them about the abortion?
Sonya:	What do you mean?
Counselor:	Did you imagine what your parents looked like when you told them?
Sonya:	No, I pictured myself sitting at a table with them and telling them that I had something to tell them and that it was horrible.
Counselor:	And then what?
Sonya:	I saw my mother standing over me, real angry and scowling down at me.
Counselor:	Anything else?
Sonya:	No.
Counselor:	Did you imagine what your mother would look like if you told her your reasons for having an abortion?
Sonya:	No.
Counselor:	Can you imagine that? Can you picture going up to her and telling her? When would you approach her? What would you say . . .
Counselor:	Okay, you are telling me that you think it's terrible to not be able to give birth to another child. And no one will respect you if you don't. Where did that idea come from?
Sonya:	From my mother, who's very religious . . . and the

church ... I go to church ... No contraceptives ... no abortion ... It's murder ...

Counselor: Does everyone think like your mother?

Sonya: No.

Counselor: Who doesn't?

Sonya: My sister Anita.

Counselor: So no one respects her.

Sonya: Oh, no. Everyone thinks Anita is perfect. A perfect wife ... perfect mother ...

Counselor: So she's learned different beliefs.

Sonya: Oh, yes ... I guess ...

Counselor: And your mother? She doesn't respect Anita.

Sonya: Oh she does. She never criticizes her. She always goes to her for advice.

Counselor: Well, the bad news is that your current set of beliefs is causing you a lot of conflict and the good news is that you learned this current set of beliefs and can unlearn it, if you want. How would that feel to you?

Counselor: What is the advantage of believing that you must have as many children as God gives you?

Sonya: I'll be respected ... I'll follow my church's beliefs.

Counselor: So you believe that, if you have as many children as you can, you will be respected.

Sonya: Yes.

Counselor: Well, what are the disadvantages?

Sonya: I won't be able to finish college at least in the forsee-able future. I'm not sure that I can afford another child ... financially. I think the financial part would put a strain on my marriage ...

Counselor: Well you say you won't be respected ... but Anita is, despite the fact that it appears as if she has planned her family ... and you have identified many reasons for limiting the number of children that you have right now. What do you think?

Preparing the Patient for the Procedure

The counselor helps the patient prepare for the physical and psychological experience of the medical procedure. She may begin by exploring the patient's level of fear by asking, "What do you expect to feel?" "What have you heard about the procedure?" This questioning can uncover myths or horror stories, as well as help the patient identify pain-related concerns. Fear of any surgical procedure is normal. Fears regarding an abortion procedure can be compounded by other difficult emotions, such as the fear of retribution from God. Such fears can be reflected in indirect questions. For example, Sonya had an aunt who had an illegal, botched abortion and who died prior to legalization in the United States.

Sonya: Do people die from abortions?

Counselor: I think everybody feels scared when they're about to have any kind of surgery. And often we imagine the worst. When abortion was illegal, women died because it so often could not be performed safely. Today it is a safe procedure. First-trimester abortion as we perform it in this clinic with suction curettage is one of the safest surgical procedures done in this country.

For the patient who is having a first-trimester abortion procedure providing facts often eliminates the fear.

Sonya: Will this hurt the baby?

Counselor: The brain and nervous system of a 12-week-old fetus are not developed enough to feel.

Sonya: What do you do with the baby after the abortion?

The counselor is drawn to Sonya's use of the word *baby*. Although the word can suggest an expression of guilt or regret, the counselor avoids responding on the basis of that assumption. Instead of responding on the basis of an assumption, the counselor asks for clarification.

Counselor: A lot of women ask about that. Can you tell me more about what concerns you?

Sonya: I want to know where they take the baby. I don't want it to be treated as trash.

Although Sonya's concern appears to be that the fetus is dealt with respectfully, other patients have other concerns or wishes. The patient may be asking if it will be used for medical purposes. It may simply be stated that a doctor examines the fetal tissue to make sure that the procedure is complete and nothing is left within the patient's uterus. If that information does not satisfy the patient, then she can be told that the tissue can be used to contribute to research that helps advance medical treatment of diseases, if she wishes.

General Fears About Surgery

Some patients, particularly adolescents, are very anxious about *pain*. An honest acknowledgment about its possibility is required.

> Counselor: I can't promise that you won't feel any pain. I can tell you that the physician and the procedure room assistant will do everything they can to make the procedure as gentle and comfortable as possible. The doctor will give you an injection of anesthesia. She or he will show you how to breathe slowly during the procedure. That will help you relax, and when you relax, it lessens the pain.

By identifying the patient's past method of pain management in other situations and encouraging her to use those techniques, if appropriate (e.g., deep and focused breathing), it reinforces the idea that the patient can manage the pain and have some control over the abortion procedure.

Many patients seem to be more afraid of the cervical *injection* than of the procedure itself. To relieve this kind of anxiety, the counselor describes how the injection might feel and then states that the local anesthetic blocks some of the nerve endings.

> Counselor: There are far fewer nerve endings in the cervix than in the arm or leg so that an injection in the cervix for most women is less painful than, say, a flu shot— you will most likely feel a slight pinch or pressure— something like a pin prick.

Concluding the Counseling Session

The counselor summarizes in two ways throughout the session. The first is a brief restatement when a section of the session has been completed so that both she and the patient have a clear understanding of what they accomplished and what they will do next.

> Counselor: Okay, we've finished discussing how you can relax and we've agreed you will practice the relaxation exercises at home this week [or while waiting today]. I will tell the procedure room assistant to help you through these exercises. Next, is it okay if we go back to something you said about _____?

The second is summarizing the content of what the patient has presented. The key points of the patient's statements are reiterated using her specific words. The summary ensures that the counselor has correctly identified what is most troublesome to the patient and it is presented in a more concise and clear way. The patient's own words are used as much as possible to convey an accurate understanding and to help maintain focus on the key issues.

The final summary also ties together the threads of the session and reinforces important points. A review of the patient's decision is included. The final element of the session is feedback and the establishment of next steps. Here the patient is asked, "What else are you concerned about? What other questions do you have?" This gives her the opportunity to state and then test her decision.

Counseling in the Procedure Room

The physician and the procedure room assistant continue the counseling process as part of their roles in the procedure room. The patient's emotional state is quickly assessed and the staff answer her questions. If the patient has not satisfactorily resolved her feelings about the abortion, those feelings may reemerge soon after the patient meets the physician. At this point, the physician and staff continue the process established by the counselor to build up the patient's confidence in her decision and help her to relax. Sonya's level of fear may be explored by asking her what concerns she has. The physician can address the patient's expressed concerns or further probe the basis of her questions, which may elicit beliefs, attitudes, values, myths, or misinformation. The physician can also identify additional important information that the patient should know.

The reality of being in the procedure room or on the table may cause a patient to reconsider her decision. If it becomes clear that the consent to abort is being called into question, it is not appropriate to try to facilitate a decision-making process while the patient is sitting or lying on the procedure table. The patient should be offered an opportunity to speak with the counselor again. If she declines, the physician may indicate the last point when the abortion procedure can be safely halted. In deciding how to proceed, physicians must trust their instincts and the information provided in pre-procedure counseling. Some patients, who do not want to assume responsibility for their decision, recant in an effort to shift responsibility from themselves to the physician or to the clinic. Under the circumstances, the physician must ask for a clear statement of the patient's intent before proceeding.

Sometimes, immediately before the procedure is to begin, a patient may display an untenable level of ambivalence or sudden and genuine questioning of the choice of abortion. This may, however, be another way of communicating her unmanageable level of fear. For example, when Sonya appeared to be inordinately anxious about pain, the physician provided an honest acknowledgment about the possibility of pain. Although

Sonya may have raised it in the counseling session, she may also want to hear about the pain involved in the procedure from the physician.

> Physician: Different women feel different things. Some feel almost nothing; others say it hurts a lot. Most are somewhere in between. What is true for most patients is that the procedure is very quick. Some feel like they are having sudden strong menstrual cramps. For most women, the cramping subsides shortly after the procedure. We can work together to help alleviate discomfort or pain. I will be administering a local anesthetic that works by blocking some of the nerves in the cervix. It will help reduce the pain. And you can also help to reduce discomfort by using some of the relaxation techniques that you have been practicing.

The presence of, and direct contact with, the procedure room assistant can reassure the patient and help her relax. Specifically, the patient should be queried as to how she has managed pain in other situations. The patient can be encouraged to use relaxation techniques during the procedure. To confirm whether the patient can use the technique, the physician may ask directly.

> Physician: The nurse (or doctor's assistant) is here to support you. She will stay near you throughout the entire procedure. Tell us if there's something you would like us to do to help you relax during the procedure.

> Doctor's assistant: I can hold your hand and talk to you. Whatever makes you most comfortable. Feel free to let me know at any time during the procedure how I can assist you. Please tell me what you are feeling throughout the process.

This is necessary because an inordinate amount of pain might indicate possible complications to the physician. Once the patient is lying on the table, the assistant remains near the patient's head as much as possible throughout the procedure. Dilation is an important time to remind the patient to relax the lower portion of her body. Support for deep breathing is especially helpful at this time, along with reminders about the amount of time needed to dilate the cervix. Patients are often surprised and grateful at how little time the process takes.

Teamwork (the collaboration among physician, doctor's assistant, and the patient) is stressed throughout the procedure. Challenging questions may also be asked by the patient during the procedure.

Sonya: Can I see it?

Physician: I can show you the fetal tissue and, if you like, I'll be glad to answer any questions you have about fetal development.

As the procedure is about the begin, the staff should ask if the patient wants to be informed about the process. Some patients want to be kept informed about what is technically occurring, whereas others do not want to know. For the latter patients, the best strategy may be diversion or distraction. For patients who want to be kept informed, the physician or the assistant can describe the procedure in a way that is appropriate to the patient's level of understanding. For example, while dilating the cervix or evacuating the uterus, the physician might say the following to Sonya:

Physician: We are going to remove the contents of the uterus by gently opening or dilating your cervix and then suctioning your uterus. The cervix is soft and will open with a little pressure. Feeling the pressure means that the cervix is opening and that we are near the end.

The patient should be told approximately how long the procedure takes. Having a sense of the amount of time involved also gives the patient a greater sense of control and makes the anticipated experience feel more manageable. Staff can also mention how many minutes are left for each portion of the procedure.

After the procedure is completed, the physician moves to the head of the table to let the patient know her physical status. A brief touch on the hand or shoulder may offer reassurance that the procedure has been completed safely. Although this may seem obvious—observations at clinics have shown that it is frequently ignored by the physician and staff.

Postprocedure Counseling

In the postabortion session, the counselor discusses the patient's experience with the procedure to reach closure and to move the patient from the abortion itself to reproductive health decisions (e.g., contraceptive use, the necessity of the follow-up visit).

Postabortion counseling can begin here with a discussion both of past and future contraception. Nondirective and if–then statements are particularly helpful in postabortion contraceptive counseling. In this session, the partnership between physician or counselor and patient that was established before and during the procedure can be continued. For example, rather than saying to Sonya, "You have to take your birth control pill every day," say, "If you don't want to get pregnant, then it is important to take your pill every day." This statement reflects the logical consequences of the patient's actions without making judgments or without demanding that she follow staff's orders. Life circumstances can prevent patients from complying with directives, even if they wish to. Thus, the followup is, "What might get in the way of your ability to do that?" The answer may initiate a problem-solving sequence in which the physician or counselor learns about the patient's barriers to contraceptive use. It may lead to a discussion of more appropriate contraceptive methods.

Another example encourages patients to let the physician or counselor know about the constraints that might limit their ability to comply with directives for safe and healthy behavior. Rather than, "Don't have intercourse for the next two weeks—until after you've returned for your postabortion checkup," the counselor may say, "**If** you want to reduce the risk of infection, **then** you will want to avoid sex until after you've returned for your postabortion checkup. How will this work for you? . . . for your partner?"

Rephrasing and following up with open-ended questions shows an awareness that sometimes what is best for the patient may not be within her control. An uncooperative partner may prevent the patient from taking care of herself, regardless of her best intentions. On learning that this is a possibility, the physician might decide to prescribe prophylactic antibiotics. A directive (e.g., "You must . . . You have to . . .") will seldom elicit the disclosure of such circumstances.

SPECIAL ISSUES IN ABORTION COUNSELING

Sexual Abuse, Incest, and Assault

Women who have been raped or abused may be experiencing fear and acute stress (Beresford, 1988). Because the patient had no control in the abusive situation, she is likely to feel extremely vulnerable during the procedure. Therefore, during the abortion procedure, in particular, the patient must have as much control as is possible. To ensure that this happens, the counselor should remain with the patient during the entire procedure and frequently assess her reactions to the process. Staff can acknowledge the difficulty of the procedure and, throughout the procedure, ask the patient how they can be helpful. Prior to the abortion procedure, staff can support the patient by using language such as, "This isn't your fault." "I'm sorry this has happened to you." "It must be hard for you to talk about this. I'm going to do everything I can to help you. I'm glad you told me." "You're brave to do that. Most people who have experienced this feel that they are alone. We are here to help you so that you don't have to be alone with this."

Patients should be given the option of choosing between a male and female physician. If only a male physician is available, then the counselor discusses with the patient her feelings about it. Male physicians must recognize that their gender might make the procedure more difficult for the patient. Before the procedure begins, the patient should be informed about what will happen. During the procedure, the patient should also be informed of changes in touch in advance so that she can anticipate them. Physicians may ask the patient for permission to touch her.

Regardless of the sensitivity of the staff, because of the trauma of the abuse and the abortion experience for someone who has been violated, the patient may have strong emotional reactions to the procedure. Staff must make an effort to prevent "personalizing" the negative reactions of the patient—to remain caring toward the patient. The patient may need follow-up counseling so that she has an opportunity to obtain closure of the situation. Referral to rape or sexual abuse counseling is essential, and local reporting laws will determine any legal action the staff is required to take.

Repeat Unintended Pregnancies

Many women indicate that they did not use contraception because they did not expect to have sex or that the side effects from the contraceptives resulted in inconsistent or discontinued use (Beresford, 1988, Luker, 1976). Sometimes, feelings related to major life changes, depression, loneliness, and anger may cause women to risk pregnancy (J. S. Beck, 1995; Russo & Zierk, 1992).

Women have a variety of responses to choosing an abortion again, ranging from no feelings or mild feelings of regret or disappointment to stronger feelings of guilt, anger, fear, or sadness. It is important to note that circumstances that resulted in a previous abortion, or feelings about it, may differ from current circumstances or feelings. By exploring the current circumstances, staff can help a patient to assess the behavior that led to this current situation.

Repeat unintended pregnancy appears to be one of the most difficult issues for clinicians and counselors (Hern, 1990). Feeling frustrated, reproductive health care professionals may perceive it as their own failure to bring about behavioral change in the patient. Rather than showing frustration or anger, the goal is to help patients become aware of the decisions they make or have made. By inquiring as to how a patient decides whether to use contraception, staff can help make the patient more conscious of her decision making. For example, "If you decide not to use contraception, can you say to yourself, 'This time I choose to risk pregnancy?'" Rather than focusing on failure, counselors may discuss how problems can be solved. Difficulties the patient had with contraception in the past can be explored. The patient is then helped to consider her commitment to fertility control, and the counselor can follow up with questions about making a change in contraceptive use. This intervention is designed to clarify problems the patient may have had with contraception. And when a patient expresses a clear wish or desire to avoid future unintended pregnancy, the counselor may ask the patient how she might do that.

> Counselor: Do you feel ready to make a change in the way you handle this? **OR** What would you need to be ready for a change? When would you like to have a child? **OR** What would you imagine you would do if you had another pregnancy in the coming year? How might you do that?

Patient-centered counseling of women with repeat unintended pregnancies requires a dramatic change in the criteria used to evaluate a successful interaction with a patient. The counselor's role is one that helps to strengthen a patient's ability to act on her decision. The counseling focus must be consciously shifted from trying to prevent another unintended pregnancy and abortion to helping the patient build up her sense of self-worth and self-control. Clinicians can feel successful with patients who have repeat unintended pregnancies when they provide patients with information they need and want, help them work on the problem and make the decision they choose, and reaffirm the acceptability of terminating a pregnancy that is unwanted.

Religious Women

Many of the emotional reactions of women who hold religious beliefs that are opposed to abortion are similar to those of other women (Beresford, 1988, 1991). Sometimes, however, specific sensitivities are required in counseling religious women. For example, a religious woman may intellectualize her decision and block herself from expressing her feelings. If she is not helped to examine her emotions prior to the abortion, afterward she may become depressed.

> Counselor: You've said this seems the right thing to do . . . sometimes what seems right can also feel difficult or frightening or make us anxious . . . Could you tell me a little more about your feelings about this?

> Patient: I just feel awful. In my family, it's like I am committing a sin.

> Counselor: Having those feelings is not unusual. How can you cope with them?

Most women with religious beliefs opposed to abortion are less conflicted about the abortion itself than about sexual behavior; using birth control; being traditional or "feminine;" or being respectful of parents, elders, or religious authorities. Counseling can help women identify the source of their "guilt." Rather than labeling it *guilt*, counselors may reframe it as *regret*.

Although the educated religious woman may use *sin*, *hell*, and *damnation*, or *punishment* in her description of her fears, her decision-making processes may be similar to other women who do not have religious sanctions about abortion. She might be able to say, "Although the church opposes abortion, my life situation makes it absolutely necessary for me to have one." On the other hand, the less educated religious woman may be more dependent on concrete answers and unable to handle ambiguity and uncertainty. Notions of hell, sin, damnation, and punishment may permeate her decision-making process. She may, therefore, need more intensive counseling to help her distinguish between her individual or personal beliefs and formal religious tenets of her faith group. A. Baker and Clark's (1997) counseling material emphasizes the "forgivingness aspect of God" for religious women who feel conflict between spiritual beliefs about abortion and their certainty that abortion is the best decision.

Special Situations and Issues

When a sonogram or postprocedure examination of fetal tissue reveals that the pregnancy was multiple, the patient deserves to have that information. Compassionate health professionals call it a double pregnancy rather than "twins." Similarly, if a pregnancy appears to be threatened (due to bleeding or other physical indications) and it is most likely that the patient would have spontaneously aborted, she should be told (Garrity & Castle, 1996).

CONCLUSION

What are the chief implications of the preceding discussion for women who have unintended pregnancies and for their health care professionals? For physicians, counselors, and procedure room staff who perform abortions in the context of short-term clinical encounters, the cognitive approach to patient-centered abortion care provides a quick assessment of a patient's emotional needs and guides their appropriate response. This allows for the development of trust, rapport, and cooperation. Techniques such as open questioning, role playing, imagery, and relaxation are used to assist patients to problem solve and make decisions. Basic communication skills involve use of paraphrasing, using if–then statements, and reflecting and normalizing the patient's feelings that allow her to examine her present perception of reality.

A cognitive approach can help a patient feel capable of making a decision that is in her best interest and reduce insecurities, anxieties, and fears during the medical procedure. As a result a patient may be more able to relax during the abortion procedure and to cooperate with the medical team throughout the surgery. In turn, the surgery may proceed more quickly and without complications. Patients who confront and resolve the emotional conflicts surrounding their abortion are also less likely to experience postabortion psychological sequelae.

Engaging in a cognitive approach to patient-centered abortion counseling also provides a woman with skills that she can generalize to other decision-making situations. Moreover, relaxation techniques that patients learn can be applied to other stressful medical experiences, for example, during a routine gynecological examination, endometrial biopsy, and so forth (Planned Parenthood of New York City, 1997).

The cognitive approach encourages a patient to take credit for gains and successes and feel stronger when she manages a problem. Physicians and other health care professionals who have used this approach report improvements in ease of performing abortion with local anesthesia and increased levels of patient compliance with postabortion recommendations (e.g., return for follow-up examinations and choice of more effective contraception; Boyd & Halvorson-Boyd, 1986).

Patients' emotions are not evaluated as deviant or behavioral disturbances that must be stopped. By applying a patient-centered approach to counseling abortion patients, reproductive health care professionals help patients make decisions and cope with them. For vulnerable women who may have limited control over their sexual lives such an approach can be empowering as patients learn that they can effectively resolve their problems. Clinicians can help them to view the experience as an opportunity for change and growth.

An important implication of the patient-centered approach is that cognitive theory can conceptualize and integrate clinical and counseling tasks to achieve the full potentialities of a humane, holistic practice of abortion care. That is the perspective that we hope this chapter communicates to those who are responsible for educating the next generation of health care clinicians and counselors.

REFERENCES

Adler, N. E. (1992). Unwanted pregnancy and abortion: Definitional and research issues. *Journal of Social Issues, 248,* 40–49.

Adler, N. E., David, H. P., Major, B. N., Roth, S. H., Russo, N. F., & Wyatt, G. E. (1992). Psychological factors in abortion. *American Psychologist, 47,* 1194–1204.

Atrash, H. K. (1987). Legal abortion mortality in the United States: 1972–1982. *American Journal of Obstetrics and Gynecology, 156,* 605.

Baker, A. (1995). *Abortion and options counseling: A comprehensive reference.* The Hope Clinic for Women, Granite City, IL.

Baker, A., & Clark, A. P. (1997). *Spiritual comfort: Before and after an abortion.* The Hope Clinic for Women, Granite City, IL.

Baker, A., Garrity, J. M., Beresford, T., & Halvorson-Boyd, G. (in press). Counseling, informed consent and patient preparation. In M. Paul et. al. (Eds.), *A clinician's guide to medical and surgical abortion.* New York: Harcourt Brace.

Beck, A. (1964). Thinking and depression: II. Theory and therapy. *Archives of General Psychiatry, 10,* 561–571.

Beck, A. (1970). The role of fantasies in psychotherapy and psychopathology. *Journal of Nervous and Mental Disease, 150,* 3–17.

Beck, A., & Emery, G. (with Greenberg, R.). (1985). *Anxiety disorders and phobias: A cognitive perspective.* New York: Basic Books.

Beck, J. S. (1995). *Cognitive therapy: Basics and beyond.* New York: Guilford Press.

Belsey, E. M. (1977). Predictive factors in emotional response to abortion: King's Termination Study: IV. *Social Science and Medicine, 11(2),* 71–82.

Beresford, T. (1988). *Short term relationship counseling.* Baltimore: Planned Parenthood of Maryland.

Beresford, T. (1991). *Repeat unintended pregnancies.* Unpublished manuscript.

Brashear, D. B. (1973). Abortion counseling. *Family Coordinator, 22,* 429–435.

Boyd, C., & Halvorson-Boyd, G. (1986, April). *Relaxation techniques and guided imagery for pain management.* Paper presented at National Abortion Federation Risk Management Seminar, Washington, DC.

Burnell, G. M., & Norfleet, M. A. (1991). Women's self-reported responses to abortion. *The Journal of Psychology, 121,* 71–76.

Chavkin, W. (1994). Medicine and abortion. *Journal of the American Medical Women's Association, 49,* 130.

Comas-Diaz, L., & Greene, B. (Eds.). (1994). *Women of color: Integrating ethnic and gender identities in psychotherapy.* New York: Guilford Press.

Ellis, A. (1962). *Reason and emotion in psychotherapy.* New York: Lyle Stuart.

Gameau, B. (1993). Termination of pregnancy: Development of a high risk screening and counseling program. *Social Work in Health Care, 18,* 179–191.

Garrity, J. M., & Castle, M. A. (1996). *A physician's guide to patient-centered care: Providing support to women during first-trimester abortion procedures.* New York: Planned Parenthood of New York City.

Gibb, G. D., & Millard, R. J. (1982). Divergent perspective on abortion counseling. *Psychological Reports, 82(3, Pt. 1),* 819–822.

Hern, W. (1990). *Abortion practice.* Philadelphia: J. B. Lippincott.

Hildebrand, J. (1977). Abortion: With particular reference to the developing role of counseling. *British Journal of Social Work, 7,* 3–24.

Johnson, K., & Hoffman, E. (1993). Women's health: Designing and implementing an interdisciplinary specialty. *Women's Health Issues, 3(2),* 115–120.

Kaminsky, B., & Shecter, L. A. (1979). Abortion counseling in a general hospital. *Health & Social Work, 4(2),* 92–103.

Khan-Edrington, M. (1979). Abortion counseling. *Counseling Psychologist, 8,* 37–38.

Lewis, S. Y. (1994). Cognitive–behavioral therapy. In L. Comas-Diaz & B. Greene (Eds.), *Women of color: Integrating ethnic and gender identities in psychotherapy,* (pp. 223–238). New York: Guilford Press.

Loader, B. (1995). Unplanned pregnancies and abortion counseling. *Psychodynamic Counseling, 1,* 363–376.

Luker, K. (1976). *Taking chances: Abortion and the decision not to contracept.* Berkeley: University of California Press.

Major, B., Mueller, P., & Hildebrandt, K. (1985). Attributions, expectations, and coping with abortion. *Journal of Personality and Social Psychology, 48,* 585–599.

Mathews, S. A. (1971). Psychological approach to the investigation of desensitization and related procedures. *Psychological Bulletin, 76,* 83–91.

Meichenbaum, D. (1977). *Cognitive–behavior modification: An integrative approach.* New York: Plenum Press.

Meichenbaum, D. (1986). *Cognitive behavior modification: An integrative approach.* New York: Plenum Press.

Mueller, P., & Major, B. (1989). Self-blame, self-efficacy, and adjustment after abortion. *Journal of Clinical Psychology, 37,* 276–279.

National Abortion Federation. (1998). *Obtaining abortion training: A guide for informed decision making.* Washington, DC: Author.

Ness, M. (1976). An appraisal of abortion counseling. *British Journal of Guidance and Counseling, 4(1),* 79–87.

O'Leary, V. E., & Ichovics, J. R. (1995). Resilience and thriving in response to challenge: An opportunity for a paradigm shift in women's health. *Women's Health: Research on Gender, Behavior, and Policy, 1,* 121–142.

Pinderhughes, E. (1994). Foreword. In L. Comas-Diaz & B. Greene (Eds.), *Women of color: Integrating ethnic and gender identities in psychotherapy* (pp. xi–xiii). New York: Guidford Press.

Planned Parenthood of New York City. (1997). *Clinician training initiative* (Final Evaluation Report). New York: Metis Associates.

Poettegen, H. (1988). The physician's counseling tasks in problem pregnancies. *Praxis der Psychotherapie und Psychosomatik, 33,* 70–76.

Roe v. Wade, 410 U.S. 113 (1973).

Romans-Clarkson, S. E. (1989). Psychological sequelae of induced abortion. *Australian and New Zealand Journal of Psychiatry, 23,* 555–565.

Russo, N., & Zierk, K. (1992). Abortion, childbearing, and women's well-being. *Professional Psychology: Research and Practice, 23,* 269–280.

Scheirer, M. F., & Carver, C. S. (1987). Dispositional optimism and physical well-being: The influence of generalized outcome expectancies on health. *Journal of Personality, 55*, 169–210.

Solomon, L. J., & Rothblum, E. D. (1986). Stress, coping and social support in women. *Behavior Therapist, 9*, 199–204.

Speckhard, A., & Rue, V. (1993). Complicated mourning: Dynamics of impacted post abortion grief [Special issue: Abortion and unwanted pregnancy]. *Pre and Peri-Natal Psychology Journal, 8(1)*, 5–32.

Stanton, A., Danoff-Burg, S., Cameron, C. L., & Ellis, A. P. (1994). Coping through emotion approach: Problems of conceptualization and confounding. *Journal of Personality and Social Psychology, 66*, 350–362.

Westhoff, C., Marks, F., & Rosenfield, A. (1993). Residency training in contraception, sterilization, and abortion. *Obstetrics & Gynecology, 81(2)*, 311–314.

14

ABORTION ISSUES IN PSYCHOTHERAPY

MARIA J. RIVERA

The purpose of this chapter is to investigate the clinical issues related to the abortion experience when women patients enter psychotherapy. Consideration of these issues during psychotherapy is different from abortion counseling, which occurs prior to or immediately after the abortion with the primary focus on abortion decision making and immediate consequences. In the psychotherapeutic setting, the abortion experience is typically viewed retrospectively by both patient and clinician. The psychotherapeutic setting involves a more comprehensive focus in that the woman is often trying to understand her abortion experience and integrate it into her own self-identity, that is, how the experience has influenced her perception of herself. (For further discussion of abortion counseling see Fisher, Castle and Garrity, chap. 13, this volume.)

Because women are under a time constraint when they choose to terminate a pregnancy, clinicians who work in women's mental health are most likely to encounter women after they have undergone an abortion. Clinicians, irrespective of discipline, most often deal with only one aspect of women's abortion experience—the psychological consequences attributed to the procedure. This is an oversight that is often detrimental to the patient in that it neglects the woman's preabortion experience.

As a clinician, it has been my experience that few women regret their decisions to abort. Nonetheless, they often have mixed or ambivalent feelings about the procedure itself, the events that led to the abortion, and reactions subsequent to the procedure. For example, one women referred to her abortion as an "necessary tragedy." Moreover, many women hold mixed feelings about the events that led up to the abortion, the conceptor, the quality of the relationship, and the pregnancy. Some women report feeling that they are being punished. Although in the United States the primary focus has been on the abortion procedure itself, and the ethical issue that it encompasses, abortion is not an isolated event. It is one aspect of a process in which the woman is trying to gain control of an unplanned reproductive outcome, an unintended or unwanted pregnancy. Prior to the abortion the woman is often in a state of crisis, brought on by the unexpected or unwanted pregnancy. Many use the abortion procedure as a last resort, after undergoing a complicated decision-making process. After the procedure, a mixture of sadness and relief is frequently experienced.

When women discuss their abortions, they are not just speaking of the medical procedure; rather they speak of the context that surrounds the medical procedure. It is this context that is composed of events and psychological states both preceding and subsequent to the medical procedure that I refer to as the "abortion experience" (Rivera, 1995). Specifically, the abortion experience consists of three interdependent and possibly overlapping phases: (a) the pregnancy acknowledgment phase, which is when the woman first acknowledges the pregnancy; (b) the pregnancy resolution phase, which involves the decision-making process of deciding to terminate an unintended or unwanted pregnancy; and (c) the postabortion response phase, which includes the emotional aftermath subsequent to the procedure. The phases of the abortion experience are not distinct from one another, nor is their order invariant. For example, many women may have decided to abort should they ever experience an unwanted or unplanned pregnancy. Despite the fact that women may undergo the phases at different times, the components of the process remain the same. My primary proposition is that during psychotherapy the abortion experience should be explored fully through consideration of all three phases.

THE PHASES OF THE ABORTION EXPERIENCE

Pregnancy Acknowledgment Phase

This phase is defined as the time period during which women think about their pregnancy but have yet to consider a specific pregnancy resolution decision. Specifically, it refers to the period between the point at which a woman first perceives herself to be pregnant up to the point at which she begins the decision-making process to have the abortion, or to pursuing the abortion procedure. In this process of acknowledging the pregnancy, women will evaluate their motivation to become a mother, examine pregnancy attribution, and consider how "intended" and "wanted" the pregnancy is.

During this period women often will evaluate their own ability to mother and raise a child. Most women, when they find out that they are pregnant, think about the prospective notion of a baby and the notion of raising a child. Most women who undergo an abortion think of their future in terms of the ability to raise that child. For many women, a primary reason for undergoing an abortion is the feeling that an infant or child has the right to be wanted and loved and the realization that their current circumstances do not allow this (Burnell & Norfleet, 1987). In other words, their maternal motivation is operating, despite their choice to terminate the pregnancy.

The acknowledgment that one is pregnant also includes the attributions that a woman makes about how and why the pregnancy came about: due to her own behavior, her partner's behavior, bad luck, the situation, or even something about her character (Major, Mueller, & Hildebrandt, 1985). This allows the woman to assign "blame" to what or who specifically caused the pregnancy.

In therapy women often bring up the issue of whether they may have gotten pregnant on purpose. Some women suggest that they may have unconsciously planned to become pregnant. While in therapy women will attempt to recall and evaluate those psychological states and behaviors that occurred prior to the conception that support such a possibility. Because women generally have the majority of reproductive responsibility, including contraception, the possibility of an unconscious intention of conceiving appears reasonable. Their male partners often support this idea by suggesting that the woman "got pregnant on purpose." Pines (1990) and Loader (1995) contend that motivations and goals other than motherhood may lead to a pregnancy. Pregnancy is often seen as a validation of one's femininity, maturity, and sexuality. Many women have reported in therapy that the unintended pregnancy confirms their fertility, allowing the women some relief in knowing that they can in fact conceive.

Miller (1980a) explains that the "intendedness" of a pregnancy occurs prior to conception and is defined by the degree that a woman or a couple plans to get or not get pregnant. The intention to get pregnant consists of behavioral acts and feeling states that correspond to either the achievement or prevention of conception. In his research Miller identified seven levels of intention ranging from *conception fully intended* through *ambivalent intention* and *subintention* to *conception not intended*. Miller described ambivalence with respect to intention as "when the individual has sufficiently strong doubt and counter-motivation that the strength of intention varies considerably over time" (p. 1).

Subintention is defined as when an individual has little or no subjective experience of intention, but their beliefs and feelings suggest an acceptance of and even an interest in the event, and their behavior exposes them to a considerably increased risk of pregnancy.

In contrast to the intendedness of pregnancy, according to Miller (1980a) the "wantedness" of the pregnancy occurs after conception and is defined as the degree to which the pregnancy or child is wanted or unwanted. Specifically, it refers to the psychological states involving how a woman feels about and responds to an already identified pregnancy. Incorporated into those states is the partner's feelings, as many women consider their partner's feelings in order to further determine their own feelings of wantedness toward the pregnancy. Miller refers to five levels of the wantedness of the pregnancy or child ranging from "active desire" through "passive acceptance" to "actively unwanted or rejected."

Therapists should investigate the levels of intendedness and wantedness of a pregnancy when a patient raises the issue of abortion. It is helpful for the patient to understand the difference between intendedness and wantedness. An understanding and acceptance of the fluctuation and incongruency of intendedness and wantedness may help to alleviate the ambivalence that a woman may hold with respect to the abortion experience and decrease the blame and guilt that she may experience subsequent to the procedure.

Therapists may assume that because a woman has had an abortion she did not intend to get pregnant or want the pregnancy, that is, they see the levels of intendedness and wantedness as concrete and dichotomous. This is rarely the case, because (as discussed in the next section) most women will evaluate their pregnancy and the context surrounding the pregnancy to determine a pregnancy resolution. This evaluation will include questioning their level of intention and desire for the pregnancy and their level of maternal motivation. Because women rarely talk with others about a terminated pregnancy, asking patients to discuss their evaluation of the pregnancy will often clarify the abortion experience for them. A patient may need to distinguish current levels of intention to get pregnant with intentions for future pregnancies. Some women may need to explore the fact that intention to become pregnant is very different from wanting to raise a child. Asking a woman to describe the positive emotions she felt once learning of her pregnancy will help to explore issues related to intention.

When exploring the issue of wantedness in psychotherapy, attention should be paid to the different levels of wantedness. A patient may experience several levels of wantedness during the course of a pregnancy. The fluctuation in the levels must be validated so that it is perceived as a part of the normal abortion experience. Many women who choose abortion report feelings of ambivalence and want the pregnancy to some degree but feel that their life circumstances prohibit them from maintaining the pregnancy. These women also report feeling guilty because their reasoning and subsequent decision may appear selfish to others. The therapist needs to help the patient understand the relationship between her well-being and the quality of her parenting. Rearing a child under uncertain conditions will greatly affect the well-being of the child. The therapist can reframe the patient's guilt-laden thinking by pointing out that the woman acted responsibly and in the best interest of the potential child. The therapist should point out that the patient's awareness of her own limitations as a parent is an issue that most women entertain at some point during pregnancy. The fact that the woman determined that her limitations were too great to continue the pregnancy is a decision that incorporated the well-being of a child. This reframing allows the woman to recognize that the abortion was performed with the potential child's best interest at heart, and will decrease the level of guilt and other negative feelings.

Even women who report that they did not intend to become pregnant, nor want the pregnancy may experience some sense of guilt. This is due primarily to cultural prescriptions that the predominant role for women is childbearing and rearing. Some women experience anger, discomfort, guilt, and confusion because they have made a personal decision that they believe to be correct for them yet contradicts prevailing social mores. These women may report questioning their womanhood because they have chosen to contradict social norms.

Dovetailing the issue of the wantedness of a pregnancy is the issue of how adaptive the woman is to the new pregnancy. To some degree, most women when pregnant are aware of how a new child will impact their personal lives. Women will then evaluate and interpret for themselves what Miller (1980a) refers to as "maternal motivation." This can be defined as a process whereby a woman will evaluate the negative and positive aspects of mothering (e.g., losing income or personal time, knowing one is fertile, or becoming aware of changes in physical body). Such an evaluation process helps a woman understand the degree to which maternity and mothering will impact her life, and if she believes she is able to tolerate this impact she will accept the mothering role. For example, many students choose to terminate a pregnancy despite wanting a baby because they would prefer not to halt their studies. They see their education as a way of improving their lifestyle, and the lifestyle they expect for their future children (Rivera, 1995). As stated above, therapists can reframe any negative feelings that occur by pointing out that the woman was acting in the best interest of a "potential child."

Pregnancy Resolution Phase

This phase of the abortion experience consists of the time period from the moment a woman begins to actively consider abortion as an option to the final determination that abortion is the best solution to the unwanted pregnancy. Many clinicians assume that when a women enters therapy with abortion as an issue, she is experiencing either regret or ambivalence about her decision. This is not necessarily true. In my professional experience, most women are satisfied with their decision to abort, yet continue to experience guilt or ambivalence. Professionals should address this guilt and ambivalence by exploring the decision process itself, specifically those factors that the patient weighed in making her decision. Women often are able to understand their decisions more clearly through such exploration and thus can accept ambivalence and guilt as an aftermath of the normal decision-making process. Clinicians must acknowledge that many clients will believe that abortion is not a "good" decision or first choice; rather, they view it as the last choice in a moment of an unwanted crisis. For example, one of my patients described her decision-making process as "murder in self-defense." She explained that she felt she was in the position of having to defend herself, and she chose abortion only after investigating all the other alternatives.

Most therapists have had some training in theories of decision making. Classical decision-making theory is derived from economics and based on mathematical models that consider gains, losses, and probabilities, which yield monetary values (Bourne, Dominowski, Roger, Loftus, & Healy, 1986). The expected-utility model of decision making has dominated. In its simplest form, the value of each alternative is multiplied by the probability of that alternative occurring. The model has been modified in order to extend its cost–benefit approach beyond the economic utility of a decision. In such modifications, each alternative is evaluated by weighing its levels of pleasure or pain (i.e., perceived benefit or cost).

Abortion is often decided when a women is in crisis, yet the use of traditional models of decision making (i.e., cost–benefit analysis) when exploring the pregnancy resolution phase is overly narrow. Therapists would do better to examine pregnancy resolution within the larger context of the women's reproductive history. Questions should be asked about other pregnancies and their outcomes, and the circumstances surrounding these pregnancies. Specifically, the patient should be asked about the decision-making process, her contraceptive behavior, and prior abortions to see if any patterns exist.

Contraceptive Decision Making

The link between contraceptive choice and abortion is evident, as the latter often results from a problem with the former. In addition, attitudes and use of contraception are positively correlated with attitudes and use of abortion (Faria, Barrett, & Goodman, 1985). Although Campbell (1990) found that as the number of abortions increased for a woman, so did the probability her using contraception. Tsoi, Tay, and Ratnam (1987) and Jacobsson, von Schoultz, and Solheim (1976) reported that repeat aborters and multiple aborters were more likely to use less reliable methods of contraception than initial aborters. They also were less consistent in their regulation of those methods, despite their greater knowledge about contraception.

Because there is limited knowledge about the connection between contraceptive behavior and abortion, therapists must explore this link with caution. The therapist may be able to point out patient risk-taking behavior that increases chances for an unintended pregnancy. For example, if a woman has the financial resources and is physically able to use oral contraceptives, yet reports using a less reliable method on an intermittent basis, the therapist may want to explore the motives for the patient's decision to use the less reliable method, while taking care not to blame her for past contraceptive behavior. Many therapists see contraception as the sole responsibility of the woman, and this may be conveyed during the course of treatment. Therapists must acknowledge that contraception is a much more complicated issue due to the woman's social context, rather than just a woman's responsibility.

DECISION MAKING IN ABORTION

There are only three available choices for a woman who has an unwanted pregnancy: continue the pregnancy with impending adoption, continue the pregnancy and keep the child, or elective abortion. Many variables affect a woman's decision to have an abortion. Public acceptability, barriers to service access, and the role and status of women within a culture are a few of the macrosystems that may influence her decision (Rivera, 1995). In addition, the mixed messages that a woman may receive from her sociocultural environment will reinforce any ambivalence that she experiences (Lemkau, 1988). The reasons her culture considers acceptable for abortion also influence her decision. For example, in many cultures abortion is deemed acceptable only if a woman is raped, carrying full term is dangerous to the woman's health, or there is a strong likelihood of genetic or congenital defects in the fetus (Kenyon, 1986; Lemkau, 1988; Westoff & Ryder, 1977). Individual level variables that may contribute to a woman's decision include career, marital and financial status, religiosity, quality of relationship, family size, age, concept of physical and psychological pain, length of gestation, personal definition of life and its inception, and fetal viability and attitudes about abortion (Aguirre, 1980; Berger, Gold,   Andres,

Gillett, & Kinch, 1984; Biasco & Piotrowski, 1989; Callan, 1983; Faria et al., 1985; Kenyon, 1986; Osofsky & Osofsky, 1972; Turell, Armsworth, & Gaa, 1990).

Although a woman's belief about abortion will contribute to her decision, her belief does not have to be congruent with her personal decision to abort should she face an unwanted or unintended pregnancy. My own research (Rivera, 1995) found that women who chose to abort held some negative opinions about abortion on the moral level yet felt their decision was necessary and the right one. Therapists may want to explore the woman's ambivalence regarding the procedure, the vacillation in their feelings during the decision process, and their coping strategies under such conditions.

PARTNER'S AND OTHERS' INVOLVEMENT IN THE DECISION TO ABORT

Reproductive events such as childbearing and contraception are primarily a woman's responsibility and burden in our culture. It can be argued, however, that her decision may reflect not only her own desires about the pregnancy but also those of her partner and others such as parents. Often the decision to abort is not made in isolation, rather it is determined within the context of an intimate relationship, or with significant input from a group of friends or family members. Most women discuss their decision with someone, usually the partner, mother, friend or possibly their physician (Faria et al., 1985; Marsiglio & Menaghan, 1990). One could therefore assume that the discussion, partner's (or others') opinions, and quality of the relationship impact the woman's personal pregnancy resolution.

Miller (1980b) points out that a woman's wantedness of pregnancy is often influenced by her partner's wantedness of the pregnancy. He suggested that ambivalence in pregnancy intentions often results when another person essential to the decision is opposed to the woman's decision. Peppers (1987) suggested that if a woman has a strong external locus of control, thereby being more influenced by her partner's attitude, she may be more subject to high ambivalence. Such ambivalence can lead to social isolation and limit the influence and social support of others (Peppers, 1987). Other research (Adler, 1992; Turell et al., 1990) also supports the finding that pregnancy ambivalence is related to a greater reliance on partner influence and the decision to abort.

Little is understood about how the quality and dynamics of the relationship with the partner may influence a woman's decision. Despite this, it has been found that the male partner has a large role in shaping the pregnancy resolution, especially if the relationship is ongoing (Marsiglio & Menaghan, 1990; Stone-Joy, 1985). Turell et al. (1990) note that if the relationship is a casual one, women find the decision to abort much easier. In a comparative study of younger and older women undergoing abortions, Campbell (1988) found older women were more coerced by their partners to abort. Both groups were more aware of their parents' marital problems, and reported a more chaotic personal life than nonaborters. One could conclude that these women are aware of their environments and fear raising a child in a similar environment, or that the abortion itself is traumatic to the relationship.

While research, although limited, has demonstrated that men do have an impact on the reproductive decisions that women make, many women choose to deny or are unaware of that influence (Wilson, 1986). In my own interviews (Rivera, 1995), I found that women would often adamantly declare that their partners were not influential in the decision-making process. Yet during the course of the interview, women would describe how they would evaluate the quality of the relationship or the partner's attitude toward the pregnancy. The women would then describe how this evaluation was used in their decision to abort. It became evident that the partners of these women were influential in the decision-making process either directly or indirectly.

Whereas some women do make the pregnancy resolution decision in isolation, most women utilize outside resources in order to come to their decision. Partner influence, whether direct or indirect, is typical of the decision-making process. Therapists must also acknowledge that partners, family members, and others may have been important resources for the patient during her decision making. It would benefit the patient who consulted with significant others during this process to understand that this is a normal and frequently beneficial coping strategy during a stressful situation. Therapists, with the patient's permission, may want to invite significant others into the psychotherapy (Trad, 1995).

As explained earlier, traditional theories of decision making may prove to be inapplicable when exploring the pregnancy resolution process with women. These traditional theories evolved in a culture that praises individuality and independence. Hence, the traditional theories do not allow or even approve of outside influences. These theories are congruent with the views of many therapists trained in the United States who value the notion of independent decision making. However, such theories may not be appropriate for women, who tend to think in terms of social connection and incorporating the opinion of others.

Sociocognition theory may give greater insight into how women incorporate the assistance of others, specifically their partners in the pregnancy resolution process. The initial individual decision-making process, according to sociocognition theorists, consists of the individual attempting to make sense of social events by pooling information from their social context in order to execute their decision (Hastie & Pennington, 1991).

In the context of pregnancy this means that the quality of the relationship with the conceptor, her family, income, and her career serve as the social context surrounding the woman. These authors suggest that the individual will develop several narrative stories on the basis of the pooled information she has collected. In essence these narratives will represent all of the possible outcomes. Eventually she will settle on one overall narrative story or outcome, which will then influence and hence become her final decision. If alone, individuals will reason in a similar fashion by creating narratives that would be congruent with the opinions of significant others who would support their decision. In this form of decision making, individuals are thinking in reference to the social context of which they are a part.

Therapists need to acknowledge the social context of relationships; even if the relationship with the conceptor was discontinued after the confirmed pregnancy, it still serves as a social context. It should also be understood that some women are more likely to rely on their partner's decision, especially if they are experiencing some ambivalence during the crisis of an unwanted pregnancy.

A therapist must balance the two types of decision making (individual and relational decision making) when discussing the abortion resolution with a patient. Therapists would be wise to acknowledge and explore outside influences in the decision-making process, assessing how direct or indirect these outside influences are. Indeed many women report that they discontinued the relationship with the conceptor. What was the cause and the effect of the termination of that relationship? It may be profitable to look at the magnitude of outside influence in relation to the patient's own preference to determine whether there is an overreliance on others. If this is the case, the therapist can examine why the patient has difficulty trusting her own judgment in decision making. Clinicians need to explore the patient's relationship with the conceptor, regardless of quality and length. How does the patient feel about the partner's input in the decision-making process? Was the input direct or indirect? Was the couple in agreement in their decision, or did each want a different resolution? Of particular importance is how the abortion issue was resolved in the relationship if the woman is still with the conceptor at the time of treatment.

POSTABORTION RESPONSE

Postabortion response refers to the emotional aftermath of the abortion. Whether a psychological reaction process exists subsequent to an abortion is under much debate. This debate is influenced by the political climate surrounding the procedure's acceptance (Wilmoth, 1992). Some researchers may seek out evidence to support their personal beliefs about abortion, suggesting either minimal reactions or a psychiatric disorder occurring as a result of an abortion. The same political climate will also affect the emotional response following the abortion; a woman's reaction cannot be separated from the influence of the cultural climate in which the abortion takes place (Turell et al., 1990).

Despite the politicized nature of some abortion research, consistent results have been reported in some areas. The psychological reactions following an abortion are influenced by a woman's cultural and religious beliefs, the social and political stigma encompassing abortion, and beliefs surrounding the inception of life (Adler, 1992; Biasco & Piotrowski, 1989; Conklin & O'Connor, 1995; Corsaro & Korzeniowsky, 1983; Kenyon, 1986; Olley, 1971; McGraw, 1989; Peppers, 1987; Tentoni, 1995; Turell et al., 1990). On an individual level, the length of gestation, other current stressors in a woman's life, self-efficacy, emotional expressiveness, and perceived social support impact postabortion adjustment, especially given the cultural sanctions against abortion and pregnancy outside of marriage (Gonda & Ruark, 1984; Major et al., 1990; Olley, 1971; Wilmoth, 1992). A woman's parity also affects her response to abortion. Turell et al. (1990) found that women with children tend to cope better following an abortion than nulliparous women. In addition, the intendedness and wantedness of the pregnancy impact upon the subsequent psychological reaction (Adler, 1992).

In addition to the political influences, beliefs about postabortion responses are influenced by the medical profession. Most women have a first-trimester abortion on an outpatient basis or in a free-standing clinic, performed by a physician who probably does not know the patient and is not trained to diagnose psychological problems. Thus, the physician is unlikely to refer her to counseling (Stotland, 1985). Women who experience the greatest degree of psychological discomfort following an abortion are more likely to use psychological services, and gynecologists are more likely to refer those women with the most obvious and severe symptoms.

POSTABORTION REACTION

Some researchers believe that postabortion reaction may present itself years later and last for several years (Speckhard & Rue, 1992). Most research, however, indicates that the common negative effects and anxiety either occur before the procedure or are short-term consequences (Adler et al., 1990), and have little impact on overall psychological functioning (Robbins, 1979). Hence, postabortion reaction is typical of the normal stress and coping that one may experience in response to a stressful event (Adler et al., 1992). Speckhard and Rue (1992) proposed that what is defined as postabortion reaction is the normal response to abortion and not indicative of pathology. These authors further suggest that it is the politicization of abortion that has led to the pathological inferences rather than the recognition of what may be a normal reaction.

Most researchers agree, however, that some women experience significant negative psychopathological consequences following an abortion (Wilmoth, 1992), although there is disagreement about severity, symptomatology, time of presentation, and duration of such postabortion responses. Also under debate is what places a woman at risk for more severe pathological reactions: the abortion itself, the context surrounding the abortion, or a history of individual psychopathology. Pathological postabortion reactions are discussed more fully under postabortion syndrome.

Symptoms of postabortion reaction are typically described as mild feelings of depression (Hafez, 1984; Kenyon, 1986). McGraw (1989) stated that up to 50% of women undergoing abortion will experience some short-term depression and guilt. The general discomfort of postabortion reaction often stems from three possible areas regarding the abortion experience; (a) physical complaints and emotional stress of the pregnancy and abortion, (b) perception of loss resulting from the abortion, and (c) a role conflict resulting from the perceived conflict surrounding the abortion decision (Speckhard & Rue, 1992).

The normal postabortion reaction often includes contradictory emotions. Adler (1975) noted that it is quite possible to feel a multitude of feelings, including those that oppose each other such as regret and happiness. Burnell and Norfleet (1987), in a retrospective study, found that 50% of the women had mixed feelings of guilt, relief, confusion, and satisfaction, perhaps because the abortion served as both a coping strategy in response to an unwanted pregnancy and a stressor (Speckhard & Rue, 1992). Turell et al. (1990) reported that feelings of depression and anxiety were lower after than prior to the procedure. Both Lemkau (1988) and Adler (1975) divided the normal negative emotional reactions following an abortion into those internally based (regret, anxiety, depression, doubt, and anger) and socially based (shame, guilt, and fear of disapproval).

Positive Effects

Several researchers describe a positive psychological experience and sense of relief that occurs as part of the postabortion reaction (Adler et al., 1990; Burnell & Norfleet, 1987; Hafez, 1984; Horobin, 1973; Lemkau, 1988; Osofsky & Osofsky, 1972; Turell et al., 1990). Neubardt and Schulman (1977) found that most women feel a sense of relief and emotional "washout" (p. 41) after the procedure, primarily due to the heightened anxiety prior to the decision, and over the pending procedure. These positive reactions are more probable if the pregnancy was both unintended and unwanted (Adler, 1992). Adler (1975) reported that time since the abortion is an important factor. She found that the mild to moderate feelings of guilt and regret more often occurred immediately after the procedure, and feelings of happiness and satisfaction with the decision to abort increased over time. Ninety-eight percent of the women in the Osofsky and Osofsky (1972) sample said they would undergo the procedure again rather than go through an unwanted pregnancy. Horobin (1973) found more distress among women who were denied the procedure and carried the pregnancy to term. Finally, Najman, Morrison, Williams, Andersen, and Keeping (1991) questioned mothers 6 months after they were denied an abortion. When compared to women who had an abortion, those women who were denied the procedure had higher rates of anxiety and depression.

The above research demonstrates that most women are eventually content with their decisions to abort. These positive feelings need to be acknowledged and encouraged. Therapists should point out to the patient that these feelings of acceptance and relief are the end result of a very difficult process. For women who feel guilty a therapist should explore how the woman's decision may benefit her future children and the courage it took to acknowledge that they were unable to rear a child at the present time.

Postabortion Syndrome

Many researchers investigating postabortion responses look for prescribed severe psychiatric sequelae rather than symptoms of self-reported distress. This possibly is because, historically, prior to the 1973 Supreme Court decision (*Roe v. Wade*, 1973) women needed a psychiatric reason in order to undergo what was then defined as a therapeutic abortion (Stotland, 1985). Also, Freudian theorists believed that a "denial of a pregnancy would be unnatural thus resulting in severe trauma" (Turell et al., 1990, p. 49).

The literature reports conflicting findings about the psychiatric sequelae resulting from an abortion. As early as 1954 (Litz, 1954 cited in Simon & Senturia, 1966; Rosen, 1954), a postabortion syndrome was described. Its symptoms included opposing feelings such as guilt and relief; depression; feeling out of contact, especially with the feminine role and its relationship to motherhood; and an unconscious sense of guilt. Hern (1984) further expanded this description and identified several postabortion mental health problems: prolonged depression, functional incapacity, denial of procedure, sexual dysfunction, or postabortion psychosis.

PAS was suggested as a possible *Diagnostic and Statistical Manual of Mental Disorders* (3rd ed., rev.; American Psychiatric Association, 1992) psychiatric diagnosis by those against abortion (Wilmoth, 1992). The prevalence of psychiatric symptomatology varies depending on when the research was conducted and the symptoms being described. Early research indicates a much higher incidence of depression, 25% (Rovinsky, 1972). More recent evidence suggests a 2.4% occurrence of psychotic reactions, and a 1%–2% occurrence of major depression (Kenyon, 1986, p. 188). McGraw (1989) reported a 5% incidence of severe psychiatric disturbance. The consensus amongst researchers is that if the woman had psychiatric or psychological problems prior to the abortion then her postabortion psychological symptoms tend to be greater (Adler, 1975; Dagg, 1991; Jacobsson et al., 1976; Kenyon, 1986; McGraw, 1989).

Presently, research on PAS-type symptoms uses the diagnosis of posttraumatic stress disorder as the operationalization of PAS (Bagarozzi, 1994; Gannon, 1994; Speckhard & Rue, 1992). This is primarily because PAS is not recognized as a disorder within the psychiatric community (Wilmoth, 1992). Symptoms include the perception of the abortion as traumatic, reexperiencing aspects of the abortion (in the form of flashbacks or nightmares), grief and anniversary reactions, avoidance or denial of the abortion, and symptoms of guilt not present prior to the abortion (Speckhard & Rue, 1992).

The Effect of the Conceptor on Women's Postabortion Responses

Little is understood about the impact of the partner or the dynamics of the relationship with the conceptor on women's postabortion responses. Turell et al. (1990) and Dagg (1991) found that women who maintained a strong relationship with their partners were more likely to experience regret over the abortion 1 year later. Contrary to this, McGraw (1989) felt that a woman would experience more problems if her relationship with her partner were unstable, or if she lacked general social support. Aguirre (1980) suggested that because many women aborted as a result of their unmarried status, this relationship was worthy of further investigation.

A common postabortion phenomenon is ambivalence toward the relationship that produced the pregnancy, often resulting in termination of the relationship (Bracken, Hachamovitch, & Grossman, 1972; Francke, 1978). Simon and Senturia (1966) and Stone-Joy (1985) found many women reported mixed emotions or dislike for the conceptor after their abortion. Prior to the procedure, they believed that they loved the man. Further analysis revealed that of those women who reported mixed emotions, approximately half soon ended their relationship. Moreover, women who felt guilty about their abortion, often felt that their relationship would have continued had they maintained the pregnancy (Stone-Joy, 1985). In addition, many repeat aborters see their own fathers as magical (Fisher, 1986). A psychodynamic explanation as to why sexual relationships tend to dissipate after an abortion is that in some cases the partner may be associated with the magical father. Because the woman feels ambivalent and disappointed about the conceptor, he then loses his status of the magical father as a result of the abortion.

The conceptor's view of the impending abortion and his capacity to support his partner will impact the woman's emotional response to the procedure. Major et al. (1990) found that women adjusted better if they simply perceived their partner as supportive as opposed to those who told their partner about the procedure and the partner was unsupportive. In addition, there is evidence to indicate that the more conflict a woman has with the conceptor surrounding the abortion the more angry and depressed the woman is after the procedure (Turell et al., 1990). Dagg (1991), however, found women who told their partners about the procedure had a worse adjustment than those women who chose not to tell anyone. On the other hand, other researchers report a more severe grief response among women who did not discuss or involve anyone in their abortion experience (Kenyon, 1986; Stone-Joy, 1985).

MOURNING AFTER AN ELECTIVE ABORTION

Grieving is a normal response to any loss (Berson, 1988). Grief refers to the sudden acute state that is composed of somatic symptoms, preoccupation with the deceased, guilt, hostility, and possible erratic behavior. Mourning occurs later and is the more prolonged stage of the grieving process. The mourning stage is the initial step of the healing process that serves as a way of obtaining closure and facilitates the person's return to normal functioning. Regardless of its voluntary status, abortion can still be viewed as a loss followed by a grief reaction as presented in some of the literature (Peppers, 1987; Speckhard & Rue, 1992; Stone-Joy, 1985). The patient may be mourning not only the loss of a potential child but also the potential role of motherhood. This may be especially true if the level of maternal motivation for the pregnancy was high.

Little investigation has been done with regard to the emotional response of loss and mourning after a elective abortion. Gonda and Ruark (1984) discussed the notion of anticipatory grief in terminally ill patients, stating that once the involved individuals are aware of the terminal nature of the illness a mourning process has already begun on the unconscious level. These authors assert that the anticipation itself allows for more successful coping. I believe that this anticipatory mourning might also be occurring for women who have decided to terminate their pregnancies. Once they have made the decision to abort, women will begin a process of letting go, as the abortion is viewed as an anticipated albeit necessary loss. Evidence for this belief is found in the work of Peppers (1987), who found that women grieved both before and after their abortions. The grief related to abortion was very similar to grief as a result of involuntary loss.

The women in his study showed a greater amount of grief just prior to the procedure. He concluded that grieving began when the decision to abort was made, not at the time of the actual procedure, and women who grieved recognized their pregnancies as a fetus and a potential child.

Maternal bonding begins in the prenatal period (Peppers, 1987). One would suspect that if the woman wants the pregnancy in any way (reflected in the level of ambivalence), she may in fact experience a loss when she aborts the pregnancy. The loss is experienced because the bonding is cut short. Peppers (1987) noted that we acknowledge maternal bonding and the resulting maternal grief in the cases of miscarriage, stillbirth, and sudden infant death syndrome, but we do not acknowledge maternal bonding and grief with respect to a voluntary abortion.

It has been my experience as a psychotherapist that women who have aborted report a full array of emotions. They report feeling relieved that the pregnancy and procedure are over, yet they often report feeling sad about "what might have been." The ambivalence seems very disquieting and is a common complaint expressed during therapy. It is this very range of emotions and ambivalence that brought these women into psychotherapy. The acknowledgment and analysis of this ambivalence in the postabortion response is crucial for the woman to fully integrate her abortion experience.

Many women who terminate a pregnancy do feel some sense of loss. Yet the idea that women who have aborted experience maternal grief is prohibited, due to the covert notion that aborters are selfish because they consider their own well-being before that of the potential child's. The therapist can use a paradoxical intervention and reframe the sadness of the postabortion response as maternal grief. The woman had the "maternal instinct" to protect her potential child or future children by not continuing the pregnancy. Often, people will try to avoid the discomfort of the grief stage by not talking about the deceased, which will inhibit the bereavement process (Berson, 1988). Corsaro and Korzeniowsky (1983) suggested that if women continue to feel depressed after an abortion they should mourn the loss by using a self-selected ritual. They point out that Japan has a funeral service for the deceased fetus. McAll and Wilson (1987) used a communion procedure in their study of mourning after an abortion. They found that most of their patients' psychological and psychosomatic symptoms halted after the ritual. Interestingly, American culture sanctions mourning rituals for those who have undergone spontaneous abortion, but this has not been instituted for those who have undergone voluntary or therapeutic abortions.

The possibility of a delayed emotional response occurring years later is also suggested (Speckhard & Rue, 1992; McGraw, 1989; Stone-Joy, 1985). Kenyon (1986) noted that a reactive depression may manifest itself during the "birthday" of the child, or the "anniversary" date of the abortion. Stone-Joy (1985) found that many women who report symptoms of depression are actually experiencing a delayed and unresolved grief reaction. These women tend to come in for psychological treatment around the time the baby would have been born.

It is important for the therapist to identify any delayed or unresolved grief issues. Therapists should allow the treatment to serve as the sanctioned mourning by offering the treatment room as the place where the patient can explore her feelings of loss. The therapist can suggest that the patient create a private ritual for herself, acknowledging her mourning. There are several ways of determining the level and phase of mourning. If the intendedness and wantedness of the pregnancy both are positive or high, or if they are incongruent, the patient may experience severe mourning. If vacillation and ambivalence during the pregnancy acknowledgment and pregnancy resolution phases were high, the therapist also should examine the possibility of mourning. This may be a good point to bring the partner into the therapy session, especially if there was some disagreement about the decision. The couple may be able to unite in the mourning phase or in the mourning ritual.

THE GUILT

Clinicians should remind patients that the feelings of guilt are part of the postabortion response. This guilt may not be readily apparent to clinicians. It has been my experience that many women have learned that initially it is socially acceptable to speak assertively of their abortions when they are in treatment. This serves as further validation of their decision. Some of these same patients will speak about pregnancy, their own future pregnancies, and children frequently. Stone-Joy (1985) reported that many women report that their earlier abortions were the cause of current fertility problems. These manifestations of guilt need exploration. Gonda and Ruark (1984) suggested that guilt can be the sign of a pathological grief response, that is, when the person feels somehow responsible for the deceased person's death. When it comes to abortion, many women do believe that they did "kill someone" despite the need for the procedure.

THE LINK AMONG THE PHASES

I have defined the abortion experience in three phases: pregnancy acknowledgment, pregnancy resolution, and postabortion response. On the basis of the work of others (Adler, 1992; Miller, 1980a; Peppers, 1987; Turell et al., 1990), a major premise of this chapter is the interdependency of the three phases. How a woman perceives her abortion experience is contingent on this interdependency, that is, problems in one phase will cause problems in another phase, thus affecting the entire abortion experience. Prior research has often isolated variables into areas that are categorized as pre- or postprocedure, often neglecting the temporal, cognitive, and emotional connections between the knowledge of conception and the postabortion reaction. Actually, it is very difficult to separate the postabortion reaction from the conditions of the conception. The perceived social and emotional contexts of a pregnancy will affect a woman's decision to abort and the psychological reaction to that abortion (Rivera, 1995).

On a personal level, the emotional context as well as the individual circumstances surrounding the pregnancy will affect the decision regarding pregnancy outcome (Adler, 1975; Bracken, 1978; Faria et al., 1985). The emotional context includes the degree of intendedness and wantedness of the pregnancy, the incongruence between the two states, and the level of ambivalence. It has been found that if the woman has ambivalent feelings about the pregnancy, she may delay her pregnancy resolution (Peppers, 1987). Adler (1992) and Major et al. (1985) found that women who felt their pregnancy was meaningful and wanted coped much worse immediately after the abortion procedure than those women who did not describe their pregnancy as meaningful. In addition, those women who intended to become pregnant, and then decided upon the abortion were more depressed 3 weeks after their abortion. Women who aborted because of fetal anomalies had a more difficult emotional reaction since they fully intended to have, and wanted, a child (Dagg, 1991; Kenyon, 1986). It is evident that women who intentionally become pregnant value their pregnancy more than those who did not intend a pregnancy.

The link between pregnancy resolution and the response to the procedure appears evident: "A woman's decision making process appears to be the variable that best explains such differences in emotional response" (Turell et al., 1990, p. 50). If a woman is dissatisfied, ambivalent, or has had difficulty making her decision to undergo an abortion, the emotional response following the abortion is more severe (Adler, 1992; Adler et al., 1990; Osofsky & Osofsky, 1972; Stone-Joy, 1985). Turell et al. (1990) reported that those women who were uncertain in their decision experienced a great deal of regret, anxiety, depression, doubt, and anger. Women who made the decision independently and took responsibility for their action were reported to suffer less trauma. Overall, women who "own" their decision to abort, and utilize effective decision-making skills such as talking about the abortion decision and seeking support experience less distress after the procedure.

Women at greatest risk for psychological distress after an abortion were those who were extremely ambivalent about the procedure and those who experienced high anxiety upon first hearing about the pregnancy (Kenyon, 1986; Turell et al., 1990). Peppers (1987) found that the ambivalence in the decision making also can affect the grief and mourning experienced after the abortion. McGraw (1989) found that women who based their decision on what parents or the partner wanted were at greater risk for a postabortion reaction. Stone-Joy (1985) reported that women who decided to abort in haste, secrecy, and isolation had the greatest desire to stop thinking about the event as quickly as possible and were more likely to experience a greater degree of loss after the abortion. Finally, Adler (1975) reported that those women who had difficulty deciding to abort reported stronger internally based emotions (regret, anxiety, depression, doubt, and fear) following the procedure.

The interdependency among the phases has multiple implications for therapists. The interconnections presented above are just a minute presentation of the dynamics that may occur. The therapist should listen carefully to the patient as they explore her abortion experience. Inquiry should be used in order to determine how the dynamics of each of the three phases play themselves out in current reproductive behaviors. The therapists should be cautious in using probing questions that would reflect their own personal biases on abortion and women's issues.

THERAPIST BIAS

Clinicians are subject to the same social influences that contribute to personal opinions about abortion as are other segments of society. Clinicians' personal opinions, whether for or against abortion, can influence their perceptions of and therapeutic interactions with women who have had abortions, particularly repeat and multiple aborters. Fueling the biases concerning abortion are the prevailing biases against women. Some psychotherapists have been found to hold views of women that are based on traditional gender roles, which are reinforced by their training, and affect the diagnoses and treatment they provide (Teri, 1982; Waisberg & Page, 1988; Weiner & Boss, 1985; "Summary and Recommendations," 1984). Sherman, Koufacos, and Kenworthy (1978) found psychotherapists held stereotypical attitudes and information about women that were often contradictory to the attitudes and information provided by their women patients. Male therapists were the least informed on issues regarding the "psychology of female bodily functioning" (Sherman et al., 1978, p. 310), which includes issues of women's health and reproduction. When asked about abortion, male therapists were inclined to believe that women should not make the decision alone without some professional help. To further confuse matters, Sherman et al. (1978) found stereotypical feminine behaviors such as passivity and dependency were considered signs of pathology. These findings suggest that some forms of therapy work to maintain the traditionally lower status of women by viewing those behaviors that vary from the male dominant status quo as either deviant or pathological. When looking at abortion, many conclude (including women themselves) that the procedure is a deviation from the traditionally passive role of women.

The decision and act of abortion is clearly a positive step in actively controlling reproduction. Yet, women are often ashamed of having to resort to abortion and "often fear contempt, censure, rejection or hostility from their doctor" (Kenyon, 1986, p. 163). The repeat or multiple aborter is in a more precarious and scorned position, often forced to hide the number of procedures she has undergone (Gibb & Millard, 1981). Many women who have undergone several voluntary abortions tend to feel that hospital and counseling staff treat them negatively (Jacobsson et al., 1976). Therapists must be aware of women's fear of ridicule and censure. It is in understanding this fear that the therapist may improve the transference in the treatment and hence improve the quality of the therapy. Issues of mistrust and dislike are likely to be confronted and assuaged if this fear is openly discussed. Professionals, especially those who are personally opposed to abortion, should be clear of their own biases toward women, abortion, and especially multiple aborters. In addition, if a clinician vacillates on their opinion of abortion, she or he should be aware of how this will affect diagnosis and treatment.

CONCLUSION

The concepts and treatment suggestions presented in this chapter serve as a guide for therapists treating women who raise abortion as an issue during psychotherapy. The goal of this chapter is to remove the assumptions of an underlying psychopathology that is frequently perceived by many aborters and to integrate their abortion experience as part of their sense of self. Therapists should investigate the entire abortion experience from the pregnancy acknowledgment phase to the postabortion response phase. In addition, each woman's abortion experience must be placed within her political, cultural, and social context and the larger sociopolitical context of the abortion debate in the United States. Indeed, the studies cited in this chapter represent a host of different ethnic and social groups and demonstrate the volatile nature of the issue, regardless of ethnicity, race, age, or other sample characteristics. (For a more specific review of the effects of culture and class in the abortion experience see Rivera, 1995.) Finally, the level of influence of the conceptor and significant others on the abortion experience should be explored. By addressing the entire abortion experience and its psychological components therapists can provide a safe therapeutic environment and a therapeutic alliance that will help women patients to integrate this experience.

When a patient raises her abortion experience as a therapeutic issue, there are several strategies that the therapist must entertain. The therapeutic alliance is a delicate relationship subject to conscious and unconscious influences. As demonstrated, the abortion experience is also subject to these same influences. The therapist's goal is to explore the issues surrounding the patient's abortion experience in order for the patient to balance and integrate the abortion experience in a manner that is optimal for her mental health.

REFERENCES

Adler, N. E. (1975). Emotional responses of women following therapeutic abortion. *American Journal of Orthopsychiatry, 45*(3), 446–454.

Adler, N. E. (1992). Unwanted pregnancy and abortion: Definitional and research issues. *Journal of Social Issues, 48*(3), 19–35.

Adler, N. E., David, H. P., Major, B. N., Roth, S. H., et al. (1992). Psychological factors in abortion: A review. *American Psychologist, 47*, 1194–1204.

Adler, N. E., David, H. P., Major, B. N., Roth, S. H., Russo, N. F., & Wyatt, G. E. (1990). Psychological responses after abortion. *Science, 48*, 41–44.

Aguirre, B. E. (1980). Repeat induced abortion: Single, married and divorced women. *Journal of Biosocial Science, 12*, 275–286.

American Psychiatric Association. (1992). *Diagnostic and statistical manual of mental disorders* (3rd ed., rev.). Washington, DC: Author.

Bagarozzi, D. (1994). Identification, assessment and treatment of women suffering from post traumatic stress after abortion. *Journal of Family Psychotherapy, 5*(3), 25–54.

Berger, C., Gold, D., Andres, D., Gillett, P., & Kinch, R. (1984). Repeat abortions, is it a problem? *Family Planning Perspectives, 16*(2), 70–75.

Berson, R. J. (1988). A bereavement group for college students. *Journal of American College Health, 37*, 101–108.

Biasco, F., & Piotrowski, C. (1989). College students' attitudes toward abortion. *The College Student Journal, 23*(3), 194–197.

Bourne, L. F., Dominowski, R. L., Roger, L., Loftus, E. F., & Healy, A. F. (1986). *Cognitive processes* (2nd ed.). Englewood Cliffs, NJ: Prentice Hall.

Bracken, M. B. (1978). A causal model of psychosomatic reactions to vacuum aspiration abortion. *Social Psychiatry, 13*(3), 135–145.

Bracken, M. B., Hachamovitch, M., & Grossman, G. (1972). Correlates of repeat induced abortions. *Obstetrics and Gynecology, 40*, 816–825.

Burnell, G. M., & Norfleet, M. A. (1987). Women's self-reported responses to abortion. *The Journal of Psychology, 121*(1), 71–76.

Callan, V. J. (1983). Repeat abortion seeking behaviour in Queensland, Australia:

Knowledge and use of contraception and reasons for terminating the pregnancy. *Journal of Biosocial Science, 15,* 1–8.

Campbell, T. A. (1990, August). *Women who have abortions: A retrospective study.* Paper presented at the 98th Annual Convention of the American Psychological Association Convention, Boston, MA.

Conklin, M. P., & O'Connor, B. P. (1995). Beliefs about the fetus as a moderator of post-abortion psychological well-being. *Journal of Social and Clinical Psychology, 14*(1), 76–95.

Corsaro, M., & Korzeniowsky, C. (1983). *A woman's guide to a safe abortion.* New York: Holt, Rinehart & Winston.

Dagg, P. (1991). The psychological sequelae of therapeutic abortion: Denied and completed. *American Journal of Psychiatry, 148,* 578–585.

Faria, G., Barrett, E., & Goodman, L. M. (1985). Women and abortion: Attitudes, social networks, decision making. *Social Work in Health Care, 11*(1), 85–99.

Fisher, S. (1986). Reflections on repeated abortions: The meanings and motivations. *Journal of Social Work Practice, 2,* 70–87.

Francke, L. B. (1978). *Ambivalence of abortion.* New York: Random House.

Gannon, K. (1994). Psychological factors in the etiology and treatment of recurrent miscarriage: A review and critique. *Journal of Reproductive and Infant Psychology, 12*(1), 55–64.

Gibb, G. D., & Millard, R. J. (1981). Research on repeated abortion: State of the field 1973–1979. *Psychological Reports, 48,* 415–424.

Gonda, T. A., & Ruark, J. E. (1984). *Dying dignified: The health professional's guide to care.* Reading, MA: Addison-Wesley.

Hafez, E. S. (Ed.). (1984). *Spontaneous abortion.* Boston: MTP Press Limited.

Hastie, R., & Pennington, N. (1991). Cognitive and social processes in decision making. In L. B. Resnick, J. M. Levine, & S. D. Teasley (Eds.), *Perspectives on socially shared cognition* (pp. 308–330). Washington, DC: American Psychological Association.

Hern, W. (1984). *Abortion practice.* New York: J. B. Lippincott Co.

Horobin, G. (Ed.). (1973). *Experience with abortion: A case study of North–East Scotland.* Cambridge, England: Cambridge University Press.

Jacobsson, L., von Schoultz, B., & Solheim, F. (1976). Repeat aborters—a social–psychiatric comparison. *Social Psychiatry, 11,* 75–86.

Kenyon, E. (1986). *The Dilemma of Abortion.* London: Faber & Faber Limited.

Lemkau, J. P. (1988). Emotional sequelae of abortion: Implications for clinical practice. *Psychology of Women Quarterly, 12,* 461–472.

Loader, B. (1995). Unplanned pregnancies and abortion counseling: Some thoughts on unconscious motivations. *Psychodynamic Counseling, 1*(3), 363–376.

Major, B., Cozzarelli, C., Sciacchitano, A., Cooper, M. L., Testa, M., & Mueller, P. M. (1990). Perceived social support, self-efficacy and adjustment to abortion. *Journal of Personality and Social Psychology, 59*(3), 452–463.

Major, B., Mueller, P., & Hildebrandt, K. (1985). Attributions, expectations, and coping with abortion. *Journal of Personality and Social Psychology, 48*(3), 585–599.

Marsiglio, W., & Menaghan, E. (1990). Pregnancy resolution and family formation. *Journal of Family Issues, 11*(3), 313–333.

McAll, K., & Wilson, W. (1987). Ritual mourning for unresolved grief after an abortion. *Southern Medical Journal, 80,* 817–821.

McGraw, R. K. (1989). Obsessive compulsive disorder apparently related to abortion. *American Journal of Psychotherapy, 43*(2), 269–276.

Miller, W. (1980a). *The intendedness and wantedness of conception and induced abortion.* Palo Alto, CA: American Institutes for Research.

Miller, W. (1980b). [*Rating the intendedness of a conception and the wantedness of a pregnancy and child.*] Unpublished raw data.

Najman, J. M., Morrison, J., Williams, G., Andersen, M., & Keeping, J. D. (1991). The mental health of women six months after they give birth to an unwanted baby: A longitudinal study. *Social Science and Medicine, 32*(3), 241–247.

Neubardt, S., & Schulman, H. (1977). *Techniques of abortion.* Boston: Little Brown & Co.

Olley, P. C. (1971). Personality factors and referral for therapeutic abortion. *Journal of Biosocial Science, 3*(1), 106–115.

Osofsky, J. D., & Osofsky, H. J. (1972). The psychological reaction of patients to legalized abortion. *American Journal of Orthopsychiatry, 42*(1), 48–60.

Peppers, L. G. (1987). Grief and elective abortion: Breaking the emotional bond? *Omega, 18*(1), 1–12.

Pines, D. (1990). Pregnancy, miscarriage, and abortion. A psychoanalytic perspective. *International Journal of Psychoanalysis, 71,* 301–307.

Rivera, M. J. (1995). Conception, pregnancy, decision making, and postabortion response among women who have undergone single, repeat and multiple voluntary first trimester abortions (Doctoral dissertation, City University of New York, 1994). *Dissertation Abstracts International, 56-10B,* 5780.

Robbins, J. M. (1979). Objective versus subjective responses to abortion. *Journal of Consulting and Clinical Psychology, 47,* 994–995.

Roe v. Wade, 410 U.S. 113 (1973).

Rosen, H. (1954). *Therapeutic abortion.* New York: Julian Press.

Rovinsky, J. J. (1972). Abortion recidivism. *Obstetrics and Gynecology, 39*(5), 649–659.

Sherman, J., Koufacos, C., & Kenworthy, J. A. (1978). Therapists: Their attitudes and information about women. *Psychology of Women Quarterly, 2*(4), 299–313.

Simon, H., & Senturia, A. G. (1966). Psychiatric sequelae of abortion. *Archives of General Psychiatry, 15,* 378–389.

Speckhard, A., & Rue, V. M. (1992). Post abortion syndrome: An emerging public health concern. *Journal of Social Issues, 48*(3), 95–119.

Stone-Joy, S. (1985). Abortion, an issue to grieve. *Journal of Counseling and Development, 63*, 375–376.

Stotland, N. L. (1985). Contemporary issues in obstetrics and gynecology for the consultation–liason psychiatrist. *Hospital and Community Psychiatry, 36*(10), 1102–1108.

Summary and recommendations: Eliminating sexist treatment. (1984). *Women and Therapy, 3*, 109–120.

Tentoni, S. C. (1995). A therapeutic approach to reduce post-abortion grief in university women. *Journal of American College Health, 44*(1), 35–37.

Teri, L. (1982). Effects of sex and sex-role style on clinical judgment. *Sex Roles, 8*(6), 639–649.

Trad, P. V. (1995). Adolescent girls and their mothers. *American Journal of Family Therapy, 23*(1), 11–24.

Tsoi, W. F., Tay, G. E., & Ratnam, S. S. (1987). Psychosocial characteristics of repeat aborters in Singapore. *Biology and Society, 4*(2), 78–84.

Turell, S. C., Armsworth, M. W., & Gaa, J. P. (1990). Emotional response to abortion: A critical review of the literature. *Women and Therapy, 9*(4), 49–68.

Waisberg, J., & Page, S. (1988). Gender role nonconformity and perception of mental illness. *Women and Health, 14*(1), 3–16.

Weiner, J. P., & Boss, P. (1985). Exploring gender bias against women: Ethics for marriage and family therapy. *Counseling and Values, 30*(1), 9–23.

Westoff, C. F., & Ryder, N. (1977). *The contraceptive revolution.* Princeton, NJ: Princeton University Press.

Wilmoth, G. H. (1992). Abortion, public health policy, and informed consent legislation. *Journal of Social Issues, 48*(3), 1–17.

Wilson, J. B. (1986). Perceived influence of male sex role identity on female partner's life choices. *Journal of Counseling and Development, 65*, 74–77.

15

BRINGING LESSONS LEARNED TO THE UNITED STATES: IMPROVING ACCESS TO ABORTION SERVICES

SABA W. MASHO, FRANCINE M. COEYTAUX, AND MALCOLM POTTS

Worldwide, women are denied access to safe abortion services. The majority of women in the world live under restrictive abortion laws and as a result suffer from the hazardous health consequences of unsafe abortion. According to World Health Organization (WHO) estimates about 50% of maternal deaths related to pregnancy and delivery are caused by unsafe abortions and most of these deaths occur in developing countries (Armstrong, 1989; WHO, 1985). Even in countries like the United States where abortion laws are liberal, the political pressure emanating from the growing moral and ethical controversies has greatly restricted access.

The United States has recently experienced a significant decline in the availability and accessibility of abortion services and continues to face threats to overturn the existing liberal abortion law. Presently, the main barriers of access to safe abortion are a sharp reduction in services, a dwindling number of providers willing and trained to perform abortions, state by state attempts to restrict the laws, and a reduction in government fund-

We thank Judith Tyson for her helpful comments and corrections.

353

ing of abortion services. According to a survey done by the Alan Guttmacher Institute, in 1992 there were only 2,380 health institutions, including hospitals, clinics, and physician's offices, providing abortion
services in the entire country and these institutions were declining at a
rate of 65 per year (Henshaw & Van Vort, 1994). For detailed information
on trends in abortion rates see Henshaw (chap. 3, this volume).

The number of health professionals trained and willing to perform
abortions is declining rapidly. Abortion providers have been harassed,
threatened, and even killed. As a result, many trained providers no longer
perform abortions and fewer new providers are being trained. The number
of residency programs that offer or require abortion training has fallen
dramatically, and currently only about 12% of the United States obstetrics
and gynecology residency programs require learning the procedure (Rosenblatt, Mattis, & Hart, 1995). Even in parts of the United States such as
California and New York where abortion is widely practiced, the number
of medical residents trained to perform abortion is very limited. For example, a survey conducted among chief obstetrics and gynecology residents
in Southern California showed that 47% of the surveyed residents had
never performed a first-trimester abortion and 43% had never done a dilatation and evacuation procedure (Westhoff, Marks, & Rosenfield, 1993).

With the current number of institutions and trained health providers
in the United States, it is increasingly difficult to meet the demand for
abortion services, where about half of the pregnancies are unintended and
approximately 40% of these pregnancies end in abortion (Forest, 1994).
The experience of some developing countries suggests ways to reverse this
trend. Although most developing countries suffer from restrictive laws and
as a result the priority concern is to reduce morbidity and mortality resulting from illegal and usually unsafe abortions, some of the experiences
gained from these countries regarding how to improve the availability of
and access to abortion services could be applied in the United States. The
purpose of this chapter is to highlight what we can learn from experiences
gained from the international arena and suggest ways in which they could
be applied in the United States to increase the number of providers, expand access to services, and prevent mistakes that would be made by restricting existing abortion laws.

LESSONS LEARNED

Many Southern country programs, although operating under very restrictive abortion laws, have struggled for years to increase the number of
trained providers who can treat incomplete abortions, decentralize the services so that rural areas are better served, and generally increase both access
to and the quality of abortion services. And they have done so in an era

of diminishing resources. Lessons learned from the international experience that could be relevant inform the United States situation as we seek to improve access to safe abortion services include (a) the integration of abortion training into existing training curricula, (b) how to increase the number and distribution of providers through the training of non-MDs, (c) decentralizing services through the use of manual vacuum aspiration (MVA), and (d) the use of new technologies to improve care and increase options. Finally, the international experience can shed some light on what we can expect in the United States if we continue to reduce access to safe abortion services.

Integrating Abortion Training Into Existing Training Curricula

Training programs are one of the most important investments in the health service delivery system today. Because of the moral and legal issues associated with abortion, most health workers lack training in safe abortion procedures. Thus, inclusion of abortion procedures in the existing curricula and training of already practicing health professionals is critical to improving the availability of abortion services.

Incorporating training programs in the existing medical school curricula and further expanding the number of trained health workers by establishing "training of trainers" programs has improved the clinical outcomes of treating incomplete abortion and reduced the cost of treatment in many countries. For example, the integration of MVA in the treatment of induced abortion within the existing training facilities proved to be effective in countries such as Kenya and Mexico (International Program Assistance Services [IPAS], 1995a, 1995c).

Although most developing countries permit abortion only under very restricted conditions, there is a great need for abortion services to treat the increasing number of incomplete abortion patients. To meet the needs of postabortion care in these countries, some teaching institutes have designed a comprehensive abortion management curriculum. The curriculum focuses on the treatment of incomplete abortion using cost-effective technology and on providing postabortion family planning counseling and services. For example, in 1989 the Nicaraguan Ministry of Health, in partnership with IPAS, developed a national program to increase women's access to abortion-related care. The program included emergency treatment of incomplete abortion with MVA, postabortion family planning counseling and services, and links to other reproductive health services. The project focused on providing treatment for incomplete abortions at secondary and tertiary levels and at rural health posts. For an effective implementation of this integrated program, training in MVA skills was offered to medical and nursing students, obstetrics and gynecology residents, physicians, and nurses throughout the country. As a result of this integrated postabortion training, trained staff now provide improved postabortion care to women in about 30 hospitals and health centers located in all of the country's local health systems, and abortion has gone from being the leading cause of maternal death in Nicaragua to the fourth cause of mortality (IPAS, 1995d).

The training of more providers in how to perform abortions is the cornerstone to improving access to safe abortion services in the United States as well. In the United States over the last decade we have witnessed a rapid reduction in the number of abortion providers and a growing number of gynecologists and obstetricians who have never performed an abortion. In fact, today most medical and nursing schools in the United States do not incorporate abortion procedures in the curricula (Westhoff, 1994). There is an urgent need to review existing curricula, and new requirements to include abortion training in obstetrics and gynecology residency programs should be encouraged.

Organizations such as the National Abortion Federation, the National Abortion Rights Action League, and Medical Students for Choice, a new national organization whose goal is to educate fellow medical students in the importance of providing abortion care, have identified training as key and are working to make the professional environment more favorable to the provision of abortion services. One model training program is the Physician Training Program undertaken by Planned Parenthood of New York City in which residents of New York City–based medical schools were assigned to Planned Parenthood abortion clinics to get the necessary training. Some of the obstacles faced in implementing this project were recruitment of medical residents, scheduling rotations, and lack of incentives for off-site education. Although the program faced a number of technical barriers, it proved to be successful in increasing the number of physicians who could perform the procedure (Castle & Hakim-Elahi, 1996).

Another important strategy that can be used to increase the number of trained providers is the training of family practice doctors and primary care physicians in abortion care. These physicians already offer a full range of medical services, including simple surgeries, to a clientele that they know relatively well, with whom they have an ongoing relationship, and who live nearby. Although providers may encounter financial and social disincentives to providing abortion care (such as higher insurance rates and harassment by antichoice groups), there are no legal or clinical barriers preventing a family practitioner with suitable training from offering abortion services as part of his or her total package of care.

If the number of family physicians providing abortions is to be increased, residency programs must offer abortion training as a more fully recognized part of the family medicine curriculum. In a study conducted among faculty and residents of eight family practices in Southern California, 62.5% of the residents believed abortion to be an appropriate procedure to be performed by family physicians, although only 19.5% had performed the procedure in the past year. Of those who believed abortion should be performed by family practitioners 48.2% showed an interest in further training to perform the procedure (Lerner & Taylor, 1994). Although the study may not be representative of the views of all family practitioners in the United States, it suggests that a significant number of family practitioners may be willing to be trained to perform the procedure in their practices. Furthermore, if the option of medical abortions using methotrexate or mifepristone becomes a reality, then individual practitioners and family doctors may once again become important abortion providers in the United States.

Training of Nonphysicians

An effective strategy explored by countries faced with a severe shortage of physicians has been the training of paraprofessional health workers. The experience of Bangladesh, where village health workers have been trained to safely perform early MVAs (referred to in Bangladesh as menstrual regulation) is particularly impressive (Greenslade, Leonard, Benson, Winkler, & Henderson, 1993). In Bangladesh, induced abortion is legal only to save the life of the mother, but menstrual regulation (performed by MVA) is legally available for women who have missed their menses. In 1979, the government of Bangladesh established a nationwide training in MVA, making menstrual regulation services available in all government hospitals and health and family planning clinics. Fourteen centers provide training in the use of MVA to government and private doctors and to female family planning auxiliary workers called Family Welfare Visitors (FWVs) who primarily serve women in rural areas. All FWVs have at least 10 years of formal education in addition to an 18-month course in family planning and maternal and child health. Between 1979 and 1990, 7,000 to 10,000 doctors and FWVs were trained to provide menstrual regulation (Maine, Karkazis, & Bolan, 1994). A 1986 survey revealed that FWVs are better candidates for MVA training than physicians because they are posted in rural areas, where 80% of the population in Bangladesh resides (International Planned Parenthood Federation [IPPF], 1993). The survey also showed that FWVs are more likely to perform menstrual regulations than doctors and less likely to emigrate than physicians.

In a country like Bangladesh where highly trained medical personnel are very scarce, it is feasible and necessary to train low level health care workers such as the FWV for the provision of specific health services like menstrual regulation and family planning. Although the utilization of such community health workers cannot be directly replicated in the United States, the availability and accessibility of abortion services can be significantly improved by allowing licensed health care providers such as physician assistants, nurse midwives, and nurse practitioners to perform abortions.

The training of physician assistants, nurse practitioners, and nurse midwives can significantly address the shortage of trained abortion providers in the United States. Training of nonphysicians to perform abortion procedures has long been contemplated by different concerned groups in the United States. The training of nongynecologists/obstetricians was even suggested by the board of the American College of Obstetricians and Gynecologists in 1994 when the board recommended the following:

> To address the shortage of health care providers who perform abortion, the college should encourage programs to train physicians and other licensed health care professionals to provide abortion in collaborative settings. (Westhoff, 1994, p. 151)

Many physician assistants have already been trained and are performing procedures under the supervision of physicians. The Vermont Women's Health Center has been allowing physician assistants to perform abortions since 1973 and has proven that physician assistants are as capable of performing abortions as physicians (Donovan, 1992). However, inconsistencies between physician-only abortion laws and physician assistant statutes have generated confusion in the medical community as to whether physician assistants, working under the supervision of physicians, can legally perform abortions. A study conducted in 1994 showed that physician assistants can perform the procedure safely, and the study concluded that the perceived conflict between physician-only and physician assistant statutes should not preclude physician assistants from providing this vital service (Lieberman & Lalwani, 1994).

The other group of licensed health workers who can also provide abortion services are nurse midwives. In 1990, a symposium was held by the American College of Obstetricians and Gynecologists and the National Abortion Federation to address the national shortage of physician abortion providers. One of the recommendations made at the symposium was that nurse midwives be trained to perform first-trimester legal abortions under the supervision of physicians (McKee & Adams, 1994). If menstrual regulation using MVA could be done with less trained providers in developing countries such as in Bangladesh, there is no reason why the relatively highly trained nurse midwives could not perform the procedure. In addition, most midwives have experience in providing abortion-related services such as abortion referrals and pre and postabortion services.

Decentralization of Abortion Services Using MVA

Providing abortion services in the first trimester has long been recognized as the most important factor in providing safe abortion care. Abortion services are provided at all levels of health care in China, Russia, and other Eastern European countries where abortion is legal. Countries like Mexico, Nicaragua, and Kenya, where abortion is legally restricted, have focused on training gynecologists, obstetricians, and other physicians in MVA to decentralize care. As the service sites in the United States have become more and more scarce, we find ourselves in a situation very similar to that of many developing countries where services are available only in limited urban areas and where large proportions of the population do not have access to care.

MVA has been proven to be a safe way of performing early abortions and less expensive than electrical suction abortions (the most commonly used procedure in the United States today). Originating in the United States and first described in 1972 (Karman & Potts, 1972), MVA has been used almost exclusively in developing countries. The procedure is performed by using a hand-held 60 cc plastic syringe with a cannula attached. It can also be used to treat an incomplete abortion and to perform late first-trimester abortions. The method is best done within the first 8 weeks of last menstrual period. The procedure can be performed under local anesthesia or without any anesthesia.

The use of MVA in the treatment of incomplete abortion in countries such as Bangladesh, Mexico, and Kenya has proven to be simpler, less time consuming, more cost effective than the commonly used dilatation and curettage (D&C), and easily handled by lower level health professionals. Studies conducted in Kenya and Mexico on the treatment of incomplete abortions using MVA showed a dramatic reduction of bed occupancy rate, patient stay, and cost of abortion (IPAS, 1995b, 1995c). Perhaps the best example of the role MVA can play in decentralizing abortion services is the experience of Kenya. As in most African countries, abortion in Kenya is allowed only when the life of the mother is in danger (IPPF, 1993). As a result, self- or illegally induced abortions resulting in incomplete abortions in 1987 accounted for up to 52% of gynecological admissions at rural hospitals and about 60% at Kenyatta National Hospital in Nairobi (IPAS, 1995a). Faced with a tremendous case load of incomplete abortions, the Department of Obstetrics and Gynecology at Kenyatta National Hospital initiated a pilot project to demonstrate the benefits and feasibility of using MVA in place of D&C for the treatment of incomplete abortions. The program reduced the cost of treating incomplete abortions at Kenyatta hospital by 66% and was expanded to both secondary and primary levels of care (IPAS, 1995a). The key to both the lowered cost and the expansion was the "low-tech" nature of the MVA equipment. No longer limited to fully equipped emergency rooms in tertiary care hospitals, incomplete abortions could be safely and effectively cared for in simple health care facilities.

Abortion services in the United States are primarily clinic based. The cost-efficiency of specializing the care and the proficiency gained from treating a greater number of clients were factors that contributed to the consolidation of services. Unfortunately, this centralization has enabled antichoice groups to target clinics such that it is now necessary to decentralize the services, not only to protect against violence but also to increase geographical access. MVA has clearly been shown to be a very effective tool in expanding services internationally, and its applicability in the United States merits exploration.

Although studies and clinical trials exploring the use of MVA over electrical suction abortion are limited in the United States, a number of the available studies have demonstrated that MVA procedures are cost-effective (Blumenthal & Remsburg, 1994; Brenner & Edelman, 1977; Freedman, Jillson, Coffin, & Novick, 1986). A time and cost analysis of management of incomplete abortion with MVA conducted in Baltimore at Johns Hopkins University showed a significant savings in both waiting times and cost compared with the use of electrical suction (Blumenthal & Remsburg, 1994). Physician unfamiliarity with, and lack of willingness to try, the method and guild issues such as the right of nonphysicians to use the equipment remain as impediments to the adoption of this technology. Paradoxically, the greatest barrier to use may be its very simplicity—a procedure completed in a few minutes with a piece of cheap plastic equipment hardly seems to count as a "proper operation."

New Abortion Technologies

Wherever abortion is illegal, there is a lively trade in pills and potions that are perceived to bring on a late period. In most of the developing world, abortifacients are sold openly from street vendors and open markets as was the case in the United States and most European countries in the 19th century (Cole, 1966; Hall & Ransom, 1906; Mohr, 1978). For example, in Chile and the Philippines, abortifacients are literally sold outside churches. Many pharmacies in developing countries also sell modern drugs without prescription either as a treatment of other illnesses or with the intention of terminating pregnancies. For example, a prostaglandin analogue known as Cytotec approved to treat gastric, and duodenal ulcer and until recently obtained over-the-counter in most Latin American countries, is being used by women in Brazil to induce abortion (Barbosa & Arilha, 1993).

The universality of natural abortifacients (most of which do not work and some of which have serious side effects, including death) justify the current scientific investigation on medical abortifacients such as mifepristone (RU486) and methotrexate. The drug known as RU486 in most of the world and as mifepristone in the United States was first marketed in France in 1988 for early first-trimester abortion and is now the method of choice for about one quarter of the women seeking abortion in France

(Editorial, 1990). Available now in England and Sweden, it has been tested in over a dozen developing countries by the WHO (Kulczycki, Potts, & Rosenfield, 1996). Unfortunately, plans to make it available in the United States have been stalled, and it is not at all clear when or whether we will ever have access to the drug in the United States.

Another drug for early first-trimester abortion that is under exploration as an abortifacient in the United States is methotrexate, a readily available drug used to treat certain cancers and other diseases. It appears to be very effective in terminating early pregnancies but has yet to be marketed for this use. The Planned Parenthood Federation of America is presently conducting clinical trials using methotrexate and plans to file for FDA labeling of the drug as an abortifacient. Methotrexate, like mifepristone is used with a second drug, a prostaglandin, which has to be taken several days to a week after the administration of the first drug. Taken in combination with the prostaglandin, methotrexate and mifepristone are between 95% and 98% effective. Because failures occur in about 5% of the cases, use of these drugs must be linked to the availability of suction abortion (David, 1992).

The advent of medical abortions is critical for both developed and developing countries because it holds the possibility of significantly increasing the accessibility to safe abortion services worldwide. Training in the safe provision of medical abortifacients, backed up by early first-trimester MVA, is much less intensive than training in later suction abortion techniques and therefore could be offered to a wider range and much greater number of health care providers. The existence of these drugs could also increase the willingness of health professionals to provide the service. For example, a survey conducted among gynecologists and obstetricians in California indicated that the majority of physicians who are not currently performing abortion would consider providing the abortifacient mifepristone if the drug is made available (Heilig, 1992).

Medical abortifacients hold the promise of increasing accessibility of safe abortion services in the United States. Abortifacients such as mifepristone and methotrexate could be supplied by local health care providers under private and confidential circumstances and can allow women the option of aborting at home (Castle & Coeytaux, 1994). This could be especially important in the United States where antiabortion harassment is rampant and the social and political environment is less and less supportive of women's choice for abortion. The irony is that many countries have more experience than the United States with the new technologies. According to research done in India and Cuba by the Population Council, approximately 90% of women felt mifepristone was satisfactory or better than the method used to induce the previous abortion (Winikoff, Coyaji, Cabezas, & Coyaji, 1992). Another study on women's preferred method of early first-trimester pregnancy termination showed that 60% to 70% of patients prefer the medical method over suction abortion. Women preferred the medical method because it afforded them greater privacy, autonomy, less invasiveness, and greater naturalness than surgery (Winikoff, 1995).

With the advent of managed care and the rise in numbers of family practice providers, these new technologies may yet be incorporated into women's reproductive health care services. If the essence of managed care is to reduce health cost by eliminating unnecessary expenses, the use of less elaborately trained health providers and more cost-effective technologies must be seriously considered. If these recommendations are put into effect, medical abortion could fit the managed care approach of providing services.

Implications of Restrictive Abortion Legislation and Laws

Perhaps the most graphic and immediate lesson one can draw from the international experience is a projection of what can happen in the United States if we continue to implement laws and policies that further restrict access to services. In the United States, approximately 20% of women who choose abortion are not able to have one because of regulatory restrictions, minimal or even absent state support, and low service and provider availability (Fried, 1994). At present, many states restrict adolescents' access to abortion services. By the end of 1995, 27 states enforced parental consent laws and 34 states restricted Medicaid for abortion. Data from 1978 to 1990 was analyzed to compare the effects of mandatory parental involvement and cuts in public funding on abortion demand among minors. Compared with the states that did not enact these laws, a reduction in the number of abortions performed was documented among minors residing in the states enforcing mandatory parental consent laws and restricting Medicaid for abortion (Haas-Wilson, 1996). Furthermore, it is estimated that if legal access to abortion is ever revoked in the United States, approximately 75,000 unwanted children will be born to American minors every year, and poor women will be most likely to be affected (Wattleton, 1990; Spitz et al., 1996).

The contemporary experience of other countries can provide useful perspectives of our future. The first clear fact is that women in all cultures and at all times in history have gone to great lengths and taken inordinate risks to terminate unwanted pregnancies. Abortion is an inescapable element in fertility control and will continue to be so for the foreseeable future (Potts, 1993). According to recent figures for Cuba, South Korea, Japan, the former Soviet Union, and several Eastern European countries, 40% of estimated pregnancies are terminated by induced abortion (Henshaw & Morrow, 1990). By the end of 1980 the estimated number of women worldwide who terminated their pregnancies through abortion was only slightly less than the number of women currently contracepting (National Research Council, 1989). Even in the United States where contraception is accessible approximately 50% of the pregnancies are unintended, of which about two out of five end up in abortion (Forest, 1994). Thus, regardless of the availability and accessibility of contraceptive methods, the need for abortion will continue to exist.

The second fact clearly proven by history is that restrictive abortion laws lead to adverse health consequences. One of the principle arguments made by people seeking to criminalize abortion is that doing so will reduce the number of abortions. Yet international experience has shown over and over again that the main effect of restrictive abortion laws is not a reduction in abortions but rather a tremendous rise in maternal morbidity and mortality (Greenslade et al., 1993). A vivid example of this is provided by Romania's experience. In 1966 when the liberal Romanian abortion law was replaced by a prohibitive enactment, the illegal abortion network reestablished itself dramatically and illegal abortion became common again. Consequently, the country experienced the highest maternal mortality in Europe (about 150 maternal deaths per 100,000 live births) and thousands of unwanted children ended up in institutions (Serbanescu, Morris, Stupp, & Stanescu, 1995). After the stringent abortion and contraception policies were repealed following the 1989 revolution, maternal mortality was reduced by almost 67% and contraceptive use rose by 20% (Remez, 1995).

If the law in the United States were ever seriously restricted it would unquestionably lead to a significant increase in maternal morbidity and mortality and an enormous amount of suffering for women and children. The lesson for the United States is that restricting abortion does not stop women from having abortion. It does however endanger women's lives and expose them to financial and sexual exploitation.

CONCLUSION

As we enter the 21st century we can be certain that abortions will remain common in the United States, as in most parts of the world. Over the past two decades abortion laws and services in the United States have been under attack, and as a result women now face a severe shortage of services to meet a need that has not diminished. Restriction of abortion services leads to higher maternal mortality, morbidity, and exploitation of women. If the current trend of restricting abortion laws continues in the United States, it will endanger women's lives and increase the number of unwanted children, with no effect on the number of women needing abortion.

The United States has much to learn from developing countries that, while operating under restrictive laws and with very low budgets, have sought to improve the availability and quality of their abortion services. Sustained efforts are required to increase the number of health institutions and practitioners willing and able to perform abortions in the United States. The inclusion of abortion training in as many existing medical curricula as possible and the training and licensing of a wide range of health providers to perform abortions would greatly augment the number of abortion providers in the United States and ensure greater access. Training of health care providers should focus on the use of MVA, medical abortifacients, and the integration of abortion services into mainstream women's health care.

REFERENCES

Armstrong, R. E. (1989). Preventing maternal deaths [Monograph]. World Health Organization, Geneva.

Barbosa, R. M., & Arilha, M. (1993). The Brazilian experience with cytotec. *Studies in Family Planning, 24,* 236–241.

Blumenthal, P. D., & Remsburg, R. E. (1994). A time and cost analysis of the management of incomplete abortion with manual vacuum aspiration. *International Journal of Gynecology and Obstetrics, 45,* 261–267.

Brenner W. E., & Edelman D. A. (1977). Menstrual regulation: Risks and abuses. *International Journal of Gynecology and Obstetrics, 15,* 177–183.

Castle, M. A., & Hakim-Elahi, E. (1996). Abortion education for residents. *Obstetrics and Gynecology, 87,* 626–629.

Castle, M. A., & Coeytaux, F. M. (1994). RU 486 beyond the controversy: Implications for health care practice. *Journal of the American Medical Women's Association, 49,* 156–164.

Cole, M. (1966). Abortifacients for sale. In *Abortion in Britain. Proceedings of conference by the Family Planning Association.* London: Pitman Medical.

David, H. P. (1992). Acceptability of mifepristone for early pregnancy interruption. *Law, Medicine & Health Care, 20,* 188–194.

Donovan, P. (1992). Vermont physician assistants perform abortion, train residents. *Family Planning Perspectives, 24,* 225.

Editorial. (1990). *Lancet, 336(8729),* 1480–1482.

Forest, J. D. (1994). Epidemiology of unintended pregnancy and contraceptive use. *American Journal of Obstetrics and Gynecology, 170,* 1485–1489.

Freedman, M. A., Jillson, D. A., Coffin, R. R., & Novick, L. F. (1986). Comparison of complication rates in first trimester abortions performed by physician assistants and physicians. *American Journal of Public Health, 76,* 550–555.

Fried, M. G. (1994). Reproductive wrongs: Women and abortion. *Women's Review of Books, 11,* 6–8.

Greenslade, F., Leonard, A., Benson, J., Winkler, J., & Henderson, V. (1993). *Manual vacuum aspiration: A summary of clinical and programmatic experience worldwide.* Carrboro, NC: International Programs Assistance Services.

Hall, A., & Ransom, W. F. (1906). Plumbism from the ingestion of diachylon as an abortifacient. *British Medical Journal, 1,* 428.

Haas-Wilson, D. (1996). The impact of state abortion restrictions on minors demand for abortions. *Journal of Human Resources, 31,* 140–159.

Heilig, S. (1992). RU 486: What physicians know, think and might do—A survey of California obstetrician/gynecologists. *Law, Medicine and Health Care, 20,* 184–194.

Henshaw, S. K., & Morrow, E. (1990). Induced abortion: A world review. 1990 Supplement. New York: The Alan Guttmacher Institute.

Henshaw, S. K., & Van Vort, J. (1994). Abortion services in the United States: 1991 and 1992. *Family Planning Perspectives, 26,* 100–108.

International Planned Parenthood Federation. (1993). Unsafe abortion: Dialogue, overview, responses, action. London: Author.

International Programs Assistance Services. (1995a). *Africa reports, Kenya.* Carrboro, NC: Author.

International Programs Assistance Services. (1995b). *Asia reports, Bangladesh.* Carrboro, NC: Author.

International Programs Assistance Services. (1995c). *Latin America reports, Mexico.* Carrboro, NC: Author.

International Programs Assistance Services. (1995d). *Latin America reports, Nicaragua.* Carrboro, NC: Author.

Karman, H., & Potts, M. (1972). Very early abortion using syringe as a vacuum source. *Lancet, I(7759),* 1051–1052.

Kulczycki, A., Potts, M., & Rosenfield, A. (1996). Abortion and fertility regulation. *Lancet, 347,* 1663–1669.

Lerner, D., & Taylor, F. (1994). Family physicians and first-trimester abortion: A survey of residency programs in southern California. *Family Medicine, 26,* 157–162.

Lieberman, D., & Lalwani, A. (1994). Physician-only and physician assistant statutes: A case of perceived but unfounded conflict. *Journal of the American Medical Women's Association, 49,* 146–149.

Maine, D., Karkazis, K., & Bolan, N. (1994). The bad old days are still here: Abortion mortality in developing countries. *Journal of the American Medical Women's Association, 49,* 137–142.

McKee, K., & Adams, E. (1994). Nurse midwives' attitudes toward abortion performance and related procedures. *Journal of Nurse-Midwifery, 39,* 300–311.

Mohr, J. C. (1978). *Abortion in America.* New York: Oxford University Press.

National Research Council. (1989). *Contraception and reproduction: Health consequences for women and children in the developing world.* Washington, DC: National Academy Press.

Potts, M. (1993). Unmet demand for family planning. *Interdisciplinary Science Review, 18,* 103–111.

Remez, L. (1995). Romanian maternal death rate fell by two-thirds after the 1989 revolution. *Family Planning Perspectives, 27,* 263–266.

Rosenblatt, R. A., Mattis, R., & Hart, L. G. (1995). Abortion in rural Idaho: Physicians' attitudes and practices. *American Journal of Public Health, 85,* 1423–1425.

Serbanescu, F., Morris, L. Stupp, P., & Stanescu, A. (1995). The impact of recent policy changes on fertility, abortion, and contraceptive use in Romania. *Studies in Family Planning, 26,* 76–87.

Spitz, A. M., Velebil, P., Koolin, L. M., Strauss, L. T., Goodman, K. A., Wingo, P., Wilson, J. B., Morris, L., & Marks, J. S. (1996). Pregnancy, abortion, and birth rates among US adolescents 1980, 1985, and 1990. *Journal of the American Medical Association, 275,* 989–994.

Wattleton, F. (1990). Teenage pregnancies and the recriminalization of abortions. *American Journal of Public Health, 80,* 269–271.

Westhoff, C. (1994). Abortion training in residency programs. *Journal of the American Medical Women's Association, 49,* 150–152.

Westhoff, C., Marks, F., & Rosenfield, A. (1993). Residency training in contraception, sterilization, and abortion. *Obstetrics and Gynecology, 81,* 311–314.

Winikoff, B. (1995). Acceptability of medical abortion in early pregnancy. *Family Planning Perspectives, 27,* 142–149.

Winikoff, B., Coyaji, K., Cabezas, E., & Coyaji, B. (1992). Studying the acceptability and feasibility of medical abortion. *Law, Medicine & Health Care, 20,* 195–198.

World Health Organization. (1985). Prevention of maternal mortality. *Report of WHO Inter-Regional Meeting.* Geneva: Author.

V

CONCLUSION

16

WHERE DO WE GO FROM HERE? RECOMMENDATIONS FOR ABORTION PRACTICE, POLICY, AND RESEARCH

S. MARIE HARVEY, LINDA J. BECKMAN, AND
SHERYL THORBURN BIRD

The chapters in this volume offer diverse perspectives on abortion. Some address issues regarding the broader sociopolitical and cultural contexts within which abortion takes place in the United States. Others address the many factors that influence women's abortion decisions and behavior. Still others discuss the provision of abortion services and abortion as an issue in psychotherapy. All of the chapters present material that has implications for research, practice, and policy. The goal of this chapter is to present key implications and recommendations that emerge from the information presented in previous chapters. We do not provide an exhaustive list of the concerns raised but attempt to highlight key issues.

PRACTICE AND POLICY RECOMMENDATIONS

Several authors acknowledge the need for strategies to address immediate service delivery problems, whereas others suggest long-term social

369

and political change. Recommendations for practice and policy are discussed in the following five sections: improving access to abortion services, improving acceptability of abortion services and practices, advocating for appropriate legislation and public policies, reducing unintended pregnancy, and promoting social change.

Improving Access to Abortion Services

Access to safe, legal abortion services decreases maternal morbidity and mortality and improves the quality of life for American women and their families (Tietze, 1984). In addition, when abortion is legal and accessible, infant mortality rates decline. This decline results from the prevention of unwanted pregnancies and a decrease in births of infants with major physical or mental defects (Corman & Grossman, 1984). Thus, ensuring that women have access to safe and legal abortion services is of paramount importance. The United States has, however, recently experienced a significant decline in the availability and accessibility of abortion services. Henshaw's findings (chap. 3) indicate that the declining number of abortion providers as well as the changes in geographic concentration and types of providers negatively impact service availability.

Several strategies could increase the number and geographic distribution of abortion providers and services. As discussed by Masho, Coeytaux, and Potts (chap. 15), abortion training needs to be a required component in medical school curricula. Similarly, training of already practicing health care providers is essential. Yet, in recent years the number of residency programs that offer abortion training has decreased substantially, and only 12% of the obstetric and gynecology residency programs require the procedure (Rosenblatt, Mattis, & Hart, 1995). In addition to targeting obstetricians and gynecologists, training physicians in family practice and primary care would help address the shortage of abortion providers. Moreover, access could be significantly increased by eliminating legal restrictions that prevent other groups of licensed health care providers (e.g., nurse practitioners, nurse midwives, and physician assistants) from performing abortions.

Abortion services have long been kept at the fringes of American medical care. Abortion practice must be brought into the mainstream of medical care with such services available in the same facilities as other reproductive health care (Henshaw, chap. 3; Radford & Shaw, 1993). Currently, the majority of abortions are performed in free-standing outpatient abortion clinics, and the percentage of abortions that occur outside of specialized clinics is declining (Henshaw, chap. 3). Decentralizing the provision of abortion and including the practice as a component of reproductive health care offered in a majority of physicians' practices would increase availability. Whereas free-standing clinics that specialize in abortion are easy targets for antiabortion violence and harassment, it is highly unlikely that the public would tolerate such harassment and violence at physicians' offices and hospitals. Moreover, without the visibility of specialized clinics, abortions could be provided under more confidential circumstances. If the threat of harassment and violence was eliminated more physicians might be willing to perform abortions. In addition, women would not be subjected to harassment by antiabortion picketers, which, as suggested by Cozzarelli and Major (chap. 4), may cause negative psychological consequences or even interfere with women's decisions to have an abortion. Furthermore, at specialized clinics women have abortions performed by physicians they usually do not know. Abortions might be less anxiety provoking for women if the service was offered at their primary health care facility.

The availability of medical methods of early abortion, such as mifepristone or methotrexate in combination with a prostaglandin, has the potential to increase the numbers, types, and geographic distribution of abortion providers and reduce other barriers (Henshaw, chap. 3; Masho, Coeytaux, & Potts, chap. 15; Chavkin, 1996). Medical abortion could be administered outside of an identified abortion clinic, under confidential circumstances, and by a wide variety of health care providers. These providers would need training in the assessment of gestational age and have backup arrangements for surgical termination, usually using vacuum aspiration. Manual vacuum aspiration (MVA) also has been proven to be safe in the treatment of incomplete abortions and the performance of early abortions (Karman & Potts, 1972). We recommend, therefore, that the Food and Drug Administration give final approval to the use of mifepristone as an abortifacient in the United States and that licensed health care providers be trained in the safe provision of medical abortifacients backed up by surgical abortion and MVA.

Improving Acceptability of Abortion Services and Practices

In addition to ensuring that women have access to safe and legal abortion services, the services provided and the abortion methods available must also be acceptable to potential users. The advent of medical abortion will give women a choice of abortion methods. Because previous studies (Henshaw, Naji, Russell, & Templeton, 1993) have suggested that choice is associated with higher levels of satisfaction regardless of the method chosen, giving women a choice among methods should increase their level of satisfaction with abortion services. Moreover, preliminary data from a sample of women who participated in the mifepristone clinical trial indicate that the overwhelming majority were satisfied with their experience of medical abortion (Beckman & Harvey, chap. 8). We recommend that women be informed of the availability of medical abortion methods. This effort may include outreach that targets different messages to different groups who may choose medical abortion for somewhat different reasons (e.g., fear of surgery vs. privacy).

To ensure that women can make a reasoned choice among methods, appropriate educational and counseling materials about medical abortion must be developed. Findings from a study of potential users of mifepristone suggest that women lack knowledge and have misconceptions about medical abortion (Beckman & Harvey, chap. 8). Moreover, women want more comprehensive information about procedures for taking pills; their chemical effects; what the conceptus will look like; and how much discomfort, pain, and anxiety they will experience. Finally, service providers need to accommodate women's diverse preferences during the period when they are waiting for the abortion to occur. A Scottish study described in Castle and Coeytaux (1994) provides a model for offering individualized options for women, including physical settings with and without beds, private areas for women who wish to be alone, arrangements for companions to be present at the clinic, and the option of going home to wait for the abortion to occur. The tailoring of medical abortion services to provide the greatest comfort and privacy for women will result in greater patient satisfaction.

Health care providers need to incorporate cultural sensitivity and linguistic competence into all delivery systems, including abortion services. As Tanjasiri and Aibe (chap. 7) suggest, such services need to consider culture-specific barriers to access, including lack of knowledge about where to get abortion services, and culture-specific perceptions of abortion and contraceptive methods (e.g., the belief among some Chinese women that sterilization causes arthritis). Inappropriate translation of English language educational materials may also create culture-specific barriers (e.g., direct translation of English language materials into Asian languages may include culturally insensitive contexts). Recommendations for improving cultural sensitivity in the provision of abortion services include the following: recruit culturally and linguistically diverse individuals into the health and medical professions, train health professionals to be culturally competent (e.g., to develop skills that will allow them to behave in a culturally appropriate and respectful way), provide interpreters for women who do not understand English; and develop counseling and educational materials that are culturally and linguistically comprehensible (Giachello, 1995).

Special efforts may be necessary for some groups such as African American women to develop a trusting relationship with abortion providers due to a long history of oppression including coercive attempts to control reproductive behavior. The theme of abortion as Black genocide is part of the ideological context of the abortion debate in African American communities and is interwoven with the struggle against racism. Indeed African American pro-life forces view abortion as a major threat to the stability of the Black family (Dugger, chap. 5). Abortion counselors and providers must have an understanding of the history and current context of the abortion debate in African American communities.

To improve women's abortion experiences, we recommend that abortion counselors and providers be educated in the use of theory-based comprehensive approaches to abortion care that have been evaluated and shown to be effective. Fisher, Castle, and Garrity (chap. 13) offer a cognitively based model for the provision of abortion counseling. These authors contend that such a cognitive approach can help a woman to feel empowered to make decisions regarding an unintended pregnancy and can reduce insecurities, anxieties, and fears related to the abortion procedure. Although the effectiveness of such models needs further evaluation, the use of theory-based educational models is more likely to result in comprehensive abortion services that are acceptable to women.

Mental health services for women who obtain abortions and for their sexual partners must be promoted. In particular, culturally sensitive pre- and postprocedure counseling is needed for women and men who may have a more difficult time with the abortion decision or its aftermath because of cultural norms, religious beliefs, or ambivalent feelings. In addition, special counseling and therapy techniques must be offered for specific groups of women, such as adolescents and victims of sexual abuse, to address their unique situations. Counseling and therapy techniques for specific post-abortion issues must also be developed and offered (Rivera, chap. 14). For example, when a medical abortion fails, the woman is at higher risk of subsequent guilt and less relief after the abortion (Miller, Pasta, & Dean, chap. 10).

Advocating for Appropriate Legislation and Public Policies

As discussed by Russo and Denious (chap. 2), much of the abortion debate has occurred in the policy and political arenas. Clearly, morality, political affiliation, and powerful special interest groups influence resource allocation and public policy related to abortion. To understand public policy concerning abortion we need to acknowledge the fact that in the United States abortion has been defined as a moral issue. According to one feminist theoretical view known as social reconstructionism or poststructuralism, positions of power enable some groups or individuals to define what is considered reality; that is, they determine what is accepted as knowledge and belief (Riger, 1992). From a poststructuralist perspective, beliefs about abortion and its morality under various circumstances are socially constructed. Different belief systems are disseminated depending on which political party or faction is in power and who their major constituency is perceived to be.

Many state legislatures have considered and passed several measures that would restrict access to safe, legal abortion services (see Gold, 1990, for a detailed description). Although much of the legislation appears to protect the interests of pregnant women, in reality it is designed to prevent women from obtaining abortions. According to Gold (1990), a yard stick against which proposed legislation should be measured is its effect on the health and safety of women and its discriminatory consequences for poor women, women of color, and women in certain geographic areas.

To ensure the health and safety of women, we must vigorously oppose state laws, government regulations, and public policies designed to curtail abortion in the United States. These include parental consent or notification for adolescents (Adler, Smith, & Tschann, chap. 12), spousal/partner consent or notification, mandatory waiting periods, specified counseling and informed-consent provisions, banning the use of federal Medicaid funds for abortion services, and banning abortions in public facilities. By increasing the cost of the procedure, imposing administrative obstacles, and requiring long distance travel, these policies delay pregnancy termination often into the second trimester, thereby increasing the health risk to women (Henshaw, chap. 3). Of particular concern is the fact that many of these policies restrict access for those women who are most likely to need an abortion: adolescents and low-income women (Chavkin, 1996). Many of these women already face numerous barriers to obtaining an abortion (e.g., no or low incomes, no health insurance, residence in an underserved area).

Reducing Unintended Pregnancy

Although some pro-life proponents believe that a woman should have as many children as she is able to or as God gives to her, both sides in the abortion debate can generally embrace the goal of preventing unintended pregnancies, especially among adolescents. The major strategy for reducing the need for abortion is to increase the proportion of pregnancies that are planned and wanted. Toward this end, the consistent use of effective contraception among those who are sexually active and do not want to become pregnant must be promoted. In particular, culturally appropriate contraceptive education, counseling, and family planning services need to be designed.

Young men and women as well as adults need to be encouraged and educated to communicate with their partners about expectations concerning sex and pregnancy prior to a pregnancy and, if possible, prior to the initiation of the sexual relationship. They must learn to communicate their views about the resolution of unwanted pregnancy to their partner before they engage in sexual intercourse. Both men and women need to be aware of the possible consequences of not using contraception and the responsibilities associated with parenthood.

Although a large segment of American society believes that sex can be separated from reproduction, a significant minority still clings to the Victorian idea that sex apart from reproduction is immoral (see Russo & Denious, chap. 2). School-based sex education that teaches adolescents and children about healthy sexuality can help prevent unwanted pregnancy and enhance sexual functioning. The debate over providing sex education in the public schools spans decades and has not abated in recent years. Opponents claim that sex/family life education increases immorality, sexual activity, pregnancy, and abortion in adolescents. However, a 1994 summary of the findings from 23 peer-reviewed studies of school-based sex education programs reports evidence that sex education does not increase sexual activity among teenagers (Kirby et al., 1994). Moreover, if information on birth control methods is presented, sex education helps prevent unintended pregnancy and abortion through the use of contraception (Kirby et al., 1994). We endorse, therefore, the recommendation of the American Medical Association and the American Public Health Association that local and state school boards of education include comprehensive sexuality education as a component of kindergarten through 12th grade school health education programs (Epner, 1996). We urge that such programs be taught in a nonjudgmental manner and that religious, ethical, or moral values not be imposed on students.

Promoting Social Change

Although many of the above recommendations focus on specific health care delivery and public policy changes, these changes must be addressed within the larger context of women in society. It must be remembered that the oppression and subordination of women are tied to denial of reproductive choice (Roberts, 1990) and that reproductive choice involves more than the choice of abortion. Policies that restrict women's access to reproductive health services, particularly family planning and abortion services; that mandate birth control use or sterilization for women; or that in any other way limit choices regarding reproduction are detrimental to women's health and well-being. Such policies promote the continued subordination of women within the political, social, and economic power structure of American society. Moreover, such restrictive and punitive policies are more likely to affect poor women and women of color. Therefore, these policies must be vigorously opposed.

The reproductive health needs of women are inextricably linked to the increasing feminization of poverty, gender inequality, sexism, and racism. Thus, long-term solutions to improving the health and well-being of women and families will require not only the implementation of changes such as those outlined in this chapter, but also the active involvement of psychologists, public health professionals, women's health advocates, and health care providers in political and social change. Social and political changes that elevate women's status and power in society and in heterosexual relationships ultimately will result in lower abortion rates. For example, the promotion of greater economic equality can reduce the abortion rate for women of color who undergo abortion most often for socioeconomic/pragmatic reasons (Dugger, chap. 5; Erickson & Kaplan, chap. 6). Also, the promotion of egalitarian power relationships between partners will enable women to refuse unprotected sex or insist on condom or contraceptive use (Amaro, 1995; Russo & Denious, chap. 9).

The public debate about abortion in the United States is dominated by two opposing perspectives: abortion as a right to attain individual freedom and social equality for women versus abortion as a threat to morality, motherhood, and social cohesion. Although it is highly unlikely that prochoice and pro-life feminists could reach a consensus position regarding the abortion debate, they might find common ground from which to work toward improving women's health and well-being. As Russo and Denious (chap. 2) suggest, we need to build bridges among pro-choice and pro-life feminists who already share many common concerns. This effort involves reframing the debate and finding areas of consensus. Both sides appear to agree that abortion is undesirable and that unintended pregnancy could be better addressed by other means. Both sides are concerned about and want to ameliorate the conditions (e.g., economic inequality for women, ineffective use of contraception, lack of adequate day care) that lead women to need abortions. They share concerns about the social, economic, and cultural contexts of abortion decisions (Callahan & Callahan, 1984). As a united and more powerful force they could work toward social reforms that would limit the need for abortion resulting from poverty, oppression of women, and lack of social support for childbearing. We urge, therefore, that pro-life and pro-choice feminists work together toward common goals that promote the health and quality of life for women and their families.

Dugger (chap. 5) described a multiracial movement for reproductive freedom that is separate from the mainstream pro-choice movement. In contrast to the one issue stance of the dominant pro-choice movement, the multiracial reproductive rights movement emphasizes basic health rights, access to primary health care services, and safeguards against reproductive abuses of women. For example, individuals involved in this movement have emphasized protection from coercive medical or legal actions against women who have AIDS or have abused drugs. The multiracial reproductive rights movement shares many common interests and goals with the dominant pro-choice movement. For example, both movements share common goals involving reproductive rights and reproductive freedom that can enhance the health and well-being of women, particularly women of color. We encourage individuals in these two movements to formulate collective objectives and unite to work on common issues.

RESEARCH RECOMMENDATIONS

Social policy and service provision can be informed by empirical data concerning issues such as subgroup differences in abortion attitudes and behavior, methods for increasing access to abortion for underserved groups, and methods for making the abortion experience more acceptable to women. The chapters in this book have highlighted several of the important gaps in the research literature on abortion. Many of these are discussed below.

The Cultural Context and Cultural Differences

As noted in the chapters addressing the cultural context of abortion, few studies have examined the abortion beliefs, attitudes, and behavior of specific racial and ethnic groups. It is insufficient to study the abortion attitudes and behavior of ethnic groups only as they compare with those of Whites. Studies that explore differing attitudes and behavior *within* ethnic populations are needed. Research that examines subgroups within broader ethnic categories (e.g., Latinos of Mexican, Cuban, or Puerto Rican heritage)—with adequate sample sizes to examine differences in abortion beliefs, attitudes, and practices *within* a subgroup—is essential. The broader social, political, historical, and economic context within which abortion occurs must be examined. Dugger (chap. 5) identified contextual factors that likely impact abortion attitudes and behavior among African Americans, including race, class, and gender relations; social and economic conditions; and inequities related to reproductive rights. These contextual factors also are likely to impact abortion attitudes and behaviors of other ethnic populations. In general, studies that examine *how* cultural, socioeconomic, and other factors affect abortion decisions, attitudes, and behavior among ethnic subgroups should be conducted. Researchers must look at the broader context of fertility behavior, including beliefs about sexuality, family and gender roles, and how each influences contraceptive and abortion behavior. In this vein, barriers to access for different racial and ethnic subgroups—access to general health care as well as access to abortion—must be identified.

Because the majority of some ethnic groups and subgroups (e.g., Asian and Pacific Islanders) are foreign born, studies that investigate how abortion-related factors of country of origin as well as how the processes of migration and acculturation influence abortion-related attitudes and practices in the United States are needed. In addition, the impact of legislation such as California's Proposition 187 on access to reproductive health services including abortion for immigrants should be assessed. This measure, which was passed in November 1994 but has not been implemented (as of December 1997) because of pending challenges in the courts, restricts access to nonemergency medical services, education, and social services to any immigrant family that cannot provide evidence of legal residency in the United States.

Finally, issues unique to racial and ethnic groups or subgroups need to be examined. If abortion is primarily a practical issue for Black and Latina women (Dugger, chap. 5; Erickson & Kaplan, chap. 6), then conceptual models and research questions must incorporate this perspective. A conceptualization of abortion as solely a matter of choice may be particularly inappropriate for African Americans. The unique historical and sociopolitical context of abortion for Black communities in the United States (e.g., abortion as genocide) needs to be taken into account when designing studies and interpreting findings involving African American samples. Erickson and Kaplan (chap. 6) report that most Latinas have abortions for socioeconomic reasons, even though data suggest that approval of abortion among Latinos is low for reasons other than health and victimization. This inconsistency also requires further investigation.

Studies that examine abortion among adolescents are also needed. Further research on the psychological sequelae of abortion among adolescents from different racial and ethnic groups and their decision making regarding abortion should be conducted. As Adler et al. (chap. 12) indicate, studies that can assess different age groups and developmental stages within adolescence will be particularly helpful.

Research that specifically focuses on men and abortion is limited. Some feminist researchers contend that men and women of similar ethnic backgrounds and social classes may be members of different cultures that have different normative values and beliefs about parenthood, gender roles, sexuality, and reproduction. As Marsiglio and Diekow (chap. 11) suggest, studies that examine men's beliefs and attitudes about abortion and fatherhood as well as their involvement in pregnancy resolution decisions are needed.

The Availability and Acceptability of Abortion Services and Practice

As Henshaw (chap. 3) reported, the number of abortion providers and abortion rates in the United States have decreased. Studies designed to provide better estimates of the extent to which the decreasing number of providers results in fewer abortions are needed. Strategies for increasing the availability of abortion must also be evaluated. For example, the extent to which health care providers other than physicians can perform abortions safely and the extent to which women are satisfied with the care offered by these other providers must be evaluated.

As noted earlier, the introduction of medical abortion in the United States may make abortion accessible to greater numbers of women. The ability of these technologies to increase access to abortion services will, however, greatly depend on provider acceptability. Thus, as new reproductive technologies become available, studies that assess their acceptability by providers are critical. We need information on what health care providers know about medical abortion and about MVA, what their experience has been in the use of these methods, and what the barriers are to providing medical abortion.

Equally important is whether women find medical abortion an acceptable method. Beckman and Harvey's research (chap. 8) on the acceptability of medical abortion to women identified several factors that could influence women's choice of abortion method (i.e., surgical vs. medical abortion). Further research on the factors that affect women's decisions about abortion method will increase understanding of the population of women who will likely use medical abortion and the circumstances under which medical abortion may be preferable. It will also provide important information about perceived and actual advantages and disadvantages of both methods that could inform the development of education materials and improve counseling about abortion. Studies that investigate the medical abortion experience (i.e., that describe women's experiences with medical abortion and how they differ from the experiences of women who have surgical abortions) will also be useful in this regard.

A vast literature exists regarding the psychological consequences of surgical abortion for women (e.g., Adler et al., 1992). Miller, Pasta, and Dean (chap. 10) have presented the first study of the psychosocial effects of medical abortion on women in the United States. Further research is needed to identify what, if any, adverse or unexpected consequences of medical abortion may occur. Studies that compare the long-term outcomes for women who have had surgical versus medical abortion could help inform abortion policy and practice.

Research is needed that evaluates methods for improving the abortion experience. Fisher, Castle, and Garrity (chap. 13) proposed a cognitive approach to patient-centered abortion care. This method must be tested with diverse populations. Other strategies for improving the experiences of women immediately before, during, and after the abortion procedure should be developed and evaluated. Cozzarelli and Major (chap. 4) discuss the potential effects of anti-abortion activities on women's decision to have an abortion and the psychosocial effects on women who enter the abortion clinic. More research is needed that examines the effects of antiabortion activities on women wanting to obtain an abortion and whether these activities result in fewer abortions. In addition, the extent to which injunctions and pro-choice escorts shield women from antiabortion activities should be studied. The extent to which restrictive abortion policies affect women's ability to obtain an abortion (e.g., the impact of varying laws about parental consent on adolescent health) must also be assessed.

Unintended Pregnancy

Abortion is one method for resolving an unwanted pregnancy. If all women had the resources and ability to prevent mistimed and unwanted pregnancies, then there would be considerably fewer abortions. Research that identifies the determinants of unintended pregnancy could inform pregnancy prevention programs and policy. In addition, studies of pregnant women that identify the predictors of abortion would improve our understanding of the characteristics of women who choose abortion, the reasons for their choices, and the factors that make obtaining an abortion difficult or impossible.

Research Methods and the Dissemination of Findings

Research methods that are used to study issues related to abortion need to be evaluated, expanded, and strengthened. Researchers must further examine how the wording of questions on surveys affects responses regarding abortion attitudes (Russo & Denious, chap. 2). In-depth qualitative studies can complement quantitative research. Qualitative research methods can lead to a better understanding of women's experiences with and attitudes toward abortion.

As we enter the 21st century it is very likely that abortion will continue to be the most divisive policy issue in the United States. Because abortion is such an emotionally charged and political issue, careful evaluation of relevant empirical research is imperative and must be shared with policy makers and women's health advocates. Such evaluation will help to assure that interpretations of research results are appropriate and that policy claims are based on solid findings rather than assumptions (Wilcox, Robbenolt, & O'Keeffe, chap. 1). Researchers in psychology, public health, medicine, and other fields should insist that their voices, expertise, and knowledge of the health and psychological consequences of abortion be included in the debate (Chavkin, 1996). We must then provide accurate up-to-date information to local, state, and national policy makers and to the media. For instance, investigators must continue to testify and provide findings from scientific research on important policy questions such as parental notification statutes, an area in which the findings to date do not support the need for legislation (see Adler et al., chap. 12).

CONCLUSION

It is important to acknowledge and be respectful of differing values about the acceptability and morality of abortion. We cannot ignore, however, the strong public health data supporting the need for access to safe, legal abortion for those women who want to terminate a pregnancy. The presence of such services reduces both maternal and infant mortality and improves the quality of women's lives. This chapter presents a number of recommendations for strengthening the availability and quality of abortion services. These include requiring abortion training as part of the curriculum in medical school, eliminating the legal restrictions that prevent qualified groups of licensed health professionals who are not physicians from performing abortions, providing abortion services at primary health care facilities rather than specialized clinics, making available to and educating women about methods of medical abortion, incorporating cultural sensitivity and linguistic competence into all delivery systems, and using theory-based comprehensive approaches to abortion care and counseling.

Feminists must advocate for legislation and public policy that both protect women who seek abortion and reduce the societal need for abortion. Recommendations include opposing laws that restrict access to safe, legal abortion; supporting programs that reduce unintended pregnancy by promoting contraceptive use, training individuals to communicate with their partners about expectations concerning sex and pregnancy, and providing sex education in the schools; opposing policies that restrict women's access to reproductive health services or that mandate birth control use for certain groups of women; and supporting social change that increases women's status and power in society and in heterosexual relationships.

It is essential that policy and advocacy efforts concerning abortion be supported by solid empirical evidence. Of particular importance is research that examines differing abortion attitudes and behaviors *within* ethnic populations; how abortion-related factors of country of origin, immigration, and acculturation affect abortion use and attitudes among immigrants to the United States; issues unique to racial and ethnic groups or subgroups; the availability and acceptability of abortion services and practices, particularly medical abortion; and issues unique to adolescents and to men. Equally essential are studies that evaluate strategies for increasing the availability of abortion and for improving the abortion experience for women, and that explore the determinants of mistimed and unwanted pregnancy.

Finally, abortion and other reproductive health services need to be considered within the larger context of women's role in society. Policies that restrict women's access to reproductive health services are linked to the continued subordination and lack of empowerment of women. The broader issues of sexism, racism, and classism must be addressed if the long-term health and well-being of women in the United States are to be improved significantly. In this endeavor the pro-choice movement must forge alliances with other feminist groups around common goals that promote women's health and improve their social, economic, and political status.

REFERENCES

Adler, N. E., David, H. P., Major, B. N., Roth, S. H., Russo, N. F., & Wyatt, G. E. (1992). Psychological factors in abortion: A review. *American Psychologist, 47*, 1194–1204.

Amaro, H. (1995). Love, sex, and power: Considering women's realities in HIV prevention. *American Psychologist, 50*, 437–447.

Callahan, S., & Callahan, D. (1984). Abortion: Understanding differences. *Family Planning Perspectives, 16*, 219–221.

Castle, M. A., & Coeytaux, F. M. (1994). RU 486 beyond the controversy: Implications for health care practice. *Journal of the American Women's Medical Association, 149*, 156–159.

Chavkin, W. (1996). Topics for our times: Public health on the line—abortion and beyond. *American Journal of Public Health, 86*, 1204–1206.

Corman, H., & Grossman, M. (1984). *Determinants of neonatal mortality rates in the United States.* Cambridge, MA: National Bureau of Economic Resources.

Epner, J. E. (Ed.). (1996). *Policy compendium on reproductive health issues affecting adolescents.* Chicago, IL: American Medical Association.

Giachello, A. (1995). Cultural diversity and institutional inequality. In D. L. Adams (Ed.), *Health issues for women of color: A cultural diversity perspective.* Thousand Oaks, CA: Sage.

Gold, R. B. (1990). *Abortion and women's health: A turning point for America?* New York: The Alan Guttmacher Institute.

Henshaw, R. C., Naji, S. A., Russell, I. T., & Templeton, A. A. (1993). Comparison of medical abortion with surgical vacuum aspiration: Women's preferences and acceptability of treatment. *British Medical Journal, 307*, 714–717.

Karman, H., & Potts, M. (1972). Very early abortion using syringe as a vacuum source. *Lancet, I(7759)*, 1051–1052.

Kirby, D., Short, L., Collins, J., Rugg, D., Kolbe, L., Howard, M., Miller, B., Sonenstein, F., & Zabin, L. S. (1994). School-based programs to reduce sexual risk behaviors: A review of effectiveness. *Public Health Reports, 109*, 339–360.

Radford, B., & Shaw, G. (1993). Beyond *Roe* and abstract rights: American public health and the imperative for abortion as a part of mainstream medical care. *Saint Louis University Public Law Review, 13*, 207–219.

Riger, S. (1992). Epistemological debates, feminist voices: Science, social values, and the study of women. *American Psychologist, 47*, 730–740.

Roberts, D. E. (1990). The future of reproductive choice for poor women and women of color. *Women's Rights Law Reporter, 12(2)*, 59–67.

Rosenblatt, R. A., Mattis, R., & Hart, L. G. (1995). Abortion in rural Idaho: Physicians' attitudes and practices. *American Journal of Public Health, 85*, 1423–1425.

Tietze, C. (1984). The public health effects of legal abortion in the United States. *Family Planning Perspectives, 16*, 26–28.

AUTHOR INDEX

Numbers in italics refer to listings in the reference section

Able, G. G., 215, *229*

Abma, J. C., 214, *228*

Abortion report Koop withheld released on Hill, 9, *22*

Acosta, E. P., 148, *151*

Acosta-Belén, E., 148, *151*

Adams, E., 358, *365*

Adams, H. P. J., 215, *228*

Adams, M. M., *230*

Adcock, A. G., 217, *232*

Adebayo, A., 36, *54*, 274, *282*

Adler, N. E., 21, *22–23*, 43, *54*, 95, *102*, 223, 225, *228*, 235, 238, 260, 264, 286–287, 290, 296, 301, 303–304, 325, 336, 339–340, 342, 345–346, *349*, 374, 379, *382*

Aguayo-Hernandez, J. R., 149, *151*

Aguirre, B. E., 335, 342, *349*

Aguirre-Molina, M., 133–134, 146, *154*

Aibe, S., 175–177, *184*

Alan Guttmacher Institute, 7, *23*, 74, *79*, 135, *151–152*, 168, *181*, 213, *228*, 285, *296*

Allman, I., 166–167, *181*

Altemeier, W. A., 47, *54*

Althaus, F. A., 71, 73, *80*

Alvarez, W., 240, *265, 266*

Amaro, H., 122, *127*, 133, 138, 145–147, *152*, 215–216, *228*, 376, *382*

Ambuel, B., 290, 292–293, *296*

American Psychological Association, *341*

American Psychological Association Public Interest Directorate, 21, *23*

American Psychological Association Task Force on Psychology, Family Planning, and Population Policy, xiii, *xiv*

Andersen, M., 341, *351*

Anderson, E. T., 215, *231*

Anderson, J., 95, *104*

Andres, D., 335, *349*

Aneshensel, C. S., 138–139, *152*

Angelini, P. J., 217, *232*

Anh, D., 167, *181*

Anzaldúa, G., 29, *57*

Arilha, M., 360, *364*

Armstrong, R. E., 353, *364*

Armsworth, M. W., 336, *352*

Asians and Pacific Islanders for Reproductive Health, 157, 174, 176, 178–180, *182*

Atkeson, B. M., 215, 220, *228–229*

Atkin, L. C., 147–148, *152*

Atrash, H. K., 301, *326*

Aviaro, H., 146, *152*

Axelrod, R. H., 271, *283*

Bachelot, A., 194, *207*

Bachman, R., 212, *229*

Back, K. W., xiii, *xiv*, 43, *54*

Bagarozzi, D., 342, *349*

Baird, D. T., 194, *209*

Baker, A., 303, 324, *326*

Baker, P., 214, *231*

Baker, T., 221, *229*

Banister, J., 165–166, *182*

Banks, J., 123, *127*

Barbosa, R. M., 360, *364*

Barnartt, S., 110, *127*

Barnett, W., 276, *283*

Barrett, E., 335, *350*

Bart, P. B., 44, *54*

Basow, S. A., 36, 47, *55*

Bass, M., 191, *207*

Bauer, G. L., 271, *283*

Baulieu, E., 51, *54*

Bean, F. D., 138, 146, *152*

Bearinger, L. H., 291, *298*

Becerra, R. M., 138, *152*

Beck, A., 305–306, 309, 322, *326*

Beck, J. S., 305, 308–310, 322, *326*

Becker, J., 92, *103*

Becker, J. V., 215, *229*

Becker-Lausen, E., 216, 220, *229*

Beckman, L. J., 193, 196, 199, *207–208*

Beebe, D. K., 214, *229*

Beilenson, P., 217, *233*

Bell, R., 224, *229*

Bellah, R. N., 271, 283
Belsey, E. M., 303, 326
Benjamin, P., 287, 296
Benson, J., 146–147, 154, 357, 364
Berenson, A. B., 217, 229
Berer, M., 194, 207
Beresford, T., 303, 321–323, 326
Berger, C., 335, 349
Berrien, J., 121–122, 127
Berson, R. J., 343–344, 349
Best, C. L., 213, 215, 231
Betzig, L., 31, 54
Biasco, F., 335, 339, 349
Binkin, E. B., 169, 183
Bisignani, J. D., 161, 182
Blake, J., 110, 127
Blanchard, D. A., 27–28, 30, 31, 35, 54,
    82–86, 102
Blank, R. H., 40, 42, 57
Blazer, D. G., 215, 230
Blum, R. W., 291–292, 296, 298
Blumenthal, P. D., 360, 364
Bobronsky, M. A., 350
Bolan, N., 357, 365
Bonavoglia, A., 47, 54
Borras, V. A., 137, 152
Boss, P., 347, 352
Bourne, L. F., 334, 349
Boyd, C., 325, 326
Boyer, D., 217, 229
Bracken, M., 95, 102
Bracken, M. B., 95, 102, 287, 289, 296,
    342, 346, 349
Brashear, D. B., 303, 326
Bray, H., 125–126, 127
Bray v. Alexandria Women's Health
    Clinic, 16, 23
Brenner, W. E., 360, 364
Brickman, E., 221, 229
Briere, J., 215, 232
Broughton, D., 230
Brown, F. D., 123–126, 127–128
Brown, L., 147, 154
Brown, S., 170, 177, 182
Brown, S. S., 114–117, 127–128
Browne, A., 214–215, 229–231
Bruce, F. C., 230
Bullock, L., 215, 231–232
Bureau of Justice Statistics, 213, 229
Burgess, A. W., 215, 229
Burke, P. J., 281, 283

Burnam, M. A., 215, 229
Burnell, G. M., 301, 326, 331, 340, 349
Bussell, D., 21, 24
Butler, J. D., 27, 54
Bygdeman, M., 194, 208
Byrne, D. M., 137, 153

Cabezas, E., 361, 366
Cabral, H., 215, 228
Calderone, M., 26, 54
Calhoun, K. S., 215, 220, 228–229
Calhoun, L. G., 95, 102
Callahan, D., 21, 23, 376, 382
Callahan, S., 376, 382
Callan, V. J., 335, 349
Cameron, C. L., 303, 328
Camp, S. L., 166, 182
Campbell, B. M., 120, 125, 128
Campbell, T. A., 335–336, 349
Cao, F. M., 183
Carmen, E., 221, 229
Carmichael, J. S., 140, 153
Carr, P., 124–126, 128
Carr, T. P., 4, 23
Cartoof, V. G., 70–71, 80
Carver, C. S., 302, 328
Cary, L., 115, 128
Castle, M. A., 196, 207–208, 302–304,
    324, 326, 356, 361, 364, 372,
    382
Cates, Jr., W., 153
Cates, W., 293, 298
Cavendish, J. C., 59
Center for Reproductive Law and Policy,
    165, 182
Centers for Disease Control and Preven-
    tion, 107, 128
Cerullo, M., 29, 54
Chancer, L. S., 33, 54
Chandra, A., 214, 228
Chavkin, W., 217, 232, 301, 326, 371,
    374, 380, 382
Chen, A. J., 165, 182
Chen, C. H. C., 168, 182
Chen, M. S., 158, 163, 169, 182
Cherlin, A. I., 280, 283
Christmas, J. J., 124, 128
Chuong, C. H., 160, 182
Cichon, J., 215, 229
Cicirelli, B., 290, 296
Clagett, A. F., 36, 58

Claire, M., 47, *54*
Clark, A. P., 303, 324, *326*
Clark, C., 31–32, 34, 37–38, *54*
Clark, J., 31–32, 34, 37–38, *54*
Clary, F., 292, *296*
Clinton, W., *18*
Cludy, L., 194, *207*
Cobos-Pons, Y., 149, *153*
Cockburn, A., 118, *128*
Coeytaux, F. M., 196, *207–208*, 361, *364*, 372, *382*
Coffin, R. R., 360, *364*
Cole, M., 360, *364*
Collins, J., *382*
Comas-Diaz, L., 303, *326*
Combs, M., 108–110, 113, *128*
Combs, M. W., 38, *54*
Committee on Unintended Pregnancy, 216, 226, *229*
Commonwealth Fund, 179–180, *182*
Condit, C. M., 30, 41, *55*
Congleton, G. K., 95, *102*
Conklin, M. P., 41, *55*, 339, *349*
Conly, S. R., 166, *182*
Conover, P., 110, *128*
Cook, E., 112, *128*
Cook, E. A., 25–26, 31, 34, 36–40, 45, 47, 49, *55*, 86, *102*
Cook, R. J., 167, *182*
Cooke, A. D. J., 48, *57*
Cooksey, E. C., 137, *152*
Cooper, M. L., 90, *103*, 223, *231*, *350*
Coppel, D. B., 92, *103*
Corman, H., 370, *382*
Corsaro, M., 339, 344, *349*
Coyaji, B., 361, *366*
Coyaji, K., 361, *366*
Coyne, J., 92, *102*
Cozzarelli, C., 28–29, *55*, 88–90, 93, 95, 97, 100, *102–103*, 223, *231*, 239, 265, 276, *283*, *350*
Craig, B. H., 25, 47–49, 52, *55*
Creinin, M. D., 190, 195, *208*
Cunningham, P. C., 29, 32, *55*
Cvejic, H., 287–288, *296*

Dagg, P., 342–343, 346, *349*
Damon, L., *230*
Daniels, J. A., 122, *128*
Danoff-Burg, S., 303, *328*
Darabi, K. F., 145, *152*

Darney, P. D., 190, *208*
David, H. P., xiv, *xiv*, xx, *xxix*, *54*, *102*, 149, *154*, 194–195, *208*, 228, *264*, *296*, 349, 361, *364*, 374, *382*
Davila, G., 293, *297*
Davis, A., 120, *128*
Davis, R. C., 221, *229*
Davis, W., 290, *297*
de Castro, L., 167, *182*
DeCrow, K., 275, *283*
Del Pinal, J. H., 110, *127*
DeMaso, D. R., 289, *297*
Denious, J. E., 223–224, *232*
Derogatis, L. R., 90, 93, *102*
Derr, M. K., 273, *283*
Des Jarlais, D., 217, *232*
Devins, N., 27, *55*
Diaz, A., 139, *152*
Diaz-Briquets, S., 148, *153*
Diggins, M., 271, *283*
Diggory, P., 167, *184*
Djerassi, C., 177, *183*
Doe v. Bolton, 3, *23*
Dominowski, R. L., 334, *349*
Donovan, J., 29, *55*
Donovan, P., 87, *102*, 358, *364*
Dugger, K., 109–110, 113, *128*
Duncan, M., *229*
Dwar, M. H., 194, *209*

Eckel, S., 28, 34, *55*
Edelman, D. A., 360, *364*
Editorial, 361, *365*
Eilenberg, J., *229*
Eisen, M., 95, *103*
Eisenberg, L., 114–117, *128*, 170, 177, *182*
Eisinger, S. H., 190, *208*
Eisman, S., 292, *298*
Elliot Institute, 27, *55*, 227, *229*
Ellis, A., 305–306, *326*
Ellis, A. P., 303, *328*
Ellis, E. M., 215, *229*
Emerson, M. R., 287, 291, *298*
Emery, G., 309, *326*
Emmanuel, S. C., 165, *182*
Epner, J. E., 375, *382*
Erhardt, C. L., 139, *152*
Erickson, P. I., 139, 147, *152–153*
Esposito, C. L., 36, 47, *55*

Faria, G., 335–336, 346, *350*
Farley, C., 27, *55*
Fawcett, J. T., xiii, *xiv–xv*
Federal Bureau of Investigation, 213, *230*
Feingold, L., *234*
Fennelly, K., 138, 146, *152*
Fergusson, D. M., 216, *230*
Feringa, B., 121, *128*
Ferree, M. M., 38, *56*, 109–110, 112–113, 124, *129*
Fielder, E. P., 138, *152*
Figueira-McDonough, J., 276, *283*
Fine, D., 217, *229*
Finkelhor, D., 216–217, 220, *230*
Finken, L., 290, *296*
Fiore, J., 92, *103*
Fischoff, B., 290, *297*
Fisher, E. R., 226, *230*
Fisher, S., 342, *350*
Fitzgerald, L., *231*
Flavier, J. M., 168, *182*
Flitcraft, A., 215, *233*
Flowers, M. J., 41, *55*
Forero, J., 87, *103*
Forest, J. D., 354, 363, *364*
Forrest, J., xix, *xxix*
Forrest, J. D., 28, 46–47, *55*, 59, 83, 87, *103*, 120, *130*, 137, *153*, 155, 285, 292, *298*
Forsythe, A. B., *229*
Forsythe, C. D., 29, 32, *55*
Foster, V., 292, *296–297*
Francke, L. B., 342, *350*
Francoeur, R. T., 271, *283*
Franks, F., 190, *208*
Freedman, M. A., 360, *364*
Freeman, E. W., 33, *55*, 239, *264*
Frejka, T., 147–148, *152*
Freudenberg, N., 276, *283*
Fried, L. W., 215, *228*
Fried, M. G., 38, *55*, 119–121, 123, 127, *128*, 362, *364*
Friedman, J. S., 138, *154*
Friedman, P., 217, *232*
Friedrich, W. N., 220, *230*
Frieze, I. H., 214, 226, *230*
Fuegen, K., 93, *102*
Fullilove, M., *229*
Furstenberg, F. F., Jr., 280, *283*

Gaa, J. P., 336, *352*

Gamble, V. N., 119, *128*
Gameau, B., 302, *326*
Gan, D., 174, 176, *182*
Gannon, K., 342, *350*
Gardner, R. W., 180, *182*
Gardner, W., 290, *297*
Garrity, J. M., 196, 207–208, 302–304, 324, *326*
Gay, D., 38, *57*, 112–113, 124, *129*
Gazmararian, J. A., 215–216, *230*
Gelles, R., 215, *230*
George, L. K., 215, *230*
Gerardo, M., 146, *153*
Gershenson, H. P., 220–221, *230*
Gerson, K., 124, *128*
Giachello, A., 372, *382*
Gibb, G. D., 304, *326*, 348, *350*
Gilbert, S., 27, *56*
Gillett, P., 335, *349*
Gillette, L. S., 139, *152*
Gilovich, T., 258, *265*
Ginsburg, F. D., 30, 32, *55*
Glei, D., 214, *230*
Glendon, M. A., 48, *56*
Gold, D., 335, *349*
Gold, E. M., 139, *152*
Gold, R. B., 373–374, *382*
Golding, J. M., *229*
Goldscheider, C., 147, *152*
Goldsmith, S., 293, *297*
Gonda, T. A., 339, 343, 345, *350*
Gondolf, E., 226, *230*
Goodkind, D., 166–167, *182*
Goodman, K. A., *366*
Goodman, L. A., 211, 214, 227, *230–231*
Goodman, L. M., 335, *350*
Gordon, L., 26, 31, 34–35, 38, 44, *56*, 110, 115–116, *128*
Gorsuch, R. L., 240, *265*
Gough, H., xii, *xv*
Grambsch, P., *230*
Granberg, B., 110, *129*
Granberg, D., 110, *128–129*
Gray, V., 110, *128*
Green, J. C., 85, *103*
Greene, B., 303, *326*
Greenslade, F., 357, 363, *364*
Griffin-Carlson, M. S., 291, *297*
Grimes, D. A., 61, 80, 190, 194–195, *208*
Grossman, G., 287, *296*, 342, *349*

Grossman, M., 370, *382*
Gschneidinger, E., 48, *58*
Guest, F., *153*
Gump, P., 113, *129*
Gurel, L., 140, *153*
Guth, J. L., 85, *103*
Guthrie, D., 216, *234*

H. Rep. No. 101–392, 8, *23*
Haas-Wilson, D., 362, *365*
Hachamovitch, M., 287, 296, 342, *349*
Hafez, E. S., 340, *350*
Haji, S., 263, *265*
Hakim-Elahi, E., 356, *364*
Hall, A., 360, *365*
Hall, E., 109–110, 112–113, 124, *129*
Hall, E. J., 38, *56*
Halvorson-Boyd, G., 303, 325, *326*
Hardee-Cleaveland, K., 165–166, *182*
Harding, S., 110, *129*
Harris, R., 110, *127*
Harris, T. R., 218, *233*
Harrison, M., 27, *56*
Hart, L. G., 354, 366, 370, *382*
Hartmann, B., 115–116, *129*
Harvey, M. R., 215, *231*
Harvey, S. M., 193, 196–197, 199, 207–208
Hass, P. H., 149, *153*
Hastie, R., 337, *350*
Hatcher, R. A., 150, *153*
Hatcher, S., 287–288, *297*
Hausknecht, R. U., 190, *208*
Hawaii Department of Health, 170, *182*
Hawks, B., 158, 163, 169, *182*
Health Action Information Network, 159, 168, *182–183*
Healy, A. F., 334, *349*
Hee, S., 162, *184*
Heilig, S., 361, *365*
Hein, D., *229*
Heinrich, J. F., *350*
Heise, L., 212, 217, *230–231*
Helton, A., 215, *231*
Hemsell, D. L., 215, *233*
Henderson, V., 357, *364*
Henshaw, R., 263, *265*
Henshaw, R. C., 371, *382*
Henshaw, S. K., xix, *xxix,* 28, 36–37, 41, 43, *55–56,* 62–67, 71–73, 75, 77, 80, 81, 83–84, 86–88,

103, 120, 122, *129,* 133, 136–137, 142, 147–148, *153,* 169, *183,* 285, 287, 291, 296, 297, 354, 362, *365*
Hern, W., 322, 326, 341, *350*
Hern, W. M., 92, 97–98, *103*
Heslet, L., 214, *231*
Hewitt, S. K., *230*
Hildebrand, J., 303, *326*
Hildebrandt, K., 302, *327,* 331, *350*
Hillard, P. J., 216, *231*
Himmelstein, J., 86, *103*
Hirsch, M. B., 287, 291, *298*
Ho, B., 175, 178, *183*
Hoffman, E., 303, *327*
Holck, J. C., 138, *154*
Hollerbach, P. E., 147–148, *153–154*
Hollis, H. M., 36, *56*
Holmes, M. M., 213, *231*
Holmstrom, L. L., 215, *229*
Holzapfel, S., 214, *231*
Hong, S., 164, *183*
Honigman, B., 293, *297*
Horn, J. D., 46–47, *58,* 285, 222, *233,* 298
Horobin, G., 340, *350*
Horowitz, M., 240, *265, 266*
Horwood, L. J., 216, *230*
Houck, J. A., 119, *128*
Houskamp, B. M., 215, *232*
Howard, M., *382*
Huang, S. M., 165, *183*
Huber, J. J., 48, *56*
Hull, G. T., 29, *56*
Hull, J. E., 87, *103*
Hunter, A., 110, *128*
Hyde Amendment, *129*

Ichovics, J. R., 304, *327*
Idelson, H., 18, *23*
Iden, S., 121, *128*
Ifill, S., 124, *130*
Infante-Castañeda, C., 149, *153*
Innes, L., *229*
International Planned Parenthood Federation, 357, 359, *366*
International Programs Assistance Services, 355–356, 359, *365*
Ivins, M., 51, *56*

Jackson, J., 125–126, *129*

Jacobs, J., 290, *296*
Jacobsson, L., 335, 342, 348, *350*
Jacobziner, H., 139, *152*
Jefferson, M., 126, *129*
Jelen, T. G., 25, 55, 86, *102*, 112, *128*
Jenkins, S., 36, 56, 124, *130*
Jensen, J. M., 160, *183*
Jillson, D. A., 360, *364*
Jitsukawa, M., 177, *183*
Joffe, C., 28, *56*
Johnson, C. H., *230*
Johnson, D. P., 147, *154*
Johnson, K., 303, *327*
Jones, E. F., 137, *153*
Jones, J. M., 22, *23*, 286, 293, 295, *297*
Jöreskog, K. G., 245, *265*
Josephs, R. A., 259, *265*
Joyce, T., 138, 140, *153*

Kallail, K. J., 47, *59*
Kalton, G., 48, *58*
Kaltreider, N. B., 293, *297*
Kaminsky, B., 303, *327*
Kantorwitz-Gordon, S. B., *234*
Kaplan, C. P., 139, *153*
Kaplan, L., 25, 42, 44, *56*
Kapp, M. B., 275, *283*
Karkazis, K., 357, *365*
Karman, H., 359, *365*, 371, *382*
Karoly, P., 92, *104*
Karrasch, A., 93, *102*
Kaufman, M., 273, *283*
Kay, M. A., 147, *153*
Keeping, J. D., 341, *351*
Keita, G. P., *231*
Kellstedt, L., 85, *103*
Kelty, M. F., xiii, *xv*
Kendall-Tackett, K., 221, *231*
Kennedy, F., 114, *130*
Kenworthy, J. A., 347, *351*
Kenyon, E., 335–336, 339–344, 346–347, *350*
Kerns, D., 213, *233*
Kershaw, K. L., 216, *230*
Khan-Edrington, M., 303, *327*
Kilpatrick, D. G., 215, *231*
Kim, S. S., 190, *208*
Kimmel, M. S., 273, *283*
Kinch, R., 335, *349*
Kinch, R. A., 287, *296*

King, R. H., 137, *153*
Kirby, D., 375, *382*
Klassen, A. D., 218, *233*
Klerman, L. V., 70–71, *80*, 95, *102*
Klitenick, P., 140, *153*
Klitsch, M., 294, *297*
Kodagoda, N., 164, *183*
Kolata, G., 72, *80*
Kolbe, L., *382*
Koocher, G. P., 289, *297*
Koolin, L. M., *366*
Koonin, L., *169*
Koonin, L. M., 36, *56*, 64, *80*, 133, 136, *153*, 285–286, *297*
Koop, C. E., 8, *23*, 235, *265*
Korzeniowsky, C., 339, 344, *349*
Koss, M. P., 211, 214–215, 217, *230–231*
Koss, P. G., 214, 217, *231*
Kost, K., xix, *xxix*, 291, *297*
Koufacos, C., 347, *351*
Koverola, C., *230*
Kowal, D., *153*
Kravitz, A., 95, *104*
Krishnan, V., 36, *56*
Kulczycki, A., 361, *365*
Kurth, A., 150–151, *153*
Kwa, S. B., 165, *182*

Lacay, R., 271, *283*
Lader, L., 26–27, 40, 51, *56*
Lalwani, A., 358, *365*
Lang, R. A., *230*
Larrick, R. P., 259, *265*
Lau, O. W. K., 194, *209*
Laufer, D., *234*
Lee, F. R., 121, 125–126, *129*
Leege, D. C., *59*
Lehman, D., 92, *102*
Lehman, S., 92, *104*
Lemkau, J. P., 94, *103*, 335, 340, *350*
Leonard, A., 357, *364*
Lerner, D., 357, *365*
Lewin, T., 28, *56*, 118, *129*
Lewis, C. C., 292, *297*
Lewis, S. Y., 304, 307, *327*
Lewit, S., 26, *59*
Li, P. Q., *183*
Li, V. C., 165, *183*
Lieberman, D., 358, *365*

Lieh-Mak, F., 165, *183*
Lin-Fu, J. S., 158, 163, 169, *183*
Ling, S. L., 165, *182*
Linn, M. W., 140, *153*
Linstedt, S., 87, *103*
Lipper, I., 287, *296*
Littlewood, T. B., 114, 116–117, *129*
Liu, W. T., 169, *185*
Loader, B., 304, *327*, 331, *350*
Loftus, E. F., 334, *349*
Lombardo, L. H., 31, *54*
Ludwig, J., 49, *58*
Luker, K., 31, 34, 40, 44, 56, 82, 85, 98,
    103, 110, 113, 125, *129*, 269,
    272, 274, 283, 322, *327*
Lunneborg, P., 33, *56*
Lushene, R. E., 240, *265*
Lynxwiler, J., 38, *57*, 112–113, 119–120,
    124, *129*

Mackin, K. J., 291, *297*
MacNair, R., 273, *283*
Macro International, 168, *183*
Madsen, R., 271, *283*
Madsen v. Women's Health Center, 17,
    23
Magee, V., *230*
Maine, D., 357, *365*
Major, B., 28–29, *54–55*, 88–90, 93, 95,
    97, 100, *102–103*, 223, *231*, 239,
    265, 276–277, *283*, 302, 304,
    327, 331, 339, 342, 346, *350*
Major, B. N., *102*, 228, 264, 296, 349,
    374, *382*
Maloy, K., 47, *57*
Malveaux, J., 115, 125, *129*
Man, V. D., 166–167, *181*, *184*
Maracek, J., 22, *23*
Margolis, A., 293, *297*
Marin, B. V., 146, *153*
Marks, F., 301, 328, 354, *366*
Marks, J. S., 230, *366*
Marsiglio, W., 270, 273–274, 276, 278–
    279, 283–284, 336, *350*
Martin, J. A., 161, 170–171, *183*
Martins, R., 214, *231*
Martorana, S., 139, *152*
Mathews, S. A., 309, *327*
Mattis, R., 354, 366, 370, *382*
Mayer, K., *234*
McAll, K., 344, *350*

McFarlane, J., 215, *231–232*
McGraw, R. K., 339–342, 344, 346, *350*
McKeachie, W. J., xii, *xv*
McKee, K., 358, *365*
McLouth, G., 274, *284*
Medical and psychological impact of abor-
    tion, 8, *23*
Medvee, V. H., 258, *265*
Meichenbaum, D., 306, *327*
Melendy, H. B., 159–160, *183*
Mellers, B. A., 48, *57*
Mellman, L., *229*
Melton, G. B., 22, *23*, 292, *297*
Menaghan, E., 278–279, 283–284, 336,
    350
Merrick, J. C., 40, 42, *57*
Mertus, J. A., 27, *57*
Meyerding, J., 217, *232*
Millard, R. J., 304, 326, 348, *350*
Miller, B., *382*
Miller, J. B., 207, *208*
Miller, J. E., 47, *57*
Miller, P. G., 47, *57*
Miller, W., 331–333, 336, 345, *351*
Miller, W. B., 235–237, 237, 239, 261,
    265
Mishell, D. R., 194, *208*
Mohr, J., 43, *57*
Mohr, J. C., 360, *365*
Molina, C. W., 133–134, 146, *154*
Moore, K. A., 31, *57*
Moore, K. S., 214, *232*
Moore, P. J., 290, *296*
Moraga, C., 29, *57*
Morris, K. T., 220, *228*
Morris, L., 363, *366*
Morris, T. M., 36, *56*
Morrison, J., 341, *351*
Morrow, E., 362, *365*
Mosher, W. D., 147, *152*, *154*, 214, *228*
Muecke, M. A., 159, *183*
Mueller, P. M., 302, 304, *327*, 331, *350*
Mukai, T., 215, *231*
Murray, J., 193, *207*
Musick, J. S., 221, 230, *232*
Myers, S. C., 137, *153*

Nagy, M. C., 217, *232*
Nagy, S., 217, *232*
Naji, S. A., 263, *265*, 371, *382*
Najman, J. M., 341, *351*

Namerow, P. B., 145, *152, 154*
Naranjo-Huebl, L., 273, *283*
Nasman, V. T., 91, 99, *103*
National Abortion and Reproductive
    Rights Action League Founda-
    tion, 79, 80
National Abortion Federation, 304, *327*
National Asian Women's Health Organi-
    zation, 161, 180, *183*
National Center for Health Statistics, 66,
    79, 80
National Center for Men, 275, *284*
National Council of Negro Women,
    178–179, *183*
National Institute of Child Health and
    Human Development, 171, *184*
National Organization for Women, Inc.
    v. Scheidler, 17, *23*
National Research Council, 363, *365*
National Victim Center, 213, *232*
Nelson, F., 139, *154*
Nelson, F. G., 139, *152*
Ness, M., 303, *327*
Neubardt, S., 340, *351*
Neumann, D. A., 215, *232*
New York Times, 25, *39*
Newcomb, M., 221, *234*
Newman, R., 274, *284*
Newman, S. H., xiii, *xv*
Ng, S., 165, *183*
Nhan, V. Q., 166, *181*
Nisbett, R. E., 259, *265*
Noonan, J. T., 42, *57*
Nord, C. W., 214, *232*
Norfleet, M. A., 301, *326*, 331, 340, *349*
Notgrass, C. M., 216, *234*
Notman, M., 95, *104*
Novick, L. F., 360, *364*
Nsiah-Jefferson, L., 119, 121–122, 124,
    129
Nuñez-Fernández, L., 146, 149, *154*
Nuttall, E. V., 140, *154*

O'Brien, D. M., 25, 47–49, 52, *55*
O'Connor, B., 41, *55*
O'Connor, B. P., 339, *349*
O'Connor, S., *54*
O'Keeffe, J. E., 22, *23*, 286, 293, 295,
    297
O'Leary, V. E., 304, *327*
Olley, P. C., 339, *351*

Ong, P., 162, *184*
Ortiz, C. G., 140, *154*
Osofsky, H. J., 95, *103–104*, 287, 297,
    336, 340, 346, *351*
Osofsky, J. D., 95, *103–104*, 287, 297,
    336, 340, 346, *351*
Ovalle, B., 139, *152*

Padilla, A. M., 146, *153*
Page, S., 347, *352*
Palmer, E. A., 18, *23*
Panzer, P., *229*
Paone, D., 217, *232*
Parducci, A., 48, *57*
Park, M., 195, *208*
Parker, B., 215, *231–232*
Parker, J., 139, *154*
Pasta, D. J., 237, *265*
Patterson, M. J., 47, *57*
Pavich, E. G., 146, *154*
Paxman, J. M., 147–149, *154*
Payne, E., 95, *104*
Payne, R., 34, *57*
Payne, W., 48, *56*
Peel, J., 167, *184*
Pennington, N., 337, *350*
Peppers, L. G., 336, 339, 343–346, *351*
Petchesky, R. P., 26, 30–33, 38, 43, *57*,
    86, *104*, 110, 114, 117, *129*
Petersen, J., 293, *297*
Peterson, J. L., 214, *232*
Peterson, L., 214, *228*
Philliber, S. G., 145, *152, 154*
Phipps-Yonas, S., 292, *297*
Piccinino, L., 214, *228*
Pick de Weiss, S., 149, *154*
Pierson, V. H., 294, *297*
Pinderhughes, E., 304, *327*
Pines, D., 331, *351*
Ping, T., 165, *184*
Piotrowski, C., 335, 339, *349*
Planned Parenthood of Central Missouri
    v. Danforth, 270, *284*
Planned Parenthood of New York City,
    325, *327*
Planned Parenthood of Southeastern
    Pennsylvania v. Casey, 271, *284*
Pliner, A. J., 286, 292–293, *297*
Plutzer, E., 113, *129*, 278, *284*
Poettegen, H., 302, *327*
Policar, M. S., *153*

Pollock, V. E., 215, *232*
Polonko, K., 273, *284*
Pope, L., 212, 222–224, *233*
Population Council, 192, *208*
Potts, M., 167, *184*, 359, 361, 362, *365*,
    371, *382*
Powell-Griner, E., 124, *130–131*
Pratt, W. P., 216, *233*
Presser, S., 49, *58*
Prewitt, T. J., 28, *54*
Puto, C., 48, *56*

Qiu, S.-H., *183*
Quadrel, M. J., 290, *297*

Radford, B., 370, *382*
Rajan, R., 95, *103–104*
Ramachandran, P., 164, *184*
Ramick, M., 133, *153*, 286, *297*
Ramirez de Arellano, A. B., 148, *154*
Randall, T., 214, *232*
Ransom, W. F., 360, *365*
Rappaport, J., 290, 292–293, *296*
Ratnam, S. S., 335, *352*
Raymond, E., 291, *298*
Reagan, R., *8*
Reardon, D. C., 27, *57*, 88, *104*, 227,
    232
Redmond, P., 120–121, 123, *129*
Rees, M., 118, *129*
Reeves, J., 28, *57*
Register, C. A., 137, *155*
Reinholtz, C., 217, *232*
Reitzes, D. C., 281, *283*
Remez, L., 363, *365*
Remsburg, R. E., 360, *364*
*The Report of the International Conference
    on Population and Development*, xi,
    xv
Reproductive Health Technologies Pro-
    ject, 191–192, *208*
Resick, P. A., 215, *232*
Resnick, H. S., 213, *231*
Resnick, M. D., 291–292, 296, *298*
Richards, C., 90, *103*, 223, *231*
Rickel, A. U., 216, 220, *229*
Rieker, P. P., 221, *229*
Riger, S., 207, *208*, 373, *382*
Rivera, M. J., 330, 333, 335–337, 345,
    348, *351*

Rizo, A., 147, *154*
Robbins, J. M., 339, *351*
Roberts, D. E., 121–122, *130*, 375, *382*
Robey, B., 180, *182*
Robinson, M., 28, *57*
Rochat, R. W., 138–139, *154*
Rodman, H., 114, *130*, 294, *298*
Rodrigue, J. M., 123, *130*
Roe v. Wade, xii, *xv*, 3, 22, 23, 25, *57*,
    124, *130*, 145, *154*, 270, 282,
    284, 301, 327, 341, *351*
Roger, L., 334, *349*
Rogers, R. R., 31, *59*
Romans-Clarkson, S. E., 302, *327*
Rook, K. S., 92, *104*
Rooks, J., 293, *298*
Roosa, M. W., 217–220, *232*
Rosen, A. S., 194, 199, *208*
Rosen, H., 341, *351*
Rosenberg, D., *230*
Rosenberg, M., 240, *265*
Rosenblatt, R. A., 354, 366, 370, *382*
Rosenblum, M., 51, *54*
Rosenfield, A., 121, *128*, 301, 328, 354,
    361, *365–366*
Ross, L. J., 117, 119, 123–125, *130*
Rossi, A. S., 35, *58*, 145, 147, *154*
Roth, S., *54*
Roth, S. H., 102, 228, 264, 296, 349,
    374, *382*
Rothblum, E. D., 304, *328*
Rovinsky, J. J., 341, *351*
Rovner, J., 9, *23*
RU486 transforming the abortion debate,
    192, *208*
Ruark, J. E., 339, 343, 345, *350*
Rubin, E. A., 25, *58*
Rubino, K. K., *230*
Ruch-Ross, H. S., *230*
Rue, V., 302, *328*
Rue, V. M., 239, *265*, 286, *298*, 339–
    340, 342–344, *351*
Ruehlman, L. S., 92, *104*
Ruggs, D., *382*
Russell, D., 221, *232*
Russell, I. T., 371, *382*
Russell, L., 263, *265*
Russo, N., 322, *327*
Russo, N. F., 22, 23, 31–33, 43, 46–47,
    54, *58*, 102, 211–212, 215–217,
    222–225, 227–228, 228, 230,

Russo, N. F. (*continued*)
    231–233, 256, 264–265, 285,
    296, 298, 349, 374, 382
Rust v. Sullivan, 9, 23
Ruth, S., 39, 58
Ryan, B., 278, 284
Ryder, N., 335, 352
Ryff, C. D., 94, 104

Sachdev, P. I. P. S, 163–164, 184
Saftlas, A. F., 213, 233
Saltzman, L. E., 212, 215, 229–230, 233
San Miguel, V. V., 217, 229
San, P. B., 166, 181
Sandler, H., 54
Santelli, J. S., 217, 233
Santos, R. A., 180, 184
Sarvis, B., 114, 130
SAS Institute, Inc., 240, 265
Sasao, T., 171, 184
Satin, A. J., 215, 233
Scanzoni, J., 271, 273, 284
Schaff, E., 190, 208
Scheidler, J. M., 88, 104
Scheirer, M. F., 302, 328
Scherer, D., 290, 297
Schneider, W., 15, 23
Schnicke, M. R., 215, 232
Schulder, D., 114, 130
Schulman, H., 340, 351
Schuman, H., 48, 58
Schur, E. M., 35, 58
Schwartz, R., 46, 58, 222, 233, 285, 298
Schwartz, R. A., 43, 58
Schwarz, N., 48, 58
Sciacchitano, A., 350
Scott, J., 48, 58
Scott, J. R., 118, 121, 130
Scott, P. B., 29, 56
Scrimshaw, S. C. M., 147–148, 152, 154
Sears, D. O., 113, 130
Seipp, C., 148, 154
Senanayake, P., 164, 183
Seng, L., 274, 284
Senturia, A. G., 341–342, 351
Serbanescu, F., 363, 366
Serpe, R. T., 281, 284
Serrano, R. A., 84, 104
Sessions, D. N., 137, 155
Shain, R. N., 237, 265
Shannon, F. T., 216, 230
Shapiro, T., 114, 116–117, 130

Shaw, G., 370, 382
Shecter, L. A., 303, 327
Shedlin, M. G., 147, 154
Shehan, C., 274, 276, 284
Sherman, J., 347, 351
Sherrod, K., 54
Shibata, K., 163, 184
Shifman, P., 271, 276, 284
Shinn, M., 92, 104
Short, L., 382
Shostak, A. B., 274, 276–280, 284
Shrader-Cox, E., 146, 154
Siegel, J. M., 229
Silverman, J., 37, 56, 133, 136–137, 153
Simmons, P. D., 34–37, 58
Simon, A., 221, 231
Simon, H., 341–342, 351
Sitaraman, B., 31, 37, 40–41, 44, 50, 58,
    145, 147, 154
Skinner, L. J., 215, 229
Slusser, M. M., 220, 233
Small, S. A., 213, 233
Smidt, C. E., 85, 103
Smith, B., 29, 56, 125, 130
Smith, H. B., xiii, xv
Smith, H. L., 165, 184
Smith, J. C., 36, 56, 64, 80, 133, 138,
    153–154, 169, 183, 285–286,
    297
Smith, P. C., 180, 182
Soeken, K., 215, 231–232
Solheim, F., 335, 350
Solinger, R., 115–118, 130
Solomon, L. J., 304, 328
Sonenstein, F., 382
Sörbom, D., 245, 265
Sorenson, S. B., 213, 229, 233
Speckhard, A., 302, 328, 339–340, 342–
    344, 351
Speckhard, A. C., 239, 265, 286, 298
Spielberger, C. D., 240, 265
Spira, A., 194, 207
Spitz, A. M., 362, 366
Sprinthall, N. A., 292, 296–297
Staggenborg, S., 29, 58
Stanescu, A., 363, 366
Stanton, A., 303, 328
Stark, E., 215, 233
Stark, P., 291, 298
Stark, T., 292, 296
Steele, C. M., 259, 265
Stein, J. A., 229

Steiner, G. Y., 3, 7, *23*
Steinhoff, P. G., 149, *154*
Stetson, D. M., 271, *284*
Stevans, L. K., 137, *155*
Stewart, F., *153*
Stewart, G. K., *153*
Stief, T. M., 31, *57*
Stone, I. C., 215, *233*
Stone-Joy, S., 336, *342–346, 351*
Stotland, N. L., 295, 298, 339, 341, *351*
Strack, F., 48, *58*
Straus, M. A., 222, *233*
Strauss, L. T., *366*
Strothers, E., 126, *130*
Stryker, S., 281, *284*
Stupp, P., 363, *366*
Sullivan, W. M., 271, *283*
Summary and recommendations: Eliminating sexist treatment, 347, *351*
Sun, J. H., *183*
Surgeon General's Workshop on Violence, 215, *233*
Swenson, I. E., 167, *184*
Swidler, A., 271, *283*
Szafran, R. F., 36, *58*

Tadiar, A. F., 167–168, *184*
Taeuber, C., 124, *130*
Takenaka, C., 170, *184*
Takeuchi, D. T., 163, *185*
Tam, Y. K., 165, *183*
Tang, G. W., 194, *209*
Tanjasiri, S. P., 163, 171–173, *173, 175–177, 184*
Tay, G. E., 335, *352*
Taylor, F., 357, *365*
Teachman, J., 273, *284*
Tein, J., 217, *232*
Telles, C. A., *229*
Templeton, A., 263, *265*
Templeton, A. A., 371, *382*
Tentoni, S. C., 339, *351*
Teri, L., 347, *352*
Testa, M., 276, *283, 350*
Tester, M., 290, *297*
Thang, N. M., 166, 167, *181, 184*
Theriot, S., 215, *233*
Thomas, S., 111–112, 114, 124, *131*
Thompson, J. J., *59*
Thompson, L., 273, *284*
Thompson, V. D., xiii, *xv*

Thong, K. J., 194, *209*
Tienda, M., 138, 146, *152*
Tietze, C., xx, *xxix*, 26, 59, 370, *382*
Tipton, S. M., 271, *283*
Torres, A., 46–47, 59, 120, *130*, 137, *155*, 285, 292, 298
Trad, P. V., 337, *352*
Trent, K., 124, *130–131*
Tribe, L. H., 30, 51, *59*
Tribe, L. W., 3, *23*
Trinh, P., 167, *184*
Tromp, S., 47, *58*
Trussell, J., *153*
Tschann, J. M., 290, *296*
Tsoi, W. F., 335, *352*
Tuan, C., 164–165, *184*
Turell, S. C., 336, *338–343, 345–346, 352*
Turner, P. A., 114, *131*

U.S. Bureau of the Census, 78, 80, 158, *161–163, 185*
U.S. Immigration and Naturalization Service, 159, 161, *185*
Uba, L., 159, *184*
Ullman, S. E., 221, *233*
United Nations Population Fund, 166, *184*
Urdaneta, M. L., 138, *155*

Valdisera, V., 124, *130*
Van Vort, J., 62, 65–67, 80, 81, 84, *87–88, 103, 120, 129, 296, 297, 354, 365*
Velebil, P., *366*
Velentgas, P., *234*
Veronen, L. J., 215, *231*
Victor, K., 8, *24*
Vietze, P., *54*
Vittinghoff, E., 190, *208*
Vogeltanz, N. D., 218, *233*
Von Knorring, K., 194, *208*
von Schoultz, B., 335, *350*

Waisberg, J., 347, *352*
Walbert, D. F., 27, *54*
Walker, J., 114, *130*
Wallace, S. P., 163, *184*

Wallin, C., 87, 97, *104*
Walling, A. D., 47, *59*
Walters, J., 113, *131*
Walters, M. F., 271, *284*
Walzer, S., *59*, 276, *284*
Wang, L. C., 159, *185*
Warren, C. W., 138, *154*
Warren, M. A., *59*
Watson, W. L., 27, *55*
Wattleton, F., 124–126, *128*, 362, *366*
Webb, N., 140, *153*
Webster v. Reproductive Health Services, 4, *24*, *131*
Weiner, J. P., 347, *352*
Weisbord, R. G., 114, 116–117, *131*
Welch, M. R., *59*
Welch, S., 38, *54*, 108–110, 113, *128*
Welter, B., 30, *59*
Wendel, G. D., 215, *233*
Westfall, J. M., 47, *59*
Westhoff, C., 301, *328*, 354, 356, 358, *366*
Westoff, C. F., 335, *352*
Wetstein, M. E., 29, 34, 36–38, 45, 47, *59*
White, J., 220–221, *233*
Wilcox, B. L., 21, *24*
Wilcox, C., 25, 38–39, *55*, *59*, 86, *102*, 110–112, 114, 124–125, *128*, *131*
Wilkinson, G. S., 217, *229*
Wille, R., 276, *283*
Willets, I., 217, *232*
Williams, G., 341, *351*
Williams, L. B., 147, *154*, 216, *233*
Williams, N., 146, *155*
Williams, R. M., Jr., 25, *59*
Willie, C., 114, *131*
Wilmoth, G. H., 21, *24*, 285, 298, 338–339, 341–342, *352*
Wilner, N., 240, *265*, *266*
Wilsnack, S. C., 218, *233*

Wilson, J. B., 337, *352*, *366*
Wilson, M., 119–120, *129*
Wilson, W., 344, *350*
Winfield, I., 215, *230*
Wingo, P., *366*
Winikoff, B., 193–194, 199, 209, 361–362, *366*
Winkler, J., 357, *364*
Wolchik, S. A., 92, *104*
Wolfe, V., *230*
Women of Color Partnership Program, 120, *131*
Wong, G. C., *183*
Wong, N. W., 92, *104*
Woodruff, W. J., 214, 217, *231*
World Health Organization, 353, *366*
Wortman, C., 92, *102*
Wright, L. S., 31, *59*
Wyatt, G., 374, *382*
Wyatt, G. E., *54*, *102*, 216–217, 220–221, 228, *234*, 264, 296, 349

Yates, S., 286, 292–293, *297*
Yip, P., 194, *209*
Young, K. N. J., 163, *185*
Yu, E. S. H., 169, *185*

Zabin, L., 287–288, 294, *298*
Zabin, L. S., 291, *382*
Zahniser, S. C., *230*
Zane, N. W. S., 163, *185*
Zelles, P., 278, *284*
Zellman, G., 95, *103*
Zierk, K., 256, *265*, 322, *327*
Zierk, K. L., 46, *58*, 215–216, 224–225, *233*
Zierler, S., 217, 220, *234*
Zubek, J., 90, *103*
Zubek, J. M., 223, *231*
Zuckerman, B., 215, *228*

SUBJECT INDEX

Abortifacients, 360–361
Abortion
  as black genocide, 114–115, 125
  as medical decision, 44
  as moral issue, 26
  occurrence, xix
  in 19th century, 40
Abortion clinics
  blockades, 83
  fake, 27
  harassment strategy, 28
  picketing, 28, 76
Abortion experience, 330–348
  conceptor's effect on women's posta-
    bortion responses, 342–343
  contraceptive decision making, 334–
    335
  decision making, 335–336
  guilt, 345
  link among phases, 345–347
  mourning after, 343–345
  partners' and others' involvement in
    decision, 336–338
  postabortion reaction, 339–342
  postabortion response, 338–339
  postabortion syndrome, 341–342
  pregnancy acknowledgment phase,
    330–333
  pregnancy resolution phase, 334
  as therapeutic issue, 348
  therapist bias, 347–348
Abortion index, 136
Abortion neutral amendment, 5–6
Abortion rate, 136
  black women, 107
  decline, 63–69
    loss of providers, 66–67
    reasons for, 65–66
  Latinas
    education and, 144
    in Latin America, 147–148
  by state, 64–65
  worldwide, 362–363
Abortion ratio, 136
Abortion services
  acceptability, 378–379

  improving, 371–373
  availability, 378–379
  isolation from mainstream medical
    care, 77
Abortion use, racial differences in, 124
Access to abortion services, 61–79
  availability, 66–67
  barriers to
    appointment availability, 72–73
    cost, 73–75, 78
    distance, 70–71
    gestation limits, 71–72
    harassment, 75–77
  improving, 353–364, 370–371
    decentralization of services using
      manual vacuum aspiration, 358–
      360
    implications of restrictive legislation
      and laws, 362–363
    integrating training into existing
      curricula, 355–357
    new technologies, 360–362
    training of nonphysicians, 357–358
Access to health care, black women, 121
Acting as if, 310
Activism, black women, 122–124
Adolescents, 285–296
  birth rate, with older partners, 214
  consulting with their parents, 291
  decision making, 289–294
  differences in reasoning ability, 292
  factors that predict competence, 293
  Hawaiian, birth rate, 170
  Latinas
    childbearing, 134
    ever-pregnant, 143
  Mexican American, 139
  parental consent requirements, 286,
    293–294
    adverse effects, 295
  pregnancy rate, 285
  psychological sequelae, 286–289
  Puerto Rican, 140
  rape incidence, 213
  sexual abuse, 217
  subsequent pregnancy, 288

Advances in Health Technology, 192
Advertising campaigns, pro-life, 28
AIDS
  impact on Latinas' abortion decisions,
    150–151
  potential of abuse, 122
Alan Guttmacher Institute, 135
  1993 Abortion Provider Survey, data
    set, 61–63
American Birth Control League, racist
    character, 115–116
American Psychological Association
  Council, approval of initial resolutions,
    xii
  Division of Population Psychology, es-
    tablishment, xiii–xiv
Anchoring-and-adjustment effects, 49
Anesthesia, availability, 75
Anger, response to anti-abortion demon-
    strators, 91, 94
Anti-abortion activities
  impact, 81–102
    effects of high personal conflict on
      response to, 95–97
    future research, 101–102
    on decision to abort, 88
    on postabortion adjustment, 92–94
    on providers, 86–88
    preabortion responses to, 90–91
    psychological effects of demonstra-
      tors, 89–97
  injunctions, 97–98
  pro-choice escorts, 98–101
  violent, 83
  who participates, 84–86
Anti-abortion organizations
  earliest, 82
  motivations to join, 85
  pro-women movement, 30
  radical, 82–83
Appropriations bill amendments
  1973–88, 6–7
  1992–96, 19–21
Asia, availability of abortion, 163–164
Asian Indians, immigration history, 160
Asian Pacific Islander Americans, 157–
    181
  abortions, 171–173
  acculturation, 174
  attitudes, 173–175
  cultural factors associated with abor-
    tion, 175–180

barriers to reproductive health care
    services, 179–180
  contraception, 176–177
  gender and family role, 178–179
  sexual health, 175–176
demographic characteristics, 164
education and income, 162–163
fertility patterns, 169–171
importance of husbands in abortion
    decisions, 178
nativity and age, 161–162
nativity and immigration history, 158–
    161
  Asian Indians, 160
  Chinese Americans, 158–159
  Filipino Americans, 159
  Pacific Islanders, 160–161
  Vietnamese Americans, 159–160
Assault, issues in abortion counseling,
    321–322
Attitudes
  of Americans, xix
  Asian Pacific Islander Americans,
    173–175
  of black women, 108–110
  black women, 124–125
  class and race, 37–39
  Latinos, 145–146
  polls, 47–48
  public, distortions, 45–46
  religious ideology, 34–37
  toward legal abortion, 31
  women's, 31–32

Bangladesh, training in manual vacuum
    aspiration, 357
Battering, 214–215
  married abortion patients, 222–223
Beliefs, core, 308
Birth control, see Contraception
Birth rate, adolescents, with older part-
    ners, 214
Black genocide, abortion as, 114–115,
    125
Black women, 107–127
  abortion rate, 107
  attitudes toward legalized abortion,
    108–110
  cultural differences hypothesis, 109–
    110
  demographic hypothesis, 108–109

differences in religiosity, 110–112
generational versus life cycle explanations, 112–114
impact of racism on reproductive lives, 108
political agenda and activism, 122–124
reproductive technologies and, 115–119
struggle for reproductive rights, 119–122
Bray v. Alexandria Women's Health Clinic, 16
Butyric acid, chemical attacks, 84

Catholic Church
Latinas' attitudes and, 148–149
opposition to abortion, 35
Catholics, pro-choice, 35
Centers for Disease Control and Prevention, 135
Cesarean deliveries, coerced, 122
Chemical attacks, 84
Child abuse
childspacing intervals and, 47
incidence in married abortion patients, 224
sexual, 217–218, 220
Childbearing
ability to time, space, and limit, 46–47
nonmarital, 66
Children
rape incidence, 213
unwanted, negative effects, xx
Child-spacing intervals, child abuse and, 47
Child support, if a woman makes unilateral decision, 275
China, abortion, 165–166
Chinese Americans, immigration history, 158–159
Christian Reconstructionism, 86–88
Civil Rights of Infants Act, 11
Civil Rights Restoration Act, 5–6
Class, attitudes and, 37–39
Clergy Consultation Service, 30
Clinton, President William, executive orders, 14
Cognitive theory, 305
Colored Women's Club Movement, 123

Competence
definition, 289
factors that predict, 293
Comstock Clean-Up Act of 1996, 18–19
Consensual sex contract, 272
Constitutional amendments
1973–88, 4–5
1992–96, 16
Contraception
Asian Pacific Islander Americans, 176–177
in China, 165
decision making, 334–335
improved use after abortion, 239
Latinas, 136–137, 148
opposition to, turn of 19th century, 38
in Philippines, 168
public acceptance, 33–34
racial issues, 117–118
reducing unintended pregnancies, 374–375
Vietnam, 167
Contract, consensual sex, 272
Controversy, xx, 25–53
beginning of human life, 41
conceptions of prenatal life, 39–42
distortion of
public attitudes, 45–46
realities of women's lives, 46–48
feminist perspectives, 29–33
government role, 39
health profession role, 42–44
other methodological issues, 48–52
pro-life agenda, 26–29
psychology's contribution, 21–22
rape as permissible reason for abortion, 212
Costs
as barrier, 73–75, 78
increased, for clinics and communities, Operation Rescue and, 87
Counseling
postprocedure, 320–321
in procedure room, 318–320
professional bias, 302–304
sexual abuse, incest, and assault issues, 321–322
techniques, 308–310
Counseling session, 302
concluding, 317–318
preabortion, 310–315

Criminalization, of abortion, toll on
    black women, 124
Crisis approach, 236, 239, 241, 247
Cuban women, abortion use, 140
Cultural context, research recommenda-
    tions, 377–378
Cultural differences, research recommen-
    dations, 377–378
Cultural differences hypothesis, 109–110
Cultural fundamentalism, 85–86

Danforth, Senator John, 5–6
Decision making, 335–336
    adolescents, 289–294
    agreement between partners, 277–278
    contraception, 334–335
    effect of relationship with partner, 336
    impact of anti-abortion activities, 88
    involvement of partner and others,
        336–338
    male authority in, 274
    sociocognition theory, 337–338
    in violent marriages, 223
Decision-making approach, 236, 239–
    241, 247
Delay laws, 24-hour mandatory, 78
Demographic hypothesis, 108–109
Department of Defense, policy on abor-
    tion, 13–14
Depression
    postabortion, 340
        impact of anti-abortion activity, 92–
        93
    reactive, 344
District of Columbia, appropriations bill
    FY90, 12–13
    FY94, 20
Doe v. Bolton, 3
Drug treatment facilities, pregnant
    women and, 121–122

Encapsulation, 31
Escorts, pro-choice, 98–101
Ethnic groups, research recommendations,
    377–378
Eugenics, 37–38, 115–116
Executive orders, President Clinton, 14

Fake abortion clinics, 27

Family, roles, Asian Pacific Islander
    Americans, 178–179
Family physicians, providing abortions,
    356–357
Family planning
    programs, foreign aid authorizations for,
        6
    support by Black community during
        1920s, 123–124
Family Welfare Visitors, 357
Fatherhood, forced, 272, 275–276
Federal Employees Health Benefits Pro-
    gram, 20
Federal financing, of abortions, 7
Feminism, definition, 29–30
Feminist
    definition, 30
    perspectives, 29–33
    pro-choice, 30, 32–33
    pro-life, 30
    reproductive agenda, 30–31
    working to promote health and quality
        of life, 376
Fetus
    pro-life constructions, 41–42
    viability, 40, 42
Filipino Americans, immigration history,
    159
Foreign aid authorizations, for family
    planning programs, 6
Foster, Henry, nomination as Surgeon
    General, 14–15
Freedom of Choice Act, 11–12

Gag rule, 10–11
Gender, roles, Asian Pacific Islander
    Americans, 178–179
Gender politics of pregnancy resolution,
    269–282
    historical context, 270–271
    ideology and interest group policies,
        271–276
    men's personal and interpersonal abor-
        tion experiences, 276–279
General Social Surveys, 45–46
Generational differences, black women's
    attitudes and, 112–114
Genocide, black, abortion as, 114–115,
    125
Gestational age, failure to define in abor-
    tion surveys, 51

Gestation limits, 71–72
  minimum, 72
Government, role in controversy, 39
Grieving, after abortion, 343–345
Guilt, 333, 345
  response to anti-abortion demonstrators, 91, 94
Gunn, Dr. David, murder, 28, 84

Harassment, as barrier, 75–77
Hatch, Senator Orrin, 4–5
Hawaiian Americans, 170
Health care
  abortion in mainstream, 370
  access to, black women, 121
Health care reforms, 17
Health professions, role in controversy, 42–44
H-HANES, 135
  estimating Latinas abortion, 140–144
Hispanic Health and Nutrition Examination Survey, see H-HANES
HIV, impact on Latinas' abortion decisions, 150–151
Hospitals, as providers, 67, 69, 77
H.R. 618, 5
Human Life Federalism Amendment, 4–5
Hyde Amendment, 120
Hyde-type amendments, 6–7, 19

Identity theory, 281
Ideologies, gender and, 271
Illegal abortions, adolescents, to avoid telling parents, 293
Illegitimacy ratio, 17–18
Illinois Policy Survey, 45
Imagery, 309
Impact of Event Scale, 266–267
Incest
  exceptions in government funding of abortion, 13
  issues in abortion counseling, 321–322
Incomplete abortion, treatment, 355, 359
Informed consent, definition, 289
Injunctions, anti-abortion activities, 97–98
Interest group politics, 271–276
Istook amendment, 19

Jericho Plan, 227
Judicial bypass, increased risk for adolescents, 293–294

Koop, C. Everett, report on health effects of abortion, 8–9

Language, as barrier to abortion and reproductive health care, 180
Late-term abortion, 18
  black women, 119–120
Latinas, 133–151
  abortion, 135–140
    Cubans, 140
    Mexican Americans, 138–139
    Puerto Ricans, 139–140
  abortion rates, in Latin America, 147–148
  age comparisons, 142–144
  birth rate, 134
  contraceptive use, 136–137, 148
  cultural perspectives, 146–149
  demographic characteristics, 141–142
  education and abortion rates, 144
  estimating abortion from H-HANES, 140–144
  impact of HIV/AIDS on abortion decisions, 150–151
Latinos
  attitudes, 145–146
  subgroups, 134
  in United States, 133–135
Lawsuits, attributing previously existing problems to abortions, 27
Learning approach, 236, 239, 241–242, 247
Legislation
  abortion-related
    1973–88, 4–8
    1989–92, 9–14
    1992–96, 15
  advocating for, 373–374
  appropriations bill amendments, 6–7, 19–21
  constitutional amendments, 4–5, 16
  19th century, 43
  parental consent, 286, 293–294
  restrictive, implications, 362–363
  statutes, 5–6

Life cycle, black women's attitudes and, 112–114
LISREL measurement model, 248–253
  changes, 252
  decision making, 250–251
  negative affect, 251–252
  stress, 248–250
LISREL structural equation model, 253–255, 259
  fit, 256
Loss approach, 236, 239, 241, 247

Madsen v. Women's Health Center, 17
Male gender role socialization, 226
Manual vacuum aspiration, 355, 357, 371
  decentralization of services by using, 358–360
Marital problems, role decision to seek abortion, 222
Maternal motivation, 333
Medicaid, exclusion of abortion, 79
Medicaid Transformations Act, 18
Medical abortion, 189–207, 360–362, 371, 378–379
  acceptability, 193–194
    international research, 194
    mifepristone, 196–204
    in U.S., 191–196
  advantages and disadvantages, 198–199
  educational and counseling materials, 372
  expectations about abortion versus experience, 203–204
  lack of knowledge and misconceptions about, 206
  public controversy, 51
  reasons for choosing, 201–202
  recommendations, 204–207
  satisfaction with, 204
  sharing experience, 203
Men
  and abortion, research agenda, 279–282
  authority in making decisions about abortion, 274
  emotional reactions to abortions, 276–277
  financially accountable for partners' unilateral decisions, 270–271
  personal and interpersonal abortion experiences, 276–279
  response to abortion, type and quality of relationship and, 279
Men's rights groups, ideology, 272
Mental health, effects of abortion, 43
Methotrexate, 190, 361, 371
Mexican American women, abortion use, 138–139, 141–144
Mifepristone, 190, 360–362, 371
  acceptability, 196–204
    focus group study, 196–199
    U.S. women's experiences, 199–204
  characteristics and history, 191–193
  delay in introduction to U.S., 191
  knowledge about, 197–198
  perceived advantages and disadvantages, 198
  see also Psychological consequences of abortion, model testing
Military facilities, abortions at, 20–21
Misoprostol, 190
Motherhood, voluntary, 30
Mourning, after abortion, 343–345

National Center for Men, 272–273
National Council of Catholic Bishops, 35
National Institutes of Health Reauthorization legislation, 16
National Longitudinal Survey, Youth Cohort, 137
National Organization for Women, Inc. v. Scheidler, 17
Negro Project, 115–116
Network support, 243–244
Neural development, prenatal, 42
Nonphysicians, training, 357–358
Norm violation approach, 236, 239, 241, 247
Norplant, as punitive and coercive measure, 118–119
Nurse midwives, performing procedures, 358

Obstetrical interventions, coerced, 122
Operation Rescue, 83
  increased costs for clinics and communities and, 87
Operation Respect, 29

Pacific Islanders, immigration history, 160–161
Pacific Islands, availability of abortion, 163–164
Parental consent legislation, 11–13, 286, 293–294
  adverse effects, 295
Partial-birth abortion, 18
Partial-Birth Abortion Ban Act of 1995, 18
Patient-centered abortion care, 301–325, 373, 379
  cognitive reframing, 305
  counseling
    concluding session, 317–318
    postprocedure, 320–321
    preabortion session, 310–315
    in procedure room, 318–320
    session, 302
    techniques, 308–310
  fears about surgery, 317
  literature review, 303–305
  preparing patient for procedure, 316–318
  principles, 306–308
  religious women, 323–324
  repeat unintended pregnancies, 322–333
  sexual abuse, incest, and assault issues, 321–322
  special situations and issues, 324
Personal conflict, high levels, effects on responses to anti-abortion demonstrators, 95–97
Personal Responsibility and Work Opportunity Act of 1996, 17
Philippines, abortion, 167–168
Physician assistants, performing procedures, 358
Physicians
  attitudes during 19th century, 43–44
  deterring from performing abortions, 27
Physician Training Program, 356
Picketing
  abortion clinics, 28, 76
  scope of activities, 82–84
Planned Parenthood of Central Missouri v. Danforth, 270
Policy, 3–22
  1989–92, 8–9
  1993–96, 14–21

appropriations bill amendments, 19–21
constitutional amendments, 16
legislation, 15
statutes, 16–19
abortion-related legislation, 1989–92, 9–14
advocating for, 373–374
appropriations bills, 1989–92, 12–14
legislation, 1973–88, 4–8
recommendations, 369–376
statutes, 1989–92, 10–12
Political agenda, black women, 122–124
Population Council, mifepristone trial, 192
Population-related workshops, history, xii–xiii
Postabortion adjustment, impact of anti-abortion activities, 92–94
Postabortion reaction, 339–342
Postabortion response, 338–339
Postabortion syndrome, 341–342
  promotion, 226–227
  risk factors, 294
Postprocedure counseling, 320–321
Preabortion counseling session, 310–315
Pregnancy
  intendedness, 331–332
  at risk for violence, 215
  unintended
    implications for violence, 225
    occurrence, xix, 216
    reducing, 374–375
    repeat, 322–333
    research recommendations, 380
  unwanted
    choices, 335
    implications for violence, 225
    repeat pattern, 304
    risk factors, 216
    wantedness, 332–333
Pregnancy acknowledgment phase, 330–333
Pregnancy rate
  abuse and, 219–220
  adolescents, 285
Pregnancy resolution phase, 334
Pregnant women, drug-addicted, 121–122
Prenatal life, conceptions of, 39–42
Prisoners, federal, access to abortion, 21
Pro-choice activism, 1960s, 44

Pro-choice escorts, anti-abortion activities impact and, 98–101
Pro-choice movement
  black advocates, 126
  contemporary, politics and racism, 119–120
  men in, 274
  white-dominated, action only when interests of white middle-class are threatened, 120
Professionals, bias, 347–348
Pro-life agenda, controversy, 26–29
Pro-life movement
  advertising campaigns, 28
  objectives, 272
Providers
  impact of anti-abortion activities, 86–88
  incorporating cultural sensitivity and linguistic competence, 372
  loss of, 66–67, 77, 87, 354
  in Philippines, 168
  types, 67–69
Psychological consequences of abortion, 235–264
  adolescents, 286–289
  discussion of results, 256–262
    acute stress response, 258–259
    decision-making approach, 259–260
    learning approach, 261
    negative affect approach, 260–261
    stress coping, 257, 259
  effects of anti-abortion demonstrators, 89–97
  factors effecting, 339
  Impact of Event Scale, 266–267
  methods, 236–245
    data analysis, 245
    data collection, 237
    design, 236
    sample, 237
    theoretical framework, 237–239
    variable measurement, 240–245
  research, clinical, and policy implications, 262–264
  results, 245–256
    independent variable total effects, 255
    individual variables, 246–248
    LISREL measurement method, 248–253
    LISREL model fit, 256

LISREL structural equation model, 253–255
  sample characteristics, 245–246
  theoretical approaches, 235–236
Psychology, contribution to abortion controversy, 21–22
Psychotherapists, bias, 347–348
Psychotherapy, see Abortion experience
Public support, for abortion, 45–46
Puerto Rican women, abortion use, 139–144

Race, attitudes and, 37–39
Racial groups, research recommendations, 378
Racism, in pro-choice movement, 119–120
Rape
  exceptions in government funding of abortion, 13
  incidence, 213
  marital, married abortion patients, 222–223
Reagan, President Ronald, anti-abortion actions, 8–9
Relationships
  effect on postabortion responses, 342–343
  social context, 338
Relief, postabortion, 340
Religiosity, differences, black women, 110–112
Religious groups
  pro-choice, 36
  pro-life, 35–36
Religious ideology, attitudes and, 34–37
Religious women, abortion counseling, 323–324
Reproductive freedom, multiracial movement, 123
Reproductive health care services, barriers to, Asian Pacific Islander Americans, 179–180
Reproductive rights affidavit, 272–273
Reproductive rights movement, 376
  black women, 119–122, 127
Reproductive technologies, 41
  black women and, 115–119
  new, 360–362
Reverse role play, 309
Right-to-life amendments, 4

Roe v. Wade, 3, 40, 270
Roussel Uclaf, 191
RU486, *see* Mifepristone
Rust v. Sullivan, 9, 10

Self-abortion
   adolescents, to avoid telling parents, 293
   Philippines, 168
Sex education, 375
Sexual abuse, 217
   children, 217–218, 220
   issues in abortion counseling, 321–322
   victims, development of precociousness, 219
Sexual behavior, high-risk, linked to violence, 217–221
Sexual health, Asian Pacific Islander Americans, 175–176
Sexual history pathways, 218
Sexuality, controlling female, 33–34
Sexual precocity, 218–220
Social change, promoting, 375–376
Sociocognition theory, 337–338
Socratic questioning, 308–309
Stalking, 84
Statutes
   1973–88, 5–6
   1989–92, 10–12
   1992–96, 16–19
Sterilization
   Asian Pacific Islander Americans, 177
   forcible, 117
Stress approach, 236, 238–240, 246–247
Stress coping, 257, 259
Strong, feeling, in response to anti-abortion demonstrators, 94
Surveys
   distortions of public attitudes, 45–46
   factorial design, 50–51
   proportion depicted as pro-life or pro-choice, manipulation by survey items, 49
   purposely biased, 49
   research recommendations, 380
   responses, effect of wording, 48

Teens, *see* Adolescents
Telecommunications Act of 1996, 19
Tiller, Dr. George, shooting, 84
Title X programs, 9–10
Training programs, 355–357, 370
   nonphysicians, 357–358
Travel, for abortion services, 70–71

Unwed motherhood, meaning in race-specific terms, 116
Vacuum aspiration method, 189–190
Victimization, cumulative, 221
Vietnam, abortion, 166–167
Vietnamese Americans, immigration history, 159–160
Violence, 211–228
   bills prohibiting at clinics, 16–17
   incidence, 212–216
      in married abortion patients, 224–225
   increasing levels at clinics, early 1980s, 83
   linked to high-risk sexual behavior, 217–221
   linked to unintended and unwanted pregnancy, 216–217
   in lives of women who have abortions, 222–225
   unwanted and unintended pregnancy, implications, 225–228
Voluntary motherhood, 30

Webster v. Reproductive Health Services, 7–8
Welfare reform, 17
Women
   attitudes, 31–32
   controlling sexuality, 33–34
   distortion of reality of life, 46–48
   promoting social change, 375–376
   providing support and outlets for stories, 53
   seeking abortion and already mothers, 46
Worse case scenario approach, 309

ABOUT THE EDITORS

Linda J. Beckman, PhD, received her doctoral degree in social psychology from the University of California, Los Angeles. She is currently a professor of health psychology at the California School of Professional Psychology in Los Angeles and an associate at the Pacific Institute for Women's Health. One of her major concerns is improving women's access to health care and the quality of reproductive health services women receive. Over the past 25 years, Dr. Beckman has published more than 80 articles and book chapters. Her work has focused on two main areas: substance abuse in women and women's reproductive health.

Dr. Beckman is the recipient of a National Institutes of Health Career Development Award (1975–1984) to study psychosocial aspects of alcoholism in women and is coeditor of the book *Alcohol Problems in Women: Antecedents, Consequences and Interventions* (1984). Her many articles in health and population psychology reflect research and theory on reproductive decision making, attitudes toward contraceptives, and partner influences on contraceptive use. Her most recent studies examine the acceptability of new contraceptive and abortion methods to women from diverse cultural groups. Dr. Beckman is currently studying the characteristics of heterosexual couple relationships, gender roles, power and communication among Latinos, and the application of this knowledge to the development and evaluation of couple-based interventions.

S. Marie Harvey, PhD, is currently the co-director of the Pacific Institute for Women's Health in Los Angeles. She is also director of research at the Center for the Study of Women in Society and an associate professor of public health in the Department of Anthropology at the University of Oregon. She has a bachelor's degree in European history from the University of Puget Sound and a master of public health and a doctor of physical health degree in population studies and family health from the

University of California, Los Angeles. Dr. Harvey is an APA Fellow in Division 34 (Population and Environmental Psychology). Throughout her career, she has focused on the reproductive health of women. She has worked on the frontlines as a social worker and family planning counselor.

For the past 20 years, Dr. Harvey has conducted research that examines the social, psychological, and cultural aspects of contraception, sexual behavior, and abortion. More recently, her research interests and writings have focused on women's attitudes toward and experience with emergency contraception and the acceptability of medical abortion among health care providers and consumers. She is currently working on a 5-year project that studies predictors of sexual risk behavior among Latino couples and designs, implements, and evaluates an intervention to reduce unprotected intercourse among young Latina women and their sexual partners. Dr. Harvey is dedicated to the use of research findings to inform policies and practices that improve women's health.